OBSESSIVE-COMPULSIVE SPECTRUM DISORDERS

*Refining the Research Agenda
for DSM-V*

OBSESSIVE-COMPULSIVE SPECTRUM DISORDERS

Refining the Research Agenda for DSM-V

Edited by

Eric Hollander, M.D.
Joseph Zohar, M.D.
Paul J. Sirovatka, M.S.
Darrel A. Regier, M.D., M.P.H.

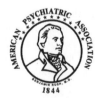

Published by the
American Psychiatric Association
Arlington, Virginia

Note: The authors have worked to ensure that all information in this book is accurate at the time of publication and consistent with general psychiatric and medical standards, and that information concerning drug dosages, schedules, and routes of administration is accurate at the time of publication and consistent with standards set by the U.S. Food and Drug Administration and the general medical community. As medical research and practice continue to advance, however, therapeutic standards may change. Moreover, specific situations may require a specific therapeutic response not included in this book. For these reasons and because human and mechanical errors sometimes occur, we recommend that readers follow the advice of physicians directly involved in their care or the care of a member of their family.

The findings, opinions, and conclusions of this report do not necessarily represent the views of the officers, trustees, or all members of the American Psychiatric Association. The views expressed are those of the authors of the individual chapters.

Manufactured in the United States of America on acid-free paper
14   13   12   11   10   5   4   3   2   1
First Edition

Typeset in Adobe's Frutiger and AGaramond.

American Psychiatric Publishing, Inc.
1000 Wilson Boulevard
Arlington, VA 22209-3901
www.appi.org

Library of Congress Cataloging-in-Publication Data
Obsessive-compulsive spectrum disorders : refining the research agenda for DSM-V / edited by Eric Hollander ... [et al.]. — 1st ed.
        p. ; cm.
    The chapters in this volume, based on presentations from the "The Future of Psychiatric Diagnosis" conference series, were originally published in Psychiatry research and CNS spectrums.
    Includes bibliographical references and index.
    ISBN 978-0-89042-659-3 (pbk. : alk. paper)
    1. Obsessive-compulsive disorder. 2. Diagnostic and statistical manual of mental disorders. I. Hollander, Eric, 1957– II. Psychiatry research. III. CNS spectrums.
    [DNLM: 1. Diagnostic and statistical manual of mental disorders. 2. Obsessive-Compulsive Disorder—diagnosis—Collected Works. 3. Obsessive-Compulsive Disorder—diagnosis—Congresses. 4. Obsessive-Compulsive Disorder—classification—Collected Works. 5. Obsessive-Compulsive Disorder—classification—Congresses.
WM 176 O1468 2011]
    RC533.O295 2011
    616.85'227—dc22
                                                                        2010006870

British Library Cataloguing in Publication Data
A CIP record is available from the British Library.

CONTENTS

CONTRIBUTORS

Paul Arnold, M.D., Ph.D., FRCP
Staff Psychologist, Scientist–Track Investigator, and Assistant Professor, Department of Psychiatry, University of Toronto, Hospital for Sick Children, Toronto, Ontario, Canada

Vasileios Boulougouris, B.Sc., M.Phil., Ph.D.
Research Associate, Experimental Psychology Laboratory, Eginition Hospital, Medical School, University of Athens; Lecturer, Department of Psychology, New York College, Athens, Greece

Ashley Braun, B.A.
Graduate Student, Department of Psychiatry, Montefiore Medical Center, University Hospital of Albert Einstein College of Medicine, Bronx, New York

Samuel R. Chamberlain, M.D., Ph.D.
Senior Visiting Clinical Research Fellow, Department of Psychiatry, University of Cambridge School of Clinical Medicine, Addenbrooke's Hospital, Cambridge, United Kingdom

Kevin J. Craig, M.B.B.Ch., M.Phil, MRCPsych
Medical Director, P1vital Ltd., Department of Psychiatry, University of Oxford, Warneford Hospital, Headington, Oxford, United Kingdom

Ygor Arzeno Ferrão, M.D., Ph.D.
Professor, Porto Alegre Federal University of Health Sciences and Psychiatry Service, Presidente Vargas Maternal-Infantile Hospital, Porto Alegre, RS, Brazil; member of The Brazilian Obsessive-Compulsive Research Consortium, São Paulo, Brazil

Naomi A. Fineberg, , M.B.B.S., M.A., MRCPsych
Professor and Consulting Psychiatrist, Department of Psychiatry, Hertfordshire Partnership NHS Foundation Trust, Queen Elizabeth II Hospital, Howlands, Welwyn Garden City, United Kingdom

Eric Hollander, M.D.
Professor and Director, Compulsive, Impulsive, and Autism Spectrum Disorders Program, Department of Psychiatry, Montefiore Medical Center, University Hospital for Albert Einstein College of Medicine, Bronx, New York

Walter H. Kaye, M.D.
Professor of Psychiatry and Director, UCSD Eating Disorders Research and Treatment Program, Department of Psychiatry, University of California, San Diego, La Jolla, California

James L. Kennedy, M.D.
Director, Neuroscience Department, Centre for Addiction and Mental Health, Toronto, Ontario, Canada

Suah Kim, M.S.
Doctoral candidate, Department of Counseling and Clinical Psychology, Teachers College, Columbia University, New York, New York

Lorrin M. Koran, M.D.
Professor Emeritus, Department of Psychiatry and Behavioral Sciences, Stanford University School of Medicine, Stanford University Medical Center, Stanford, California

Nuria Lanzagorta, BSPSY
Clinical Research Coordinator, Carracci Medical Group, Mexico City, Mexico

James F. Leckman, M.D.
Neison Harris Professor of Child Psychiatry, Pediatrics, and Psychology and Director of Research, Yale University School of Medicine, Yale Child Study Center, New Haven, Connecticut

Laura Marsh, M.D.
Executive Director, Mental Health Care Line, Michael E. DeBakey Veterans Affairs Medical Center; Professor, Departments of Psychiatry and Neurology, Baylor College of Medicine, Houston, Texas

David Mataix-Cols, Ph.D.
Senior Lecturer and Honorary Consultant Clinical Psychologist, King's College London, Institute of Psychiatry, London, United Kingdom

Hisato Matsunaga, M.D., Ph.D.
Assistant Professor, Department of Neuropsychiatry, Osaka City University Graduate School of Medicine, Osaka, Japan

Euripedes Constantino Miguel, M.D., Ph.D.
Professor, Department of Psychiatry, University of São Paulo Medical School, São Paulo, SP, Brazil; member of The Brazilian Obsessive-Compulsive Research Consortium, São Paulo, Brazil

Gerald Nestadt, M.D., M.P.H.
Professor, Department of Psychiatry and Behavioral Sciences, Johns Hopkins Medical School; Professor of Mental Health, Bloomberg School of Public Health, Johns Hopkins University, Baltimore, Maryland

Humberto Nicolini, M.D., Ph.D.
Director, Carracci Medical Group, Mexico City, Mexico

Stefano Pallanti, M.D., Ph.D.
Visiting Associate Professor, Department of Psychiatry, Mount Sinai School of Medicine, New York, New York; Istituto di Neuroscienze, Florence, Italy; Associate Professor, University of Florence, Florence, Italy

Katharine A. Phillips, M.D.
Professor, Department of Psychiatry and Human Behavior, Brown University School of Medicine, Butler Hospital, Providence, Rhode Island

Marc N. Potenza, M.D., Ph.D.
Associate Professor, Department of Psychiatry, Substance Abuse Clinic, Connecticut Mental Health Center, Yale University School of Medicine, New Haven, Connecticut

Scott L. Rauch, M.D.
Chair, Partners Psychiatry and Mental Health; Professor of Psychiatry, Harvard Medical School; President and Psychiatrist in Chief, McLean Hospital, Belmont, Massachusetts

Darrel A. Regier, M.D., M.P.H.
Executive Director, American Psychiatric Institute for Research and Education; Director, Division of Research, American Psychiatric Association, Arlington, Virginia

Trevor W. Robbins, Ph.D., FRS, FMedSci
Professor, Behavioural and Clinical Neuroscience Institute (BCNI), and Chair, Department of Experimental Psychology, University of Cambridge, Cambridge, United Kingdom

Sanjaya Saxena, M.D.
Professor in Residence, Department of Psychiatry, University of California, San Diego, San Diego, California

Soraya Seedat, Ph.D., MBChB, FCPsych
Co-Director, Medical Research Council Unit on Anxiety and Stress Disorders, Professor, Department of Psychiatry, Stellenbosch University, Tygerberg, South Africa

Daphne Simeon, M.D.
Associate Professor, Department of Psychiatry, Albert Einstein College of Medicine; Co-director, Family Center for Bipolar Disorder, Beth Israel Medical Center, New York, New York

Paul J. Sirovatka, M.S. (1947–2007)
Director of Research Policy Analysis, Division of Research and American Psychiatric Institute for Research and Education, Arlington, Virginia

Dan J. Stein, M.D., Ph.D.
Professor, Department of Psychiatry and Mental Health, University of Cape Town, Cape Town, South Africa; Professor, Department of Psychiatry, Mount Sinai School of Medicine, New York, New York

A. Ting Wang, Ph.D.
Assistant Professor, Departments of Psychiatry and Neuroscience, Seaver Autism Center for Research and Treatment, Mt. Sinai School of Medicine, New York, New York

Joseph Zohar, M.D.
Chair and Professor, Department of Psychiatry, Chaim Sheba Medical Center, Tel-Hashomer, Israel

DISCLOSURE STATEMENT

The research conference series that produced this monograph was supported with funding from the U.S. National Institutes of Health (NIH) Grant U13 MH-067855 (Principal Investigator: Darrel A. Regier, M.D., M.P.H.). The National Institute of Mental Health (NIMH), the National Institute on Drug Abuse (NIDA), and the National Institute on Alcohol Abuse and Alcoholism (NIAAA) jointly supported this cooperative research planning conference project. The conference series was not part of the official revision process for *Diagnostic and Statistical Manual of Mental Disorders*, Fifth Edition (DSM-V), but rather was a separate, rigorous research planning initiative meant to inform revisions of psychiatric diagnostic classification systems. No private-industry sources provided funding for this research review.

Coordination and oversight of the overall research review, publicly titled "The Future of Psychiatric Diagnosis: Refining the Research Agenda," were provided by an Executive Steering Committee composed of representatives of the several entities that cooperatively sponsored the NIH-funded project. Members of the Executive Steering Committee included:

- *American Psychiatric Institute for Research and Education*—Darrel A. Regier, M.D., M.P.H. (P.I.), Michael B. First, M.D. (co-P.I.; consultant)
- *World Health Organization*—Benedetto Saraceno, M.D., and Norman Sartorius, M.D., Ph.D. (consultant)
- *National Institutes of Health*—Bruce Cuthbert, Ph.D., Wayne S. Fenton, M.D. (NIMH; consultant), Michael Kozak, Ph.D. (NIMH), Bridget F. Grant, Ph.D. (NIAAA), and Wilson M. Compton, M.D. (NIDA)

NIMH grant project officers were Lisa Colpe, Ph.D., Karen H. Bourdon, M.A., and Mercedes Rubio, Ph.D.

APIRE staff were William E. Narrow, M.D., M.P.H. (co-P.I.), Emily A. Kuhl, Ph.D., Maritza Rubio-Stipec, Sc.D. (consultant), Paul J. Sirovatka, M.S., Jennifer Shupinka, Erin Dalder-Alpher, Kristin Edwards, Leah Engel, Seung-Hee Hong, and Rocio Salvador.

The following contributors to this book have indicated financial interests in or other affiliations with a commercial supporter, a manufacturer of a commercial product, a provider of a commercial service, a nongovernmental organization, and/or a government agency, as listed below:

Darrel A. Regier, M.D., M.P.H.—The author, as Executive Director of American Psychiatric Institute for Research and Education, oversees all federal and industry-sponsored research and research training grants in APIRE but receives no external salary funding or honoraria from any government or industry.

Samuel R. Chamberlain, M.D., Ph.D.—The author has received consultant fees from Cambridge Cognition and P1Vital.

Kevin J. Craig, M.B.B.Ch., M.Phil, MRCPsych—The author has received grant, research, and/or consulting support from P1vital Ltd and GlaxoSmithKline.

Ygor Arzeno Ferrão, M.D., Ph.D.—The author has received speaker support from Solvay Pharma, Eli Lilly, and Roche Laboratories.

Naomi A. Fineberg, M.B.B.S., M.A., MRCPsych—The author has received consultation fees from Lundbeck, GlaxoSmithKline, Servier, and Bristol Myers. The author has received research support from AstraZeneca, GlaxoSmithKline, Wellcome, and Lundbeck. The author has received honoraria and speaker support from Janssen, Jazz, Lundbeck, Servier, AstraZeneca, and Wyeth.

Eric Hollander, M.D.—The author has received consultation fees from Transceit, Neuropharm, and Nastech.

Walter H. Kaye, M.D.—The author has received grant, research, and/or consulting support from the National Institute of Mental Health, the National Institutes of Health, the Price Foundation, AstraZeneca, Lundbeck, and Merck.

James L. Kennedy, M.D.—The author has received consultant fees from Sanofi-Aventis.

Lorrin M. Koran, M.D.—The author has received speaking and consultant support from Forest Pharmaceuticals and Jazz Pharmaceuticals.

James F. Leckman, M.D.—The author has received research support from the NIH, Tourette Syndrome Association, and Klingenstein Third Generation Foundation. The author has received book royalties from John Wiley and Sons, McGraw Hill, and Oxford University Press.

Laura Marsh, M.D.—The author has received support from Forest Research Institute and Boehringer-Ingelheim, GbMH.

David Mataix-Cols, Ph.D.—The author has received research support from the Life Foundation, University of London, European Commission, and UK Department of Health. The author receives salary support from King's College, London.

Euripedes Constantino Miguel, M.D., Ph.D.—The author has received speaker support from Solvay Pharma and Lundbeck Laboratories.

Stefano Pallanti, M.D., Ph.D.—The author has received support from Pfizer, GlaxoSmithKline, Jazz Pharmaceuticals, Solvay International, and Transcept Pharmaceutical.

Katharine A. Phillips, M.D.—The author has received salary support or funding from Rhode Island Hospital, Butler Hospital, Alpert Medical School of Brown University, the National Institute of Mental Health, the Food & Drug Administration, the American Foundation for Suicide Prevention, Forest Laboratories, Oxford University Press, Guilford Press, and The Free Press.

Marc N. Potenza, M.D., Ph.D.—The author has received financial support from Boehringer Ingelheim, Somaxon, the National Institutes of Health, Veteran's Administration, Mohegan Sun Casino, the National Center for Responsible Gaming and its affiliated Institute for Research on Gambling Disorders, Forest Laboratories, Ortho-McNeil, Oy-Control/Biotie, and GlaxoSmithKline. The author has participated in surveys, mailings, or telephone consultations related to drug addiction, impulse control disorders, or other health topics. The author has consulted for law offices and the federal public defender's office in issues related to impulse control disorders. The author provides clinical are in the Connecticut Department of Mental Health and Addiction Services Problem Gambling Services Program.

Scott L. Rauch, M.D.—The author received research support from Cephalon, Cyberonics, Medtronics, and Northstar.

Trevor W. Robbins, Ph.D., FRS, FMedSci—The author as received consultation support from Camrbidge Cognition, Pfizer, Eli Lilly, Roche, Lundbeck, Allon Therapeutics, Pangenics, GlaxoSmithKline, Springer-Verlag, and Johnson & Johnson.

Soraya Seedat, Ph.D., MBChB, FCPsych—The author has received support from Servier.

Dan J. Stein, M.D., Ph.D.—The author has received research support and/or consultation support from AstraZeneca, Eli-Lilly, GlaxoSmithKline, Jazz Pharmaceuticals, Johnson & Johnson, Lundbeck, Orion, Pfizer, Pharmacia, Roche, Servier, Solvay, Sumitomo, Takeda, Tikvah, and Wyeth.

Joseph Zohar, M.D.—The author has received grant support from Lundbeck, Servier, and Pfizer. The author has received speaking and consultant fees from Lundbeck, Servier, Solvay, and Pierre Fagre.

The following contributors to this book do not have any conflicts of interest to disclose:

Paul Arnold, M.D., Ph.D., FRCP
Vasileios Boulougouris, B.Sc., M.Phil., Ph.D.
Ashley Braun, B.A.
Suah Kim, M.S.
Nuria Lanzagorta, BSPSY
Hisato Matsunaga, M.D., Ph.D.
Gerald Nestadt, M.D., M.P.H.
Humberto Nicolini, M.D., Ph.D.
Sanjaya Saxena, M.D.
Daphne Simeon, M.D.
A. Ting Wang, Ph.D.

PREFACE

Darrel A. Regier, M.D., M.P.H.

We are pleased to have the opportunity to present a selection of review articles that reflect the proceedings of a conference focused on an array of conditions, clustered under the rubric of "obsessive-compulsive spectrum disorders." The conference was one in a series titled "The Future of Psychiatric Diagnosis: Refining the Research Agenda," convened by the American Psychiatric Association (APA) in collaboration of the World Health Organization (WHO) and the U.S. National Institutes of Health (NIH), with funding provided by the NIH.

The APA/WHO/NIH conferences were key elements in an extensive research review process designed to assess the status of scientific knowledge that is relevant to psychiatric classification systems and to generate specific recommendations for research to advance that knowledge base. Conferees attempted to identify short-term research (e.g., reanalyses of existing datasets) that can be completed for consideration prior to publication of DSM-5, scheduled for 2013. Results of such efforts may also inform WHO's ICD-11 Mental and Behavioral Disorders section, which is due to be published approximately 4 years from now. In its entirety, the project comprised 10 work groups, each focused on a specific diagnostic topic or category, and two additional work groups dedicated to methodological considerations in nosology and classification. The chapters presented here underscore APA's interest in ensuring that information and recommendations developed as part of this process are available to scientific groups who are concurrently updating other national and international classifications of mental and behavioral disorders.

Within the APA, the American Psychiatric Institute for Research and Education (APIRE), under the direction of the author (D.A.R.), holds lead responsibility

This preface was first published as "Obsessive-Compulsive Behavior Spectrum: Refining the Research Agenda for DSM-V." *Psychiatry Research* 170:1–2, 2009 (copyright 2009; used with permission) and "Obsessive-Compulsive Behavior Spectrum: Refining the Research Agenda." *CNS Spectrums* 12:343–344, 2007 (copyright 2007; used with permission).

Support for preparation of this preface was provided by a grant (U13 MH067855) from the National Institute of Mental Health.

for organizing and administering the diagnostic research planning conferences. The Executive Steering Committee for the series included representatives of the WHO's Department of Mental Health and Prevention of Substance Abuse and of three NIH institutes that jointly funded the project: the National Institute of Mental Health (NIMH), the National Institute on Drug Abuse (NIDA), and the National Institute on Alcohol Abuse and Alcoholism (NIAAA).

Although DSM-5 is not scheduled to appear until 2013, planning for the fifth revision began in 1999 with a collaboration between APA and NIMH designed to stimulate research that would address identified opportunities in psychiatric nosology. A first product of this joint venture was preparation of six white papers that proposed broad-brush recommendations for research in key areas. Topics included Developmental Issues, Gaps in the Current Classification, Disability and Impairment, Neuroscience, Nomenclature, and Cross-Cultural Issues. Each team that developed a paper included at least one liaison member from NIMH, with the intent—largely realized—that these members would integrate many of the work groups' recommendations into NIMH research support programs. These white papers were published in *A Research Agenda for DSM-V* (Kupfer et al. 2002). This volume was then followed by a second compilation of white papers (Narrow et al. 2007) that outline diagnosis-related research needs in the areas of gender, pediatric, and geriatric populations.

As a second phase of planning, the APA leadership envisioned a series of international research planning conferences that would address specific diagnostic topics in greater depth, with conference proceedings serving as resource documents for groups involved in the official DSM-5 revision process. The NIMH, with substantial additional funding support from the NIDA and NIAAA, awarded a cooperative research planning conference grant to APIRE in 2003. The conferences funded under the grant are the basis for this monograph series and represent a second major phase in the scientific review and planning for DSM-5.

In addition to the immediate, short-term research objective just described, the research conferences had multiple aims. One was to promote international collaboration among members of the scientific community in order to increase the likelihood of developing a future DSM that is unified with other international classifications. A second was to stimulate the empirical research necessary to allow informed decision making regarding deficiencies identified in DSM-IV (American Psychiatric Association 1994). A third was to facilitate the development of broadly agreed-upon criteria that researchers worldwide can use in planning and conducting future research exploring the etiology and pathophysiology of mental disorders. Challenging as it is, this last objective reflects widespread agreement in the field that the well-established reliability and clinical utility of prior DSM classifications must be matched in the future by a renewed focus on the validity of diagnoses.

Given the vision of an ultimately unified international system for classifying mental disorders, members of the Executive Steering Committee have attached high priority to ensuring the participation of investigators from all parts of the world in the project. Toward this end, each conference in the series had two co-chairs, drawn respectively from the United States and a country other than the United States; approximately half of the experts invited to each working conference were from outside the United States, and half of the conferences were being convened outside the United States.

Two leaders in the field—Eric Hollander, M.D., from the Montefiore Medical Center of the University Hospital of Albert Einstein College of Medicine, Bronx, New York, and Joseph Zohar, M.D., from the Chaim Sheba Medical Center, Tel-Hashomer, Israel—agreed to organize and co-chair the Obsessive-Compulsive Spectrum Work Group and Conference, which convened in Arlington, Virginia, in June 2006. The co-chairs worked closely with the APA/WHO/NIH Executive Steering Committee to identify and enlist a stellar roster of participants for the conference.

The chapters in this volume, based on presentations from the "The Future of Psychiatric Diagnosis" conference series, were first published as articles in *Psychiatry Research* and *CNS Spectrums*. Although the journals ensured dissemination of the articles to the widest possible audience as well as the listing of the articles in *Index Medicus,* the monograph serves as a resource document for the DSM-5 Task Force and disorder-specific work groups. In addition, a summary report of this and other conferences in the series is available online at www.dsm5.org.

We express our appreciation to officials at NIMH, NIDA, and NIAAA who made funding available for this conference series. We hope that research recommendations coming out of these conferences in time will stimulate investigator-initiated proposals to NIH and other sources for studies that will advance psychiatric classification and diagnoses. The APA greatly appreciates, as well, the contributions of all participants in the Obsessive-Compulsive Spectrum Disorders Research Planning Work Group and the interest of our broader audience in this topic.

References

American Psychiatric Association: Diagnostic and Statistical Manual of Mental Disorders, 4th Edition. Washington, DC, American Psychiatric Association, 1994

Kupfer DJ, First MB, Regier DA (eds): A Research Agenda for DSM-V. Washington, DC, American Psychiatric Association, 2002

Narrow WN, First MB, Sirovatka P, et al (eds): Age and Gender Considerations in Psychiatric Diagnosis: A Research Agenda for DSM-V. Washington, DC, American Psychiatric Association, 2007

INTRODUCTION

Cross-Cutting Issues and Future Directions for the Obsessive-Compulsive Spectrum Disorders

Eric Hollander, M.D.

Suah Kim, M.S.

Ashley Braun, B.A.

Daphne Simeon, M.D.

Joseph Zohar, M.D.

The chapters in this volume reflect the proceedings from the research planning conference for the fifth edition of *Diagnostic and Statistical Manual of Mental Disorders* (DSM-V), entitled "Obsessive-Compulsive Spectrum Behavior Disorders: Refining the Research Agenda for DSM-V." The conference examined possible similarities in phenomenology, comorbidity, familial and genetic features, brain circuitry, and treatment response between obsessive-compulsive disorder (OCD) and several related disorders that are characterized by repetitive thoughts or behaviors. Such data support a reexamination of the DSM-IV-TR classification of OCD and the anxiety disorders, with possible inclusion of a group of obsessive-compulsive spectrum disorders (OCSDs) in DSM-V. Various disorders were systematically examined for inclusion in such a grouping, and later a smaller number were determined to meet the threshold criteria for inclusion in the OCSDs. The disorders that were originally examined included OCD, obsessive-compulsive personality disorder (OCPD), Tourette's syndrome and other tic disorders, Sydenham's chorea, pediatric autoimmune neuropsychiatric disorders associated with streptococcal infections (PANDAS), trichotillomania, body dysmorphic disorder (BDD), autism, eating disorders, Huntington's disease and Parkinson's disease, and impulse-control disorders, as well as substance and behavioral addictions.

This introduction was adapted with permission from "OCSDs in the Forthcoming *DSM-V*." *CNS Spectrums* 12:320–323, 2007 and "Cross-Cutting Issues and Future Directions for the OCD Spectrum." *Psychiatry Research* 170:3–6, 2009. Used with permission.

The developmental perspective recognizes the repetitive and somewhat compulsive behavior that normally peaks in children at 2 years and has semblance to OCD symptoms found in patients. In examining the nosology of OCD, Fineberg and colleagues describe in this volume (Chapter 1) similarities in phenomenology between this disorder and other obsessive-compulsive–related disorders (OCRDs) to support modifying the conceptualization of OCD away from anxiety disorders where differences emerge. In comparison to anxiety disorders, OCD exhibits earlier onset, with a male gender bias and chronic course of illness, as well as greater rates of comorbidity with OCRDs than with some anxiety disorders, such as social anxiety disorder and panic disorder. Pharmacological studies of OCD show differences in treatment response as compared with anxiety disorders, whereby anxiolytics, including benzodiazepines, are less effective in treating OCD.

BDD and eating disorders are most often comorbid with OCD and share intense preoccupations with OCD, usually coupled with associated compulsions, but differ in content and other features of their obsessive-compulsive–related behaviors, as illustrated by Phillips and Kaye in Chapter 2. BDD and OCD are similar in the intrusive, repetitive, persistent, and ego-dystonic nature of their obsessions. However, there are differences in the content of the obsessions, with BDD obsessions focused on physical appearance and dissatisfaction of the self, characterized by poorer insight, and almost never beleaguered by moral repulsion. The compulsions of BDD and OCD are similar in that BDD compulsions are performed knowingly, in response to obsessions, to reduce anxiety or prevent an undesired event; are repetitive, excessive, and time-consuming; and are often rigid and not pleasurable. They differ in the content of the behaviors, as BDD compulsions are sometimes not repetitive if performed once daily (i.e., camouflaging) and are less likely to reduce anxiety. On the other hand, obsessions and compulsions associated with anorexia nervosa tend to be ego-syntonic, and sufferers feel bound to perform ritualistic behaviors even if they cause further anxiety. There have also been similarities and differences found in brain and neuropsychological features between BDD or eating disorders and OCD, but there are too few studies to offer conclusive comparisons.

Ferrão, Miguel, and Stein, in Chapter 3, compare the phenomenology, psychobiology, and treatment response of OCD, Tourette's syndrome, and trichotillomania in considering their reclassification into a spectrum of related disorders. While compulsive behaviors observed in OCD in the absence of Tourette's syndrome are responses to obsessive thoughts, the repetitive behaviors in Tourette's syndrome and OCD with tics are usually exhibited to alleviate unpleasant sensations. Similarly, while the repetitive behavior of trichotillomania exclusively involves hairpulling, this behavior often follows high anxiety and results in lowered anxiety. The authors point out that OCD combined with vocal or motor tics exhibits similar frequency of repetitive behaviors as Tourette's syndrome but greater symptom frequency than OCD, and lies between these two disorders in terms of phenomenological features such as comorbidity, symptom onset, and frequency of somatic obsessions. These findings support the idea that OCD and tic disorders may lie on a continuum. Family studies show a greater prevalence of obsessive-compulsive symptoms and OCD in relatives of Tourette's syndrome sufferers, as well as higher rates of tics or Tourette's syndrome in family members of OCD patients, when compared with healthy controls. Likewise, trichotillomania and OCD are more common in relatives of trichotillomania probands.

Potenza, Koran, and Pallanti describe, in Chapter 4, both commonalities and differences in the clinical, phenomenological, and biological features between intermittent explosive disorder, pathological gambling, and OCD, with the overarching similarity being an inability to resist repetitive behaviors that may be harmful to the self or others. A distinct contrast between these disorders is the ego-dystonic nature of OCD versus the ego-syntonic nature of impulse-control disorders. However, the repetitive behaviors in impulse-control disorders may change over time and become less pleasure-driven and more driven to alleviate distress, thereby resembling those of OCD. From a phenomenological point of view, although intermittent explosive disorder and OCD are similar in their intrusiveness and repetitiveness, the behaviors seen in intermittent explosive disorder are not intended to reduce anxiety and are not in response to obsessions, as compulsions are in OCD. Other differences include a higher prevalence rate of intermittent explosive disorder than OCD, predominance of intermittent explosive disorder in males, and an association of intermittent explosive disorder with marriage and low educational level.

The dimensional approach to understanding OCD proposed by Leckman, Rauch, and Mataix-Cols in Chapter 5 is a quantitative method of assessing phenotypic traits, with aggression toward the self or others, sexual obsessions, and moral obsessions, along with related compulsions, constituting Factor I; symmetry or exactness obsessions, repetition, counting, and ordering compulsions constituting Factor II; contamination obsessions and cleaning or washing compulsions constituting Factor III; and hoarding obsessions and compulsions constituting Factor IV. This perspective of OCD offers to address the apparent heterogeneity and temporal stability of symptoms and provides an innovative method to enhance research in comorbidity, response to treatment, genetic, familial, and neurological studies. Using this approach, several studies have shown relationships between certain comorbid disorders and shared symptom domains. Because of the variability in OCD etiology, it is difficult to narrow genetic markers of the disorder. In breaking down the heterogeneous phenotypes of the disorder into symptom dimensions, this approach may facilitate new methods of tracking genetic susceptibility. While neuroimaging studies show robust data on orbitofrontal cortex involvement in obsessive-compulsive symptoms, there is less consistent information about other areas of brain circuitry. Utilization of the dimensional approach may help account for individual differences, as suggested in some studies, that show correlations between obsessive-compulsive symptoms and different neural activities, which may in turn mediate the manifestation of these symptoms.

Nicolini and colleagues provide, in Chapter 6, insights into the genetics and familial factors of OCD and related disorders. Family studies of OCD generally show that the prevalence of OCD is significantly higher in relatives, especially in the presence of comorbid tics and earlier age at onset, and also depends on the types of obsessions and compulsions exhibited by probands. Twin studies, although few in number, have suggested some significant genetic influence in the heritability of obsessive-compulsive symptoms. Family studies on the whole have supported the heterogeneity of OCD and the identification of subgroups of patients including early onset, sex-typing, symptom clustering, and treatment response. There may also be some evidence of a single major gene contributing to some OCD subtypes such as symmetry and ordering, eating disorders, early age at onset, and sex-specific subtypes.

In Chapter 7, Hollander and colleagues discuss two neurological disorders that encompass obsessive-compulsive features: autism and Parkinson's disease. Although autism, a developmental disorder, and Parkinson's disease, a degenerative disorder, may at first appear dissimilar, both disorders may be characterized by repetitive behaviors and impulsive behaviors, and similar processes may occur in both a developmental and a degenerative disorder. Autism spectrum disorders and OCD are similarly characterized by rigid observance of routines and rituals, and some autistic patients also report having obsessions and compulsions. Studies on obsessive-compulsive symptoms in Parkinson's disease are mixed. However, a condition in Parkinson's disease called *punding,* which may be due to excess dopaminergic therapy in Parkinson's disease, resembles the repetitive behaviors seen in OCD and is also often anxiety-reducing. By contrast, punding is neither rigid nor in response to obsessions or aimed at averting unpleasant events. Although autism and OCD share some similar comorbidities, autism is also significantly comorbid with seizures, epileptiform electroencephalographic abnormalities, mental retardation, genetic disorders, and speech and language disorders. Findings on comorbidities in obsessive-compulsive symptoms with Parkinson's disease are limited, but punding is associated with impulse-control disorders, psychosis, and excessive use of dopaminergic medications resembling an addiction, as well as motoric side effects such as extreme on-off fluctuations and dyskinesias. Autism is similar to early-onset OCD in its predominance in boys, prolonged course of illness, and association with tics. It is also highly heritable, and studies have suggested associations between OCD or obsessive-compulsive behaviors in parents of autistic children and repetitive behavior scales.

Boulougouris, Chamberlain, and Robbins describe, in Chapter 8, animal modeling of OCSDs as occurring on two levels—the etiological level and the symptomatic level. It is probable that several candidate genes contribute to OCD vulnerability so that difficulties in modeling arise. Furthermore, behavioral symptoms simulated in mice may not wholly reflect the subtleties of the disorder. Still, advances in understanding the neural substrates of OCD and efficacy of pharmacological treatment may validate animal models. Ethological and behavioral models have identified several repetitive behaviors in animals suggestive of OCD, such as acral lick dermatitis, hairpulling, barbering, cribbing, and wheel-running, and have tested the effects of drug therapy. Exploring what mechanisms are involved in turning habit into compulsions in these animals is of interest. Genetic models of OCD have involved the *hoxb8* mutant seen in excessive grooming and manipulations of dopamine and serotonin functioning that have elicited similar behaviors, from repetitive jumping to chewing. Boulougouris and colleagues also describe signal attenuation and extinction as behavioral models of OCD, whereby the animal receives poor feedback that a behavior has been completed, leading to perseverative compulsions that can been reduced by drugs typically used to treat OCD.

Finally, in Chapter 9, Matsunaga and Seedat report shortcomings in the descriptive data of OCD across nations are in the absence of such data from areas of southern Africa, Eastern Europe, and Central Asia, and in the inconsistency of data collection from time frame to variability in the diagnostic tools (i.e., DSM and the International Classification of Diseases) and interviewing methods used. Such variability calls for a universal approach to diagnosing OCD in order to enhance cross-cultural reliability. Some consistencies in the descriptive features of OCD have been noted. While men have an earlier age at onset of the disorder, women are more likely to develop OCD later in life, such as postpregnancy. Symptoms of OCD have shown gender differences as well across nations. Where culture may play a role in the expression of OCD is in the focus of obsessions and compulsions, such as in religion, where piety and rituals are central in some cultures. Although family studies have shown positive diagnoses of first-degree relatives of probands with OCD and related disorders, such studies have not been readily conducted multinationally.

There is growing interest in the scientific community to explore the relationships between obsessive-compulsive spectrum disorders and obsessive-compulsive disorder based on commonalities of phenomenology, comorbidity, course of illness, brain circuitry, familial and genetic factors, and treatment response. The research planning conference on OCSDs aimed to bring an international group of scientists together to gather empirical research that may inform classification for future DSM efforts. The collection of chapters in this volume present some of the findings related to genetics and OCD nosology, cross-species models of OCSDs, and the relationships between OCD and related disorders. Although findings are mixed in comparing the domains described above, future directions in research should examine OCSDs based on endophenotypic features.

Endophenotyping efforts should include the following features:

1. Clarification of OCD symptom dimensions
2. Clarification of inclusion criteria for OCSDs

3. Determination of which disorders should be included in the OCSDs
4. Clarification of subtypes
5. Use of exiting databases
6. Construction of a common endophenotype battery that includes neurocognition, genotyping, functional brain imaging, symptom scales, structured assessment for comorbidity, and treatment response
7. Development of self-administered scales for threshold diagnosis and sensitivity to change
8. Multicenter trials that include an endophenotyping project
9. Comparison of the OCSDs to the other anxiety disorders

Because OCD and especially OCSDs are underdiagnosed in patients who report a broad symptom of anxiety, a reclassification of OCD and related disorders into a broader category would promote better assessment of obsessive-compulsive symptoms, more accurate diagnoses, greater research efforts, and potentially the development of more effective treatments.

1

OBSESSIVE-COMPULSIVE DISORDER

Boundary Issues

Naomi A. Fineberg, M.B.B.S., M.A., MRCPsych
Sanjaya Saxena, M.D.
Joseph Zohar, M.D.
Kevin J. Craig, M.B.B.Ch., M.Phil, MRCPsych

The current debate about where obsessive-compulsive disorder (OCD) best belongs in psychiatric classification has highlighted an interesting paradox. Although OCD is currently classified by DSM-IV-TR (American Psychiatric Association 2000) as an anxiety disorder, a growing corpus of literature has emphasized the role of corticostriatally mediated control and reward systems in the pathophysiology of OCD (Chamberlain et al. 2005). The focus has thus shifted from learning models in which anxiety-driven obsessions entrain neutralizing compulsions to an emphasis on the primacy of obsessional thoughts and compulsive behaviors as disorders of basal ganglia dysregulation. Moreover, the serotonin (5-HT) hypothesis for OCD (Insel et al. 1985), derived largely from clinical psychopharmacological response data, has not been satisfactorily substantiated by a growing body of molecular imaging and genetic evidence that points to dopaminergic dysfunction as a

This chapter was first published as "Obsessive-Compulsive Disorder: Boundary Issues." *CNS Spectrums* 12:359–375, 2007. Copyright 2009. Used with permission.

candidate etiological factor (Denys et al. 2004, 2006; Pooley et al. 2007). In turn, this has prompted the move toward conceptualizing OCD as a prototype disorder for a group of "obsessive-compulsive spectrum disorders" (OCSDs; Hollander and Wong 1995), for which failures of behavioral (cognitive and motor) inhibition constitute a key characteristic.

In DSM-IV-TR, OCD is categorized as an anxiety disorder. A central role for anxiety in mediating symptoms was argued: obsessions were considered to contribute to escalating anxiety and compulsions performed to avoid or reduce this anxiety (Marks 1987). Moreover, the observation that OCD frequently coexisted with other anxiety disorders (simple phobia [22%], social phobia [18%], and panic disorder [12%]) (Pigott et al. 1994; Rasmussen and Eisen 1990) was thought to reflect a common etiological basis. In contrast to DSM-IV-TR, ICD-10 (World Health Organization 1992) recognizes anxiety, with and without autonomic arousal, to be a common but not essential feature of OCD and separates OCD from other anxiety disorders, placing it as a separate illness within the group of neurotic, stress-related, and somatoform disorders.

Mental disorders can be difficult to define on the basis of phenomenological grounds, owing to substantial overlap between the content and form of symptoms across so many disorders (Shapiro and Shapiro 1992). The comorbidity argument is also limited by diagnostic systems based on phenotypic symptoms (similarities in phenomenology and comorbidity rates could argue equally well for inclusion of OCD into affective disorders, psychotic disorders, and even addiction). Endophenotypes, representing measurable intermediate markers on the pathway between the phenotype and the distal genotype, have been proposed to be more biologically meaningful than phenotypes and have so far shown promise in identifying specific inherited aspects of nonpsychiatric illness, such as heart disease (Gottesman and Gould 2003). Arguably, the identity and relationship between OCD and other neuropsychiatric disorders may be better understood by mapping the disorders across a number of key endophenotypic domains, including outcomes on tests of neurocognition, brain imaging, and molecular mechanisms (Hollander et al. 2007). By so doing, an endophenotype profile or "grid" for each individual disorder can be constructed (Table 1–1) and used as a benchmark against which the other disorders can be compared.

The aim of this review is to map out the nosological boundaries of OCD. Using OCD as the prototypic disorder and applying the endophenotype-grid model as systematically as possible within the limitations of available data, we attempt to identify important cognitive, imaging, and molecular findings that link or distinguish OCD from other neuropsychiatric disorders, including anxiety disorders, depression, schizophrenia, and putative OCSDs such as body dysmorphic disorder (BDD), hypochondriasis, grooming disorders, Tourette's syndrome, obsessive-compulsive personality disorder (OCPD), and poststreptococcal neuropsychiatric syndromes.

TABLE 1–1. Endophenotype grid

Category[a]	Example
Clinical characteristics	Subtypes of obsessions/compulsions defined
Course of Illness	Biphasic onset (childhood and early adulthood)
Comorbidities	Depression (66% lifetime prevalence)
Epidemiology	Male:female ratio = 1.5:1
Family history	OCD in 10% first-degree relatives of probands
Genetic factors	COMT met:met genotype in males
Brain circuitry	Lateral orbitofrontal-ventral striatal circuit dysfunction
Neuropsychology	Breakdown of inhibitory mechanism
Pharmacological dissection	No effect of tryptophan depletion
Biomarkers	↑ Basal ganglia antibodies in some pediatric cases
Treatment response	Preferential response to selective serotonin reuptake inhibitor medication
Cross-species models[b]	D_2/D_3 stimulation (quinpirole) induced checking behavior in rats

Note. COMT=catechol-O-methyltransferase; D_2/D_3=dopamine type 2/dopamine type 3 receptors; OCD=obsessive-compulsive disorder.
[a]Potential categories for an OCD endophenotype with some examples from the literature.
[b]Hwang et al. 2000; Szechtman et al. 1998.

Comparison Between Obsessive-Compulsive Disorder and Other Mental Disorders

OBSESSIVE-COMPULSIVE DISORDER VERSUS AXIS I DISORDERS: ANXIETY DISORDERS

Epidemiology

Whereas in clinical samples the gender ratio of OCD is roughly equal, females predominate in community populations (~1.5:1), although not to the same extent as in other anxiety disorders (2–3:1), perhaps reflecting greater illness severity in males. Males predominated in a sample of clinical cases of early onset OCD (Rasmussen and Eisen 1990), whereas in the large-scale epidemiological analysis by Wittchen and Jacobi (2005) there was an equal gender ratio in individuals 35–49 years of age, but females predominated in the 18–34 years of age and 50–65 years of age ranges. Lochner et al. (2004) compared clinical and genetic data across gender and found that males with OCD showed an earlier onset and a trend toward more tics and poorer outcome, different symptom profiles, and different genetic polymorphisms. The meta-analytic study by Pooley et al. (2007) also identified sexual dimorphism in relation to catechol-O-methyltransferase *(COMT)* gene polymorphisms, implying that gender contributes to the clinical and biological heterogeneity of OCD. The earlier age of onset and stable course of OCD also differentiate OCD from other anxiety disorders (Table 1–2).

Comorbidity

In epidemiological samples, comorbid OCD is twice as common (1.4%) as noncomorbid OCD (0.7%) (Hollander et al. 1996). Table 1–3 shows the disorders that most commonly coexist in individuals with clinical cases of OCD. Although comorbidity with anxiety disorders is relatively common (Pigott et al. 1994), Richter et al. (2003) found greater lifetime rates of comorbid OCSDs, such as tic disorders, BDD, trichotillomania, skin-picking, and eating disorders in OCD patients (37%) compared with patients with panic disorder and social anxiety disorder, suggesting specificity for cosegregation of OCSDs above anxiety disorders in general.

Family Studies

Family studies (Nestadt et al. 2001) have shown that in families with an OCD proband, there are higher-than-expected rates of anxiety disorders, including panic disorder, generalized anxiety disorder (GAD), agoraphobia, separation anxiety, and recurrent major depressive disorder (MDD), implying either a common cause or a consequential link. In some studies (Carter et al. 2004; Fyer et al. 2005), GAD and agoraphobia occurred more frequently, even in case relatives who did not have OCD, suggesting that these disorders share a familial etiology. However, other studies found no increased rate of anxiety disorders in unaffected relatives of OCD patients compared with relatives of control subjects, calling into question the idea of a familial association between OCD and anxiety disorders. In a study by Carter et al. (2004), rates of panic disorder, GAD, and MDD were higher only among case relatives with OCD but not in those without OCD, leading the authors to suggest that anxiety and depression may have occurred in these relatives as a consequence of having OCD rather than due to a shared inherited etiology.

Neurobiology

Functional brain imaging research has led to a greater understanding of the neurobiological mediation of OCD. Various positron emission tomography (PET) studies of OCD (Saxena 2003) have found elevated glucose metabolic rates in the orbitofrontal cortex, anterior cingulate gyrus, caudate nuclei, and thalamus that

TABLE 1–2. Obsessive-compulsive disorder (OCD) and anxiety disorders, major depressive disorder, and schizophrenia: similarities and differences systematically examined

	OCD	GAD	SAD	PD	MDD	Schiz
Prevalence	2%–3%	3%	2%–7%	2%	20%	1%
Male:female ratio	1:1[a]	2–3:1	2:1	2–3:1	2–3:1	1:1?
Early age of onset	+++	+	+++	+	–	++
Chronic course	++	++	++	++	–	+++
Functional impairment	+++	+++	+++	+++	+++	+++
Comorbid with depression	+++	+++	++	+++	+++	+++
Comorbid with eating disorder	++	+	+	+	++	?
Comorbid with OCSD	+++	++	+	+	+++	–
Comorbid with other anxiety disorders	++	+++	+++	+++	+++	++
Inherited in OCD families	+++	++	++	++	?	–
Corticostriatal circuit abnormalities	+++	–	–	–	–	++
Limbic circuit abnormalities	+	+++	+++	+++	+++	++
Decreased cognitive flexibility	+++	–	–	–	++	+++
Cognitive disinhibition	+++	–	–	–	–	+
Disordered emotional processing	+	+++	+++	+++	+++	++
Preferential response to SSRIs[b]	+++	–	–	–	–	–

Note. ?=insufficient evidence; +=limited evidence or small effect size; ++=strong evidence or large effect size; +++=strong evidence and large effect size; –=evidence of no effect; GAD=generalized anxiety disorder; MDD=major depressive disorder; OCD=obsessive-compulsive disorder; OCSD=obsessive-compulsive spectrum disorder; PD=panic disorder; SAD=social anxiety disorder; Schiz=schizophrenia; SSRIs=serotonin reuptake inhibitors.
[a]Male>female in early-onset OCD.
[b]Compared with antidepressants with other modes of action.

TABLE 1–3. Reported comorbidity rates for obsessive-compulsive disorder

Comorbid disorder	Rate
Depression	66%
Simple phobia	22%
Social phobia	18%
Eating disorder	17%
Alcohol dependence	14%
Panic disorder	12%
Tourette's syndrome	7%

Source. Pigott et al. 1994.

normalize with response to treatment. Interventions that provoke OCD symptoms have been found to increase activity in these same brain regions (Breiter et al. 1996; Cottraux et al. 1996; McGuire et al. 1994; Rauch et al. 1994). These and other findings (Alexander et al. 1986; Chamberlain et al. 2005) have led to the theory that the symptomatic expression of OCD is mediated by hyperactivity along specific, frontal-subcortical circuits connecting the orbitofrontal cortex, ventromedial caudate, globus pallidus, and the medial dorsal nucleus of the thalamus.

In contrast to OCD, the brain circuits most often found to be dysfunctional in anxiety disorders are thought to involve the amygdala, which processes the emotional response to threat; the hippocampus, which is involved in fear conditioning; and more diffuse pathways subserving attention and arousal (Kent and Rauch 2003). Abnormal activation of the amygdala and hippocampus has been reported in social anxiety disorder, both in emotion-processing (Schneider et al. 1999) and symptom-provocation studies (Stein et al. 2002; Tillfors et al. 2002). In contrast, most symptom-provocation studies in OCD have not found the amygdala to be abnormally activated (see Saxena 2003 for review). Few imaging studies (Mataix-Cols and van den Heuvel 2006) have directly compared OCD with other anxiety disorders on tests of neuronal circuitry. Lucey et al. (1997) compared OCD patients with groups of patients with panic disorder, posttraumatic stress disorder, and healthy control subjects and found significant differences between OCD patients and the other three groups in cerebral blood flow to the caudate nuclei. Overall, neuroimaging research indicates that the pathophysiology of OCD differs from that of other anxiety disorders (Kent and Rauch 2003; Mataix-Cols and van den Heuven 2006).

By the same token, few studies have directly compared OCD with anxiety disorders on neurocognitive tasks. Individuals with OCD were more impaired than those with panic disorder on a range of executive tasks in four studies (Airaksinen et al. 2005; Boldrini et al. 2005; Clayton et al. 1999; Purcell et al. 1998). GAD patients were included in one study and did not separate from control subjects (Airaksinen et al. 2005). Social anxiety disorder patients showed similar or worse impairment than OCD on some executive tasks (Airaksinen et al. 2005; Cohen et al. 2003), suggesting a closer relationship between these two disorders (Table 1–4).

Psychopharmacology

The robust selectivity of the pharmacotherapeutic response for serotonergic agents has distinguished OCD from depression and anxiety disorders, for which a wider range of medications are known to be effective, and has implicated serotonin in the mechanism of the treatment effect (Fineberg and Gale 2005). Randomized, controlled trials of anxiolytic drugs, such as benzodiazepines (Crockett et al. 2004) and buspirone (Grady et al. 1993; McDougle et al. 1993), do not show efficacy in treating OCD. Anxiogenic challenges, such as yohimbine (Rasmussen et al. 1987), sodium lactate, caffeine, carbon dioxide (Griez et al. 1990), and pentagastrin and cholecystokinin (de Leeuw et al. 1996), do not exacerbate OCD symptoms.

Although the OCD phenotype shows some overlap with anxiety disorders in terms of shared symptoms, comorbidities, and family history, important differences, including age of onset, gender bias, differing functional neuroanatomy, and neuropsychological deficits cast question on its membership in the anxiety disorders group (Bartz and Hollander 2006).

OBSESSIVE-COMPULSIVE DISORDER VERSUS DEPRESSION

Depression and anxiety frequently overlap. Lifetime prevalence rates for comorbid mood disorders in OCD are reported as high as in MDD (66%), dysthymia (26%), and bipolar disorder (10%) (Pigott et al. 1994; Rasmussen and Eisen 1990). Comorbid MDD usually follows the onset of OCD and, like OCD, responds selectively to selective serotonin reuptake inhibitors (SSRIs). Comorbid depression is also characterized by different symptoms and imaging profiles from those of noncomorbid MDD (Saxena 2003), hinting it may be integral to OCD (Fineberg et al. 2005).

OCD often starts in childhood and runs a chronic course, whereas depression has a peak age of onset in adulthood and tends to be episodic. Episodic OCD, with complete interepisodic recovery, has been reported in up to 25% cases (Ravizza et al. 1997) and is thought to share a possible association with bipolar affective disorder (Perugi et al. 2002). OCD can be distinguished from MDD by its selective pharmacotherapeutic response to SSRIs (Fineberg and Gale 2005) and the tricyclic antidepressant clomipramine. These drugs are effective even when depression is rigorously excluded in the reference population, implying a specific antiobsessional effect. Antidepressant drugs lacking these properties, such as other tricyclics (e.g., amitriptyline, nortriptyline) and monoamine oxidase inhibitors (e.g., clorgyline, phenelzine), have been found to be ineffective for OCD (Hoehn-Saric et al. 2000).

TABLE 1–4. Obsessive-compulsive disorder (OCD) shows more impairment than anxiety disorders on neurocognitive tests of executive function

Study	Sample	N	Test	Results
Cohen et al. 2003	OCD, SP, and control subjects	114	Trails B	SP>OCD
Purcell et al. 1998	OCD, PD, and control subjects	90	SWM, TOL, spatial recognition	OCD>PD
Clayton et al. 1999	OCD, PD, and control subjects	44	Sustained attention, selective attention, set-shifting	OCD>PD
Boldrini et al. 2005	OCD, PD, and control subjects	55	WCST, facial recognition	OCD>PD (not facial recognition)
Airaksinen et al. 2005	OCD, PD SP, GAD, and control subjects	55 175	Trails, episodic memory, verbal fluency	OCD, PD>control subjects SP>control subjects, episodic memory GAD=control subjects

Note. GAD=generalized anxiety disorder; PD=panic disorder; SP=social phobia; SWM=Spatial Working Memory; TOL=Tower of London; Trails B=Trail Making Test, Part B; WCST=Wisconsin Card Sorting Test.

Studies investigating lithium and electroconvulsive therapy have also not produced positive findings (Fineberg and Gale 2005).

The treatment effect is slow and gradual in OCD, with a linear, incremental pattern of improvement that also appears different from depression. Dosage-finding studies (Montgomery et al. 2001; Tollefson et al. 1994; Wheadon et al. 1993) have suggested that higher dosages are required (e.g., citalopram 60 mg/day, fluoxetine 60 mg/day, paroxetine 60 mg/day, and sertraline 200 mg/day) than those usually used to treat depression or anxiety disorders (Fineberg and Gale 2005). Unlike depression and social anxiety disorder (Argyropoulos et al. 2004), tryptophan depletion does not seem to precipitate the reemergence of symptoms in SSRI-treated cases of OCD (Barr et al. 1994) nor do changes in cortisol secretion (Vielhaber et al. 2005), casting doubt on the essential role of serotonin in the mechanism of treatment effect.

Trait-like deficits in cognitive flexibility and motor inhibition have been consistently demonstrated in nondepressed patients with OCD and their unaffected relatives (Chamberlain et al. 2007a). It has been suggested that these deficits may represent distinct neuropathology of the lateral orbitofrontal-subcortical circuit in OCD (Alexander et al. 1986; Chamberlain et al. 2005). Similarly, patients with bipolar disorder and MDD show deficits in cognitive flexibility (Bearden et al. 2001; Veiel 1997) and attentional set shifting (Clark et al. 2002). In affective disorders, as with OCD, these deficits seem to be trait-like in that they remain when patients are euthymic and are also found in euthymic first-degree relatives (Clark et al. 2005). These findings, along with anatomical studies in bipolar patients, suggest overlapping pathology in the lateral prefrontal cortex. Conversely, the deficits in motor inhibition on tests, such as the stop signal reaction-time task, found to be associated with OCD (Chamberlain et al. 2006b) do not seem to occur in depression, whereas verbal learning has been identified as a state marker for depression and bipolar disorder (Clark et al. 2002) but remains intact in OCD.

The relationship between OCD and depression is complex. Areas of convergence include comorbidity, response to serotonergic treatment, deficits in cognitive flexibility, and attentional set shifting. On the other hand, OCD has an earlier onset, a different mechanism of response to SSRIs, a different pattern of structural and functional brain abnormalities, and impairments in motor inhibition that distinguish it from affective disorders (Table 1–2). However, there may be a common underlying factor leading to vulnerability to both disorders (e.g., trait neuroticism or abnormal serotonin neurocircuitry) that explains the high level of comorbidity and unusual profile of the comorbid disorder.

OBSESSIVE-COMPULSIVE DISORDER VERSUS SCHIZOPHRENIA

In the past, OCD was thought to have more in common with psychotic disorders than we recognize today. For a long time, European psychiatrists held that anxiety, depression, and repetitive behaviors were less important than the delusional qualities, magical rituals, psychosocial disability, absence of insight, persistence of certain themes (religion, sex, and violence), hallucinatory experiences, and motor disorders in the understanding of OCD (Berrios 1995).

Like OCD, schizophrenia develops in early adulthood, runs a chronic course, and shows roughly equal gender ratios in clinical cohorts. Co-occurrence of OCD, bizarre grooming, and hoarding in schizophrenia is well recognized (Luchins et al. 1992; Tracy et al. 1996). It remains unclear whether the observed overrepresentation of obsessive-compulsive symptoms in schizophrenia reflects true comorbidity, more severe illness, or distinct neuropsychological substrates unique to this group.

Neurobiology

There is convergent evidence that schizophrenia involves dysfunction of the dorsolateral prefrontal cortex (Abbruzzese et al. 1997; Cavallaro et al. 2003; Goldstein et al. 1999; Meador-Woodruff et al. 1997; Silberswieg et al. 1995), whereas OCD involves overactivity of the orbitofrontal cortex (Breiter et al. 1996; Cottraux et al. 1996; McGuire et al. 1994; Rauch et al. 1994; Saxena 2003; Saxena and Rauch 2000) and perhaps also some parts of the dorsolateral prefrontal cortex (Chamberlain et al. 2005). Deficits in working memory and "cortical hypofrontality," which characterize schizophrenia, are not found in OCD.

Numerous studies (Hwang et al. 2000; Lysaker et al. 2000, 2002; Whitney et al. 2004) have compared the profiles of neurocognitive deficits in patients with schizophrenia only versus patients with both schizophrenia and OCD or obsessive-compulsive symptoms. Most, but not all, of these studies have revealed more severe neuropsychological impairments in the patients with both conditions (Table 1–5). Several studies (Hwang et al. 2000; Lysaker et al. 2000, 2002) have reported greater impairment of executive function, as measured by performance on the Wisconsin Card Sorting Test, in patients with schizophrenia and obsessive-compulsive symptoms than in those with schizophrenia only. A recent study comparing executive function in patients with both schizophrenia and OCD with that in patients with schizophrenia only or OCD only suggested that rather than having a unique pattern of neuropsychological deficits, the group with both conditions was more impaired than the other two groups across several neuropsychological domains (Whitney et al. 2004). Preliminary results from another study by Poyurovsky and colleagues (M. Poyurovsky, M.D., written communication, 2006), which attempted to match subjects for degree of illness severity, demonstrated abnormal results on the Wisconsin Card Sorting Test for those with schizophrenia only and schizophrenia with OCD but not those with OCD only, and impairment on the Iowa Gambling Task for those with schizophrenia with OCD and OCD only but not schizophrenia only. These findings support a "pathophysiological double jeopardy" in the overlap group.

Genetics

Family and genetic studies have not found any familial relationship or shared etiology between OCD and schizophrenia. Interestingly, specific genotypes of polymorphisms of the same gene may differentially confer risk for the two disorders. The COMT gene contains a functional polymorphism (Val/Met; Irle et al. 1998) that determines high and low activity of this enzyme, which impacts cognition and psychiatric illness. Homozygosity for the low-activity (Met) allele is associated with a three- to fourfold reduction in the COMT activity compared with homozygotes for the high-activity valine (Val) variant, resulting in reduced degradation of synaptic catecholamines in individuals with the Met allele. Recent evidence suggests (Karayiorgou et al. 1997; Pooley et al. 2007) an association between the Met allele and males with OCD. Met (Irle et al. 1998) alleles may also be associated with an advantage in memory and attention but have also been linked with increased pain sensitivity and hoarding (Lochner et al. 2005; Zubieta et al. 2003). Conversely, those with Val (Irle et al. 1998) alleles have increased COMT activity and lower prefrontal extracellular dopamine compared with those with the Met substitution. Val homozygotes perform poorly on measures of working memory and have an increased incidence of schizophrenia. However, Val alleles may be associated with an advantage in the processing of aversive stimuli, set switching, and cognitive flexibility where rapid disengagement from stimuli is beneficial. Thus, Val alleles may confer protection against OCD and pain susceptibility, whereas Met alleles may confer protection against schizophrenia (although the data remain controversial) (Stein et al. 2006).

In summary, obsessive-compulsive symptoms are common in schizophrenia, and there are clear similarities in terms of natural history and endophenotypic factors (Table 1–2). Both conditions respond to antipsychotics (Fineberg et al. 2006), although only as an adjunct to SSRI treatment in the case of SSRI-resistant OCD. However, the disorders differ considerably in phenomenology, neurobiology, genetics, and treatment response. Important differences in *COMT* polymorphisms that may confer reciprocal cognitive vulnerability to OCD or schizophrenia merit further exploration across these disorders.

OBSESSIVE-COMPULSIVE DISORDER VERSUS ADDICTIVE DISORDERS

Compulsive behavior has much in common with addictive disorders. A central feature in both is the loss of control over behavior, which significantly impairs everyday functioning. However, in contrast to compulsive drug use, the compulsions of OCD are not inherently pleasurable to perform. Moreover, the compulsions of substance dependence are driven by craving rather than obsessive fears. Drug addiction has been characterized as a transition from voluntarily initiated recreational

TABLE 1–5. Published controlled studies comparing neurocognitive tests of executive function in patients with schizophrenia, obsessive-compulsive disorder (OCD), or schizophrenia with OCD

Study	Task	Neural system	N	Outcome
Berman et al. 1998	Visual memory	Frontostriatal	30	Schiz+OCS>Schiz
	WCST	Frontal		Schiz+OCS=Schiz
	Trails A/B			
Lysaker et al. 2000	WCST	Frontal	46	Schiz+OCS>Schiz
Hwang et al. 2000	WCST	Frontal	20	Schiz+OCS>Schiz
Lysaker et al. 2002	WCST	Frontal	63	Schiz+OCD>Schiz
	CPT	Attention		Schiz+OCD>Schiz
	Visual reproduction	Frontostriatal		Schiz>Schiz+OCD
Borkowska et al. 2003	Trails	Frontal	60	Schiz>Schiz+OCD
	Stroop	Attention		>OCD>control subjects
	Verbal fluency			
Ongur and Goff 2005	WCST	Frontal	118	Schiz+OCS=Schiz
	Verbal learning	Attention		
	Stroop			
	Trails A/B			
Hermesh et al. 2003	WCST	Frontal	40	Schiz+OCD=Schiz
	Alternation learning	Orbitofrontal cortex		Schiz+OCD=Schiz

TABLE 1–5. Published controlled studies comparing neurocognitive tests of executive function in patients with schizophrenia, obsessive-compulsive disorder (OCD), or schizophrenia with OCD *(continued)*

Study	Task	Neural system	N	Outcome
Whitney et al. 2004	WCST Attention Iowa Gamble	Frontal Attention Orbitofrontal cortex	65	Schiz+OCS>Schiz >OCD (not significant)

Note. >=more impaired on cognitive task; CPT = Continuous Performance Task; OCS = obsessive-compulsive symptoms; Schiz = schizophrenia; Trails A/B = Trail Making Test, Parts A and B; WCST = Wisconsin Card Sort Test.

drug use to a maladaptive pattern of compulsive drug seeking and uncontrolled drug intake (Everitt and Robbins 2005). Chronic drug users experience compulsions in the form of intense urges to consume the drug, which they fail to resist, even in face of the adverse consequences precipitated by further drug use.

Brain imaging studies have found some overlap in dopaminergic abnormalities in the two conditions. Studies using PET in medication-naïve OCD patients (Denys et al. 2004; Hesse et al. 2005) and chronic drug users (Volkow et al. 1993, 2001) revealed reduced levels of dopamine D_2 receptors in the striatum in both patient groups compared with healthy volunteers. These data are compatible with the notion that compulsive and addictive behaviors may be driven by abnormal function of the same underlying brain systems, namely the ascending dopaminergic projections into frontostriatal circuitry (Volkow and Fowler 2000). PET radioligand studies in medication-naïve OCD patients (van der Wee et al. 2004) have also shown higher dopamine transporter binding in the striatum. These data are consistent with a model of compulsive and addictive behavior sharing dopamine overactivity in ascending pathways involving $D_{2/3}$ receptors. On the other hand, OCD is characterized by increased orbitofrontal corticostriatal activity (Baxter et al. 1987; Breiter et al. 1996; Cottraux et al. 1996; McGuire et al. 1994; Rauch et al. 1994; Saxena 2003; Saxena and Rauch 2000), whereas substance use disorders are typically associated with decreased orbitofrontal activity (Volkow et al. 2004).

Chronic drug use is harmful to the brain and can be associated with a range of neuroadaptive and neurotoxic effects in the prefrontal cortex and limbic system (Wilson et al. 1996). One putative effect of these changes is a progressive breakdown of inhibitory control implemented by this circuitry (Nestler 2001). There is significant overlap in impaired performance in measures of inhibitory control between chronic drug users (Fillmore and Rush 2002; Moeller et al. 2002) and individuals with OCD (Chamberlain et al. 2006b).

In conclusion, different forms of compulsive behavior are central to OCD and addictive disorders. Dopaminergic dysfunction in frontostriatal circuits has been found in both, as has impaired performance on neurocognitive tests of behavioral inhibition. However, baseline abnormalities in brain function differ markedly between the conditions. Furthermore, there is no familial or genetic association between OCD and substance use disorders, and they differ greatly in their psychopharmacology. Dopaminergic drugs can both exacerbate and remediate compulsive behaviors in the context of several therapeutic areas. Compulsive gambling is considered a behavioral addiction. It shares many characteristics with substance addiction and a suggested comorbidity with OCSDs (Grant et al. 2006; Potenza et al. 2003; Siever et al. 1999). A survey of cases of compulsive gambling induced by dopamine agonist medications in Parkinson's disease revealed a close link between occurrence of gambling and D_3-preferent medications (Dodd et al. 2005). Conversely, the selective D_3 antagonist SB-277011-A has been shown to successfully attenuate drug-seeking behavior on a rodent model (see Di Ciano et al. 2003). The behaviorally opposite effects of agonist and antagonist drugs acting at D_3 receptors may thus be understood in terms of their opposing modulatory effects on frontostriatal systems.

OBSESSIVE-COMPULSIVE DISORDER VERSUS HYPOCHONDRIASIS, BODY DYSMORPHIC DISORDER, AND GROOMING DISORDERS

Obsessional fears and compulsive checking are central features of hypochondriasis and BDD. Grooming disorders, such as trichotillomania, skin picking, and nail biting, are characterized by a loss of motor control over irresistible urges and are associated with a prior buildup of tension that is temporarily relieved by enacting the behavior. There is significant comorbidity in clinical cohorts between patients with OCD as a primary diagnosis and these disorders (e.g., trichotillomania [12.9%], hypochondriasis [8.2%] and BDD [12.9%]) (du Toit et al. 2001). Of those with a primary diagnosis of BDD, 30% also fulfilled criteria for OCD (Gunstad and Phillips 2003). In trichotillomania, females outnumber males by three to one (Chamberlain et al. 2007b). These disorders seem to share a specific familial relationship with OCD. Bienvenu et al. (2000) found increased rates of hypochondriasis, BDD, and grooming disorders in families of OCD probands relative to control subjects. However, there was no familial association between eating disorders or impulse-control disorders and OCD (Grados et al. 2001).

In contrast to OCD, these disorders have higher rates of poor insight, overvalued ideation, delusions, and ideas of reference (Fontenelle et al. 2006; Phillips et al. 2007). Hypochondriasis and BDD have a similar profile of selective responsivity to high-dose SSRIs (Heimann 1997; Perkins 1999) and cognitive-behavioral therapy (CBT) utilizing exposure- and response-prevention techniques (Barsky and Ahern 2004; Castle et al. 2006); the CBT method with the best results for trichotillomania and skin picking is habit reversal (Ninan et al. 2000; Rapp et al. 1998).

Trichotillomania and hypochondriasis may also differ significantly from OCD in their neurobiology and pathophysiology. A neurocognitive study comparing trichotillomania with OCD (Chamberlain et al. 2006a) suggested more limited and specific failures of behavioral inhibition in the former using tests sensitive to cortical function. In contrast to OCD, for which the major neuroimaging findings have implicated the caudate and orbitofrontal cortex, imaging studies in trichotillomania have reported decreased activity and volume in the putamen (Kent and Rauch 2003; O'Sullivan et al. 1997) and cerebellum (Keuthen et al. 2007; Swedo et al. 1991). Rauch et al. (2002) reported enlarged white matter volume and altered asymmetry in the caudate nucleus—an area implicated in OCD—in patients with BDD. A study by van den Heuvel et al. (2005) compared OCD with hypochondriasis and panic disorder using an emotional Stroop task. Although all disease groups showed activation of the amygdala relative to control subjects, only OCD showed decreased performance on color-related words, which was accompanied by activation of posterior brain regions and a specific neural response in mainly ventrolateral brain regions and the amygdala. In contrast, patients with panic disorder and hypochondriasis displayed no interference for incongruent versus congruent words but showed a more generalized attentional bias for negative stimuli (panic-related and OCD words), involving both ventral and dorsal brain regions. Patients with panic disorder also showed amygdala activation limited to panic-related words. Thus, although there is evidence that these body-focused symptoms cluster together in patients with OCD, they seem to have different cognitive substrates (Carey et al. 2004; Stein 2000).

OBSESSIVE-COMPULSIVE DISORDER VERSUS TOURETTE'S SYNDROME

Tics are involuntary movements or vocalizations driven by premonitory urges. They constitute the core feature of Tourette's syndrome, a relatively rare juvenile-onset disorder that emerges in childhood (2–18 years of age) and affects males more than females at a ratio of 1.5–3:1. In contrast to tics, the compulsions of OCD are goal directed and aimed at preventing or reducing distress or a dreaded event. Tourette's syndrome and chronic tic disorders are frequently comorbid with OCD and associated with symmetry and hoarding compulsions in particular (Baer 1994; Leckman et al. 1997; Mataix-Cols et al. 1999). Tourette's syndrome occurs in roughly 7% of patients with OCD as a primary diagnosis (Pigott et al. 1994). Conversely obsessive-compulsive symptoms are common in patients with Tourette's syndrome, with rates as high as 50% in children (Park et al. 1993). Tic disorders, including Tourette's, are also more common in first-degree relatives of patients with OCD (Grados et al. 2001) and vice versa (Pauls et al. 1986b).

Juvenile-onset OCD with symmetry and hoarding symptoms, male gender, and the presence of tics have been proposed as a poor prognosis subtype of OCD (Rosario-Campos et al. 2001; Samuels et al. 2002). Leckman et al. (2001) found evidence for at least three subsets of OCD with differing family histories: OCD with a family history of tic disorders, OCD with a family history of OCD, and OCD with no family history of tics or OCD. The close relationship between Tourette's syndrome and OCD has also been reflected in candidate gene studies (Pauls et al. 1986a, 1986b). Zhang et al. (2002) investigated compulsive hoarding (a subtype of OCD) in a study of 77 sibling pairs concordant for Tourette's syndrome. Hoarding in Tourette's was associated with regions on chromosomes 4q, 5q, and 17q. However, sibling pairs were not concordant for the hoarding phenotype, suggesting a separate etiology.

Converging evidence suggests that Tourette's syndrome involves abnormal corticostriatal circuitry. Tourette's has been associated with small striatal volumes

(Peterson et al. 2003). Functional imaging studies using PET and functional magnetic resonance imaging have implicated corticostriatal pathways similar to OCD (Braun et al. 1995; Stern et al. 2000). A cognitive study (Watkins et al. 2005) comparing Tourette's syndrome with OCD found that both showed deficits in set-shifting tasks compared with control subjects. However, there were also important differences between the cognitive profiles of the two groups in the areas of recognition memory and decision making.

Tourette's syndrome is associated with increased dopaminergic innervation in the striatum (Albin and Mink 2006; Albin et al. 2003; Freeman et al. 1994). Dopamine receptor antagonists are effective in the treatment of the disorder (Gilbert 2006; Gilbert et al. 2004, 2006), whereas dopamine agonists exacerbate it (Goodman et al. 1990). SSRIs also have a role in treating the obsessive-compulsive symptoms associated with Tourette's syndrome (George et al. 1993). Although dopamine antagonists are currently considered ineffective as monotherapy in OCD, they are effective as adjuncts to SSRIs in SSRI-resistant cases.

There are significant overlaps between early onset SSRI-resistant OCD and Tourette's syndrome in terms of phenomenology, comorbidity, family history, functional imaging, and pharmacological treatment. This overlap supports the argument for juvenile-onset, male, tic-related OCD as a clinically relevant subgroup (Rosario-Campos et al. 2001).

OBSESSIVE-COMPULSIVE DISORDER AND AXIS II DISORDERS

In clinical cohorts, up to 75% of individuals with OCD meet criteria for at least one comorbid Axis II (personality) disorder (Bejerot et al. 1998). Several clinical studies have shown a predominance of Cluster C personality disorders (avoidant, dependent, OCPD) (Baer and Jenike 1992; Bejerot et al. 1998; Diaferia et al. 1997; Mataix-Cols et al. 2000; Matsunaga et al. 1998, 2000; Mavissakalian et al. 1990; Samuels et al. 2000). Norman et al. (1996) reported that 35%–50% of OCD patients have schizotypal traits, reinforcing the view that there is an association between OCD and schizophrenia-spectrum symptoms. Among those with OCD, the prevalence of individual categories of Axis II disorder seems to vary between the sexes. Males with OCD are more likely to meet diagnostic criteria for antisocial personality disorder (Matsunaga et al. 2000), schizotypal personality disorder (Matsunaga et al. 2000), or OCPD (Thomsen and Mikkelsen 1993), whereas borderline and dependent disorders appear more frequently among females (Matsunaga et al. 2000).

Clinical cohorts may be biased by the effects of the comorbid personality disorder on their likelihood to present for treatment for OCD. In an epidemiological sample (Kolada et al. 1994), OCD was associated with antisocial personality disorder in 10% of cases. However, this was the only type of personality disorder assessed in that survey. In a community study by Nestadt et al. (1994), compulsive, borderline, and histrionic were the only categories of personality disorder significantly associated with OCD.

OBSESSIVE-COMPULSIVE DISORDER VERSUS OBSESSIVE-COMPULSIVE PERSONALITY DISORDER

The fundamental symptoms of OCPD comprise orderliness and perfectionism. Conscientiousness, indecisiveness, and rigidity have also been considered integral at times. Samuels et al. (2000) reported that OCPD stood out from other Axis II disorders by being overrepresented in never-married high school graduates, drawing parallels with the high celibacy rates reported for individuals with OCD. Some OCPD features seem indistinguishable from OCD (e.g., hoarding). However, hoarding severity does not correlate with the severity of OCPD symptoms (Black et al. 1993), and of the eight diagnostic criteria for DSM-IV-TR OCPD, hoarding was found to have the lowest specificity and predictive value (Alnaes and Torgersen 1988). In addition, the obsessional fears and repetitive behaviors that characterize OCD distinguish it from OCPD.

Family studies have found that relatives of OCD patients also frequently had obsessional personality traits. However, the occurrence of personality traits in relatives of non-OCD control groups was not reported (Pfohl et al. 1990). Some studies (Baer and Jenike 1992; Baer et al. 1990; Diaferia et al. 1997; Joffe et al. 1988; Pfohl et al. 1990; Ravizza et al. 1997; Stanley et al. 1990) that used standardized personality disorder assessment instruments found a relatively high comorbidity of DSM-III-R (American Psychiatric Association 1987) OCPD in OCD patients, ranging from 16% to 44%. In contrast, other similar studies found a low co-occurrence (2%–6%; Dinn et al. 2002; Eisen 2004; Mavissakalian et al. 1990) and a high frequency of avoidant, dependent, and passive-aggressive personality disorders (classified with OCPD in the DSM-III-R "anxious" cluster). Schizoid, schizotypal, paranoid, histrionic, narcissistic, and borderline personality disorders have also been reported by multiple studies to be present in individuals with OCD.

In a carefully controlled community study (Samuels et al. 2000), DSM-IV-TR OCPD was found in around 32% of OCD probands, compared with 6% of control probands, and in 12% of case relatives, compared with 6% of control relatives. Of personality disorders, only OCPD occurred significantly more often than expected in the case relatives, suggesting a shared heritability linking the two disorders. Case relatives also scored significantly higher on dimensional scale measures of neuroticism, including anxiety, self-consciousness, and vulnerability to stress, suggesting a common inherited temperament.

Although most studies have suggested that OCPD occurred more frequently in cases of OCD than in non-OCD control subjects, OCPD as defined by DSM-IV-TR criteria was not found in most OCD cases. Thus, OCPD is not a prerequisite for OCD. The issue of underreporting is relevant, not least because of the secretiveness and lack of insight associated with OCPD and problems with the categorical DSM-IV-TR "threshold model," which may miss relevant cases. It may be more appropriate to consider, instead, individual OCPD traits or dimensions. Eisen (2004) investigated the traits most commonly occurring in OCD cases with comorbid OCPD. Preoccupation with details, rigidity, reluctance to delegate, and perfectionism all occurred in roughly one-third of cases. These comorbid patients had higher compulsion scores, were more socially impaired, and had earlier onset of illness than those with uncomplicated OCD. Interestingly, there were no gender differences. Two factors within OCD (hoarding and symmetry) have been reported to be more frequently associated with OCPD (Mataix-Cols et al. 2000). Suggestions that "incompleteness" rather than "harm avoidance" is the core cognitive feature separating this group from the other forms of OCD and that comorbid cases are more treatment refractory need to be confirmed in controlled studies.

There have been no studies investigating brain abnormalities in uncomplicated OCPD. Irle et al. (1998) retrospectively assessed the long-term outcome in 16 patients with treatment-refractory OCD who had undergone neurosurgery involving ventromedial frontal leucotomy performed in 1970. Three patients with comorbid OCPD had improved significantly less. These findings hint that OCPD may be associated with a more refractory form of OCD that might involve different neural pathways.

There have been no studies specifically examining neurocognitive function in OCPD. A study of university students identified associations between performance deficits on measures of frontal executive function and obsessive-compulsive traits (Murphy et al. 2006). OCD is associated with prominent executive dysfunction involving frontostriatal circuitry (Chamberlain et al. 2006a). A preliminary, unpublished analysis by the authors suggested similar executive impairments in OCD cases with and without OCPD, but the OCPD-positive group was significantly more impaired on measures of cognitive flexibility.

OCPD overlaps with OCD on many phenomenological factors (see Table 1–6). Converging evidence from family studies points to a link between OCPD, neuroticism, and OCD. Endophenotypic evidence is, however, still scanty. Further exploration of this relationship using imaging and neurocognitive probes is indicated.

OBSESSIVE-COMPULSIVE DISORDER AND AXIS III DISORDERS

OCSDs are more frequent in patients with active or prior rheumatic fever (Swedo et al. 1998). The prominence of obsessive-compulsive symptoms in rheumatic fever, systemic lupus erythematosus (Carapetis and Currie 1999; Slattery et al. 2004), and Sydenham's chorea has prompted studies into the possibility of an autoimmune form of OCD. There is still both debate and interest in the hypothesis

TABLE 1–6.   Obsessive-compulsive personality disorder (OCPD) and obsessive-compulsive disorder (OCD); similarities outweigh differences

	OCPD	OCD
Prevalence	0.78%	2%–3%
Ego-alien obsessions	−	++
Obsessions resisted	−	+/−
Distressing obsessions	−	++
Gender	M > F	F = M[a]
Early age at onset	+++	+++
Chronic course	++	++
Shift to psychosis	13%	15%
Functional impairment	?/−	++
Celibacy	+	+
Comorbid with depression	+++	+++
Comorbid with eating disorder	+++	+++
Comorbid with OCSD	++	+++
Comorbid with anxiety disorders	++	++
Inherited in OCD families (frequency in first-degree relatives)	++ (11.5%)	+++ (12%)
Monoamine genes	+	++
CSTC circuit abnormalities	?	++
Blunted d,l-fenfluramine responses	+	+/−
Preferential response to SSRIs	+	+++

Note.   − = evidence of no effect; + = limited evidence or small effect size; ++ = strong evidence or large effect size; +++ = strong evidence and large effect size; ? = insufficient evidence; CSTC = cortico-striatal-thalamico-cortical; OCSD = obsessive-compulsive spectrum disorder; SSRIs = selective serotonin reuptake inhibitors.
[a]M > F in early-onset OCD.

that streptococcal infections may lead to OCD and/or tic disorders in childhood without concomitant chorea (Hounie et al. 2007). Coined *pediatric autoimmune neuropsychiatric disorders associated with streptococcal infections* (PANDAS) (Dale et al. 2005), the symptoms of these disorders can include OCD, tics, and attention-deficit/hyperactivity disorder. Clinically, symptoms usually appear suddenly following a group A β-hemolytic streptococcal infection and run a fluctuating course with exacerbations. Males are more likely to develop poststreptococcal OCD-like symptoms and at an earlier age than females (Arnold and Richter 2001; Dale et al. 2005). Family studies (Asbahr et al. 2005) have demonstrated similar rates of OCD in family members of probands with PANDAS and probands with childhood-onset

OCD. For example, a recent family study by Hounie et al. (2007) found significantly higher rates of OCSDs among first-degree relatives of probands with rheumatic fever compared with control subjects.

The proposed mediators of PANDAS are anti–basal ganglia antibodies. In a study by Dale et al. (2005) positive anti–basal ganglia antibodies binding (as seen in Sydenham's chorea) was found in 42% of a cohort of 50 children with OCD compared with 2%–10% of control groups ($P<0.001$ in all comparisons), supporting the hypothesis that central nervous system autoimmunity may have a role in a significant subgroup of cases of OCD. Further study is required to examine whether the antibodies concerned are pathogenic or coincidental.

With circumstantial evidence of PANDAS accumulating slowly, there are few studies addressing possible differences in the endophenotype (apart from immunological biomarkers). Similarly, little is known about the differences between Sydenham's chorea, PANDAS, and Tourette's syndrome in terms of psychiatric symptoms (Bejerot and Humble 1999). A study by Asbahr et al. (2005) reported similar symptom clusters (violent thoughts and contamination obsession) in patients with Sydenham's chorea and primary OCD. The symptom clusters differed significantly from those who had tic disorders, in whom a preponderance of symmetry and ordering obsessions was found. The authors suggested that this may be due to a shared neurological substrate in the case of OCD and Sydenham's chorea that differs from obsessive-compulsive symptoms in tic disorders. Apart from the temporal correlation between β-hemolytic streptococcal infection and the emergence of symptoms, it does not seem likely that PANDAS can be reliably differentiated from idiopathic OCD on phenomenology alone.

Like OCD, OCSDs caused by PANDAS respond to standard treatment with SSRIs and CBT (Steketee and Frost 2003). Trials of antibiotic therapy and/or prophylaxis (Hounie et al. 2007) have shown some promising results but are hindered by small sample sizes. It is unclear whether symptoms remit after acute exacerbations or progress to chronic OCD.

Conclusion

The studies reviewed in this chapter cover a wide range of methods, from epidemiology through family studies to neuroimaging, genetics, and neurocognition. All lend support to the validity of an obsessive-compulsive spectrum of disorders discrete from anxiety disorders. OCD might be considered a prototype for this spectrum of disorders, although all OCSDs share compulsive behavior and failures in behavioral inhibition as an endophenotype. The question of which other disorders should be included within the spectrum is an empirical one requiring further work. OCD seems to share a closer relationship with BDD, grooming disorders, OCPD, Tourette's syndrome, and PANDAS in terms of comorbidity, family history, and cognitive failures and may thus be considered part of the same category. Juvenile-onset, male, tic-related OCD with associated symmetry/order/repeating/touching compulsions and poor response to SSRIs may represent a distinct subtype or variant of OCD. Studies designed to delineate cause, consequence, and common factors are a challenging but essential area for future research.

Despite high comorbidity rates, emerging evidence suggests substantial endophenotypic differences between OCD and anxiety disorders, depression, schizophrenia, and addictions, although comparative data are lacking and the picture is far from clear. Comorbidity rates are higher for other OCSDs than for disorders such as anxiety and depression. Similarly, family studies have not shown increased risk of anxiety disorders in unaffected relatives. Finally, the few cognitive and neuroimaging studies that have directly compared anxiety with OCD have indicated more differences than similarities.

Although OCD and addictions share endophenotypic similarities, such as impaired behavioral inhibition and abnormal dopamine signaling in frontostriatal pathways, they seem phenotypically and neurobiologically different, with lower-than-expected comorbidity rates and no familial or genetic association (Grilo et al. 2001). Grouping these disorders in terms of compulsive behavior has facilitated research into cognitive endophenotypes and helped to distinguish this spectrum of disorders from anxiety and depression.

Future studies that systematically investigate different OCD subgroups, compare OCD with OCSDs, and compare OCD with other major mental disorders and the patients' first-degree relatives, using a standardized battery of endophenotype markers, may help clarify the overlap and the boundaries between these disorders. These studies will inevitably require collaborative expertise integrating diverse fields (e.g., clinical, neuroimaging, pharmacological challenge, biological markers, neuropsychology, and genetics).

References

Abbruzzese M, Ferri S, Scarone S: The selective breakdown of frontal functions in patients with obsessive-compulsive disorder and in patients with schizophrenia: a double dissociation experimental finding. Neuropsychologia 35:907–912, 1997

Airaksinen E, Larsson M, Forsell Y: Neuropsychological functions in anxiety disorders in population-based samples: evidence of episodic memory dysfunction. J Psychiatr Res 39:207–214, 2005

Albin RL, Mink JW: Recent advances in Tourette syndrome research. Trends Neurosci 29:175–182, 2006

Albin RL, Koeppe RA, Bohnen NI, et al: Increased ventral striatal monoaminergic innervation in Tourette syndrome. Neurology 61:310–315, 2003

Alexander GE, DeLong MR, Strick PL: Parallel organization of functionally segregated circuits linking basal ganglia and cortex. Ann Rev Neurosci 9:357–381, 1986

Alnaes R, Torgersen S: DSM-III symptom disorders (Axis I) and personality disorders (Axis II) in an outpatient population. Acta Psychiatr Scand 78:348–355, 1988

American Psychiatric Association: Diagnostic and Statistical Manual of Mental Disorders, 3rd Edition Revised. Washington, DC, American Psychiatric Association, 1987

American Psychiatric Association: Diagnostic and Statistical Manual of Mental Disorders, 4th Edition, Text Revision. Washington, DC, American Psychiatric Association, 2000

Argyropoulos SV, Hood SD, Adrover M, et al: Tryptophan depletion reverses the therapeutic effect of selective serotonin reuptake inhibitors in social anxiety disorder. Biol Psychiatry 56:503–509, 2004

Arnold PD, Richter MA: Is obsessive-compulsive disorder an autoimmune disease? C Med Assoc J 165:1353–1358, 2001

Asbahr FR, Garvey MA, Snider LA, et al: Obsessive-compulsive symptoms among patients with Sydenham chorea. Biol Psychiatry 57:1073–1076, 2005

Baer L: Factor analysis of symptom subtypes of obsessive compulsive disorder and their relation to personality and tic disorders. J Clin Psychiatry 55(suppl):18–23, 1994

Baer L, Jenike MA: Personality disorders in obsessive compulsive disorder. Psychiatr Clin North Am 15:803–812, 1992

Baer L, Jenike MA, Ricciardi JN 2nd, et al: Standardized assessment of personality disorders in obsessive-compulsive disorder. Arch Gen Psychiatry 47:826–830, 1990

Barr LC, Goodman WK, McDougle CJ, et al: Tryptophan depletion in patients with obsessive-compulsive disorder who respond to serotonin reuptake inhibitors. Arch Gen Psychiatry 51:309–317, 1994

Barsky AJ, Ahern DK: Cognitive behavior therapy for hypochondriasis: a randomized controlled trial. JAMA 291:464–470, 2004

Bartz JA, Hollander E: Is obsessive-compulsive disorder an anxiety disorder? Prog Neuropsychopharmacol Biol Psychiatry 30:338–352, 2006

Baxter LR Jr, Phelps ME, Mazziotta JC, et al: Local cerebral glucose metabolic rates in obsessive-compulsive disorder: a comparison with rates in unipolar depression and in normal controls. Arch Gen Psychiatry 44:211–218, 1987

Bearden CE, Hoffman KM, Cannon TD: The neuropsychology and neuroanatomy of bipolar affective disorder: a critical review. Bipolar Disord 3:106–150, 2001

Bejerot S, Humble M: Low prevalence of smoking among patients with obsessive-compulsive disorder. Compr Psychiatry 40:268–272, 1999

Bejerot S, Ekselius L, von Knorring L: Comorbidity between obsessive-compulsive disorder (OCD) and personality disorders. Acta Psychiatr Scand 97:398–402, 1998

Berman I, Merson A, Viegner B, et al: Obsessions and compulsions as a distinct cluster of symptoms in schizophrenia: a neuropsychological study. J Nerv Ment Dis 186:150–156, 1998

Berrios GE: Obsessive compulsive disorders, in A History of Clinical Psychiatry: The Origin and History of Psychiatric Disorders. Edited by Berrios GE, Porter R. London, United Kingdom, Athlone Press, 1995, pp 573–598

Bienvenu OJ, Samuels JF, Riddle MA, et al: The relationship of obsessive-compulsive disorder to possible spectrum disorders: results from a family study. Biol Psychiatry 48:287–293, 2000

Black DW, Noyes R Jr, Pfohl B, et al: Personality disorder in obsessive-compulsive volunteers, well comparison subjects, and their first-degree relatives. Am J Psychiatry 150:1226–1232, 1993

Boldrini M, Del Pace L, Placidi GP, et al: Selective cognitive deficits in obsessive-compulsive disorder compared to panic disorder with agoraphobia. Acta Psychiatr Scand 111:150–158, 2005

Borkowska A, Pilaczynska E, Rybakowski JK: The frontal lobe neuropsychological tests in patients with schizophrenia and/or obsessive-compulsive disorder. J Neuropsychiatry Clin Neurosci 15:359–362, 2003

Braun AR, Randolph C, Stoetter B, et al: The functional neuroanatomy of Tourette's syndrome: an FDG-PET Study, II. Relationships between regional cerebral metabolism and associated behavioral and cognitive features of the illness. Neuropsychopharmacology 13:151–168, 1995

Breiter HC, Rauch SL, Kwong KK, et al: Functional magnetic resonance imaging of symptom provocation in obsessive-compulsive disorder. Arch Gen Psychiatry 53:595–606, 1996

Carapetis JR, Currie BJ: Rheumatic chorea in northern Australia: a clinical and epidemiological study. Arch Dis Child 80:353–358, 1999

Carey P, Seedat S, Warwick J, et al: SPECT imaging of body dysmorphic disorder. J Neuropsychiatry Clin Neurosci 16:357–359, 2004

Carter AS, Pollock RA, Suvak MK, et al: Anxiety and major depression comorbidity in a family study of obsessive-compulsive disorder. Depress Anxiety 20:165–174, 2004

Castle DJ, Rossell S, Kyrios M: Body dysmorphic disorder. Psychiatr Clin North Am 29:521–538, 2006

Cavallaro R, Cavedini P, Mistretta P, et al: Basal-corticofrontal circuits in schizophrenia and obsessive-compulsive disorder: a controlled, double dissociation study. Biol Psychiatry 54:437–443, 2003

Chamberlain SR, Blackwell AD, Fineberg NA, et al: The neuropsychology of obsessive compulsive disorder: the importance of failures in cognitive and behavioural inhibition as candidate endophenotypic markers. Neurosci Biobehav Rev 29:399–419, 2005

Chamberlain SR, Blackwell AD, Fineberg NA, et al: Strategy implementation in obsessive-compulsive disorder and trichotillomania. Psychol Med 36:91–97, 2006a

Chamberlain SR, Fineberg NA, Blackwell AD, et al: Motor inhibition and cognitive flexibility in obsessive-compulsive disorder and trichotillomania. Am J Psychiatry 163:1282–1284, 2006b

Chamberlain SR, Fineberg NA, Menzies LA, et al: Impaired cognitive flexibility and motor inhibition in unaffected first-degree relatives of patients with obsessive-compulsive disorder. Am J Psychiatry 164:335–338, 2007a

Chamberlain SR, Menzies L, Sahakian BJ, et al: Lifting the veil on trichotillomania. Am J Psychiatry 164:568–574, 2007b

Clark L, Iversen SD, Goodwin GM: Sustained attention deficit in bipolar disorder. Br J Psychiatry 180:313–319, 2002

Clark L, Sarna A, Goodwin GM: Impairment of executive function but not memory in first-degree relatives of patients with bipolar I disorder and in euthymic patients with unipolar depression. Am J Psychiatry 162:1980–1982, 2005

Clayton IC, Richards JC, Edwards CJ: Selective attention in obsessive-compulsive disorder. J Abnorm Psychol 108:71–75, 1999

Cohen Y, Lachenmeyer JR, Springer C: Anxiety and selective attention in obsessive-compulsive disorder. Behav Res Ther 41:1311–1323, 2003

Cottraux J, Gerard D, Cinotti L, et al: A controlled positron emission tomography study of obsessive and neutral auditory stimulation in obsessive-compulsive disorder with checking rituals. Psychiatry Res 60:101–112, 1996

Crockett BA, Churchill E, Davidson JR: A double-blind combination study of clonazepam with sertraline in obsessive-compulsive disorder. Ann Clin Psychiatry 16:127–132, 2004

Dale RC, Heyman I, Giovannoni G, et al: Incidence of anti-brain antibodies in children with obsessive-compulsive disorder. Br J Psychiatry 187:314–319, 2005

de Leeuw AS, Den Boer JA, Slaap BR, et al: Pentagastrin has panic-inducing properties in obsessive compulsive disorder. Psychopharmacology (Berl) 126:339–344, 1996

Denys D, van der Wee N, Janssen J, et al: Low level of dopaminergic D2 receptor binding in obsessive-compulsive disorder. Biol Psychiatry 55:1041–1045, 2004

Denys D, Van Nieuwerburgh F, Deforce D, et al: Association between the dopamine D(2) receptor TaqI A2 allele and low activity COMT allele with obsessive-compulsive disorder in males. Eur Neuropsychopharmacol 16:446–450, 2006

Di Ciano P, Underwood RJ, Hagan JJ, et al: Attenuation of cue-controlled cocaine-seeking by a selective D3 dopamine receptor antagonist SB-277011-A. Neuropsychopharmacology 28:329–338, 2003

Diaferia G, Bianchi I, Bianchi ML, et al: Relationship between obsessive-compulsive personality disorder and obsessive-compulsive disorder. Compr Psychiatry 38:38–42, 1997

Dinn WM, Harris CL, Aycicegi A, et al: Positive and negative schizotypy in a student sample: neurocognitive and clinical correlates. Schizophr Res 56:171–185, 2002

Dodd ML, Klos KJ, Bower JH, et al: Pathological gambling caused by drugs used to treat Parkinson disease. Arch Neurol 62:1377–1381, 2005

du Toit PL, van Kradenburg J, Niehaus D, et al: Comparison of obsessive-compulsive disorder patients with and without comorbid putative obsessive-compulsive spectrum disorders using a structured clinical interview. Compr Psychiatry 42:291–300, 2001

Eisen JL: Obsessive compulsive personality disorder: its treatment and relationship to OCD. Paper presented at the 157th annual meeting of American Psychiatric Association, New York, May 1–6, 2004

Everitt BJ, Robbins TW: Neural systems of reinforcement for drug addiction: from actions to habits to compulsion. Nat Neurosci 8:1481–1489, 2005

Fillmore MT, Rush CR: Impaired inhibitory control of behavior in chronic cocaine users. Drug Alcohol Depend 66:265–273, 2002

Fineberg NA, Gale TM: Evidence-based pharmacotherapy of obsessive-compulsive disorder. Int J Neuropsychopharmacol 8:107–129, 2005

Fineberg NA, Fourie H, Gale TM, et al: Comorbid depression in obsessive compulsive disorder (OCD): symptomatic differences to major depressive disorder. J Affect Disord 87:327–330, 2005

Fineberg NA, Gale TM, Sivakumaran T: A review of antipsychotics in the treatment of obsessive compulsive disorder. J Psychopharmacol 20:97–103, 2006

Fontenelle LF, Telles LL, Nazar BP, et al: A sociodemographic, phenomenological, and long-term follow-up study of patients with body dysmorphic disorder in Brazil. Int J Psychiatry Med 36:243–259, 2006

Freeman CP, Trimble MR, Deakin JF, et al. Fluvoxamine versus clomipramine in the treatment of obsessive compulsive disorder: a multicenter, randomized, double-blind, parallel group comparison. J Clin Psychiatry 55:301–305, 1994

Fyer AJ, Lipsitz JD, Mannuzza S, et al: A direct interview family study of obsessive-compulsive disorder, I. Psychol Med 35:1611–1621, 2005

George MS, Trimble MR, Ring HA, et al: Obsessions in obsessive-compulsive disorder with and without Gilles de la Tourette's syndrome. Am J Psychiatry 150:93–97, 1993

Gilbert D: Treatment of children and adolescents with tics and Tourette syndrome. J Child Neurol 21:690–700, 2006

Gilbert D, Bansal AS, Sethuraman G, et al: Association of cortical disinhibition with tic, ADHD, and OCD severity in Tourette syndrome. Mov Disord 19:416–425, 2004

Gilbert DL, Wang Z, Sallee FR, et al: Dopamine transporter genotype influences the physiological response to medication in ADHD. Brain 129:2038–2046, 2006

Goldstein JM, Goodman JM, Seidman LJ, et al: Cortical abnormalities in schizophrenia identified by structural magnetic resonance imaging. Arch Gen Psychiatry 56:537–547, 1999

Goodman WK, McDougle CJ, Price LH, et al: Beyond the serotonin hypothesis: a role for dopamine in some forms of obsessive compulsive disorder? J Clin Psychiatry 51(suppl): 36–43, 1990

Gottesman II, Gould TD: The endophenotype concept in psychiatry: etymology and strategic intentions. Am J Psychiatry 160:636–645, 2003

Grados MA, Riddle MA, Samuels JF, et al: The familial phenotype of obsessive-compulsive disorder in relation to tic disorders: the Hopkins OCD family study. Biol Psychiatry 50:559–565, 2001

Grady TA, Pigott TA, L'Heureux F, et al: Double-blind study of adjuvant buspirone for fluoxetine-treated patients with obsessive-compulsive disorder. Am J Psychiatry 150:819–821, 1993

Grant JE, Brewer JA, Potenza MN: The neurobiology of substance and behavioral addictions. CNS Spectr 11:924–930, 2006

Griez E, de Loof C, Pols H, et al: Specific sensitivity of patients with panic attacks to carbon dioxide inhalation. Psychiatry Res 31:193–199, 1990

Grilo CM, McGlashan TH, Morey LC, et al: Internal consistency, intercriterion overlap and diagnostic efficiency of criteria sets for DSM-IV schizotypal, borderline, avoidant and obsessive-compulsive personality disorders. Acta Psychiatr Scand 104:264–272, 2001

Gunstad J, Phillips KA: Axis I comorbidity in body dysmorphic disorder. Compr Psychiatry 44:270–276, 2003

Heimann SW: SSRI for body dysmorphic disorder. J Am Acad Child Adolesc Psychiatry 36:868, 1997

Hermesh H, Weizman A, Gur S, et al: Alternation learning in OCD/schizophrenia patients. Eur Neuropsychopharmacol 13:87–91, 2003

Hesse SU, Muller U, Lincke T, et al: Serotonin and dopamine transporter imaging in patients with obsessive-compulsive disorder. Psychiatry Res 140:63–72, 2005

Hoehn-Saric R, Ninan P, Black DW, et al: Multicenter double-blind comparison of sertraline and desipramine for concurrent obsessive-compulsive and major depressive disorders. Arch Gen Psychiatry 57:76–82, 2000

Hollander E, Wong CM: Obsessive-compulsive spectrum disorders. J Clin Psychiatry 56(suppl):3–6, 1995

Hollander E, Greenwald S, Neville D, et al: Uncomplicated and comorbid obsessive-compulsive disorder in an epidemiologic sample. Depress Anxiety 4:111–119, 1996

Hollander E, Kim S, Khanna S, et al: Obsessive-compulsive disorder and obsessive-compulsive spectrum disorders: diagnostic and dimensional issues. CNS Spectr 12(suppl):5–13, 2007

Hounie AG, Pauls DL, Rosario-Campos MC, et al: Obsessive-compulsive spectrum disorders and rheumatic fever: a family study. Biol Psychiatry 61:266–272, 2007

Hwang MY, Morgan JE, Losconzcy MF: Clinical and neuropsychological profiles of obsessive-compulsive schizophrenia: a pilot study. J Neuropsychiatry Clin Neurosci 12:91–94, 2000

Insel TR, Mueller EA, Alterman I, et al: Obsessive-compulsive disorder and serotonin: is there a connection? Biol Psychiatry 20:1174–1188, 1985

Irle E, Exner C, Thielen K, et al: Obsessive-compulsive disorder and ventromedial frontal lesions: clinical and neuropsychological findings. Am J Psychiatry 155:255–263, 1998

Joffe RT, Swinson RP, Regan JJ: Personality features of obsessive-compulsive disorder. Am J Psychiatry 145:1127–1129, 1988

Karayiorgou M, Altemus M, Galke BL, et al: Genotype determining low catechol-O-methyltransferase activity as a risk factor for obsessive-compulsive disorder. Proc Natl Acad Sci USA 94:4572–4575, 1997

Kent JM, Rauch SL: Neurocircuitry of anxiety disorders. Curr Psychiatry Rep 5:266–273, 2003

Keuthen NJ, Makris N, Schlerf JE, et al: Evidence for reduced cerebellar volumes in trichotillomania. Biol Psychiatry 61:374–381, 2007

Kolada JL, Bland RC, Newman SC: Epidemiology of psychiatric disorders in Edmonton: obsessive-compulsive disorder. Acta Psychiatr Scand Suppl 376:24–35, 1994

Leckman JF, Grice DE, Boardman J, et al: Symptoms of obsessive-compulsive disorder. Am J Psychiatry 154:911–917, 1997

Leckman JF, Zhang H, Alsobrook JP, et al: Symptom dimensions in obsessive-compulsive disorder: toward quantitative phenotypes. Am J Med Genet 105:28–30, 2001

Lochner C, Hemmings SM, Kinnear CJ, et al: Gender in obsessive-compulsive disorder: clinical and genetic findings. Eur Neuropsychopharmacol 14:105–113, 2004

Lochner C, Kinnear CJ, Hemmings SM, et al: Hoarding in obsessive-compulsive disorder: clinical and genetic correlates. J Clin Psychiatry 66:1155–1160, 2005

Lucey JV, Costa DC, Adshead G, et al: Brain blood flow in anxiety disorders: OCD, panic disorder with agoraphobia, and post-traumatic stress disorder on 99mTcHMPAO single photon emission tomography (SPET). Br J Psychiatry 171:346–350, 1997

Luchins DJ, Goldman MB, Lieb M, et al: Repetitive behaviors in chronically institutionalized schizophrenic patients. Schizophr Res 8:119–123, 1992

Lysaker PH, Marks KA, Picone JB, et al: Obsessive and compulsive symptoms in schizophrenia: clinical and neurocognitive correlates. J Nerv Ment Dis 188:78–83, 2000

Lysaker PH, Bryson GJ, Marks KA, et al: Association of obsessions and compulsions in schizophrenia with neurocognition and negative symptoms. J Neuropsychiatry Clin Neurosci 14:449–453, 2002

Marks I: Fears, Phobias and Rituals: Panic, Anxiety, and Their Disorders. New York, Oxford University Press, 1987

Mataix-Cols D, van den Heuvel OA: Common and distinct neural correlates of obsessive-compulsive and related disorders. Psychiatr Clin North Am 29:391–410, 2006

Mataix-Cols D, Rauch SL, Manzo PA, et al: Use of factor-analyzed symptom dimensions to predict outcome with serotonin reuptake inhibitors and placebo in the treatment of obsessive-compulsive disorder. Am J Psychiatry 156:1409–1416, 1999

Mataix-Cols D, Baer L, Rauch SL, et al: Relation of factor-analyzed symptom dimensions of obsessive-compulsive disorder to personality disorders. Acta Psychiatr Scand 102:199–202, 2000

Matsunaga H, Kiriike N, Miyata A, et al: Personality disorders in patients with obsessive-compulsive disorder in Japan. Acta Psychiatr Scand 98:128–134, 1998

Matsunaga H, Kiriike N, Matsui T, et al: Gender differences in social and interpersonal features and personality disorders among Japanese patients with obsessive-compulsive disorder. Compr Psychiatry 41:266–272, 2000

Mavissakalian M, Hamann MS, Jones B: Correlates of DSM-III personality disorder in obsessive-compulsive disorder. Compr Psychiatry 31:481–489, 1990

McDougle CJ, Goodman WK, Leckman JF, et al: Limited therapeutic effect of addition of buspirone in fluvoxamine-refractory obsessive-compulsive disorder. Am J Psychiatry 150:647–649, 1993

McGuire PK, Bench CJ, Frith CD, et al: Functional anatomy of obsessive-compulsive phenomena. Br J Psychiatry 164:459–468, 1994

Meador-Woodruff JH, Haroutunian V, Powchik P, et al: Dopamine receptor transcript expression in striatum and prefrontal and occipital cortex: focal abnormalities in orbitofrontal cortex in schizophrenia. Arch Gen Psychiatry 54:1089–1095, 1997

Moeller FG, Dougherty DM, Barratt ES, et al: Increased impulsivity in cocaine dependent subjects independent of antisocial personality disorder and aggression. Drug Alcohol Depend 68:105–111, 2002

Montgomery SA, Kasper S, Stein DJ, et al: Citalopram 20 mg, 40 mg and 60 mg are all effective and well tolerated compared with placebo in obsessive-compulsive disorder. Int Clin Psychopharmacol 16:75–86, 2001

Murphy TK, Sajid MW, Goodman WK: Immunology of obsessive-compulsive disorder. Psychiatr Clin North Am 29:445–469, 2006

Nestadt G, Samuels JF, Romanoski AJ, et al: Obsessions and compulsions in the community. Acta Psychiatr Scand 89:219–224, 1994

Nestadt G, Samuels J, Riddle MA, et al: The relationship between obsessive-compulsive disorder and anxiety and affective disorders: results from the Johns Hopkins OCD Family Study. Psychol Med 31:481–487, 2001

Nestler EJ: Molecular basis of long-term plasticity underlying addiction. Nat Rev Neurosci 2:119–128, 2001

Ninan PT, Rothbaum BO, Marsteller FA, et al: A placebo-controlled trial of cognitive-behavioral therapy and clomipramine in trichotillomania. J Clin Psychiatry 61:47–50, 2000

Norman RM, Davies F, Malla AK, et al: Relationship of obsessive-compulsive symptomatology to anxiety, depression and schizotypy in a clinical population. Br J Clin Psychol 3:553–566, 1996

O'Sullivan RL, Rauch SL, Breiter HC, et al: Reduced basal ganglia volumes in trichotillomania measured via morphometric magnetic resonance imaging. Biol Psychiatry 42:39–45, 1997

Ongur D, Goff DC: Obsessive-compulsive symptoms in schizophrenia: associated clinical features, cognitive function and medication status. Schizophr Res 75:349–362, 2005

Park S, Como PG, Cui L, et al: The early course of the Tourette's syndrome clinical spectrum. Neurology 43:1712–1715, 1993

Pauls DL, Leckman JF, Towbin KE, et al: A possible genetic relationship exists between Tourette's syndrome and obsessive-compulsive disorder. Psychopharmacol Bull 22:730–733, 1986a

Pauls DL, Towbin KE, Leckman JF, et al: Gilles de la Tourette's syndrome and obsessive-compulsive disorder: evidence supporting a genetic relationship. Arch Gen Psychiatry 43:1180–1182, 1986b

Perkins RJ: SSRI antidepressants are effective for treating delusional hypochondriasis. Med J Aust 170:140–141, 1999

Perugi G, Toni C, Frare F, et al: Obsessive-compulsive-bipolar comorbidity: a systematic exploration of clinical features and treatment outcome. J Clin Psychiatry 63:1129–1134, 2002

Peterson BS, Thomas P, Kane MJ, et al: Basal ganglia volumes in patients with Gilles de la Tourette syndrome. Arch Gen Psychiatry 60:415–424, 2003

Pfohl B, Black DW, Noyes R, et al: Axis I and Axis II comorbidity findings: implications for validity, in Personality Disorders: New Perspectives on Diagnostic Validity. Edited by Oldham JM. Washington, DC, American Psychiatric Press, 1990, pp 147–161

Phillips KA, Pinto A, Menard W, et al: Obsessive-compulsive disorder versus body dysmorphic disorder: a comparison study of two possibly related disorders. Depress Anxiety 24:399–409, 2007

Pigott TA, L'Heureux F, Dubbert B, et al: Obsessive compulsive disorder: comorbid conditions. J Clin Psychiatry 55(suppl):15–27, 1994

Pooley EC, Fineberg NA, Harrison PJ: The met(158) allele of catechol-O-methyltransferase (COMT) is associated with obsessive-compulsive disorder in men: case-control study and meta-analysis. Mol Psychiatry 12:556–561, 2007

Potenza MN, Leung HC, Blumberg HP, et al: An FMRI Stroop task study of ventromedial prefrontal cortical function in pathological gamblers. Am J Psychiatry 160:1990–1994, 2003

Purcell R, Maruff P, Kyrios M, et al: Neuropsychological deficits in obsessive-compulsive disorder: a comparison with unipolar depression, panic disorder, and normal controls. Arch Gen Psychiatry 55:415–423, 1998

Rapp JT, Miltenberger RG, Long ES, et al: Simplified habit reversal treatment for chronic hair pulling in three adolescents: a clinical replication with direct observation. J Appl Behav Anal 31:299–302, 1998

Rasmussen SA, Eisen JL: Epidemiology of obsessive compulsive disorder. J Clin Psychiatry 51(suppl):10–13, 1990

Rasmussen SA, Goodman WK, Woods SW, et al: Effects of yohimbine in obsessive compulsive disorder. Psychopharmacology (Berl) 93:308–313, 1987

Rauch SL, Jenike MA, Alpert NM, et al: Regional cerebral blood flow measured during symptom provocation in obsessive-compulsive disorder using oxygen 15-labeled carbon dioxide and positron emission tomography. Arch Gen Psychiatry 51:62–70, 1994

Rauch SL, Shin LM, Dougherty DD, et al: Predictors of fluvoxamine response in contamination-related obsessive compulsive disorder: a PET symptom provocation study. Neuropsychopharmacology 27:782–791, 2002

Ravizza L, Maina G, Bogetto F: Episodic and chronic obsessive-compulsive disorder. Depress Anxiety 6:154–158, 1997

Richter MA, Summerfeldt LJ, Antony MM, et al: Obsessive-compulsive spectrum conditions in obsessive-compulsive disorder and other anxiety disorders. Depress Anxiety 18:118–127, 2003

Rosario-Campos MC, Leckman JF, Mercadante MT, et al: Adults with early onset obsessive-compulsive disorder. Am J Psychiatry 158:1899–1903, 2001

Samuels J, Nestadt G, Bienvenu OJ, et al: Personality disorders and normal personality dimensions in obsessive-compulsive disorder. Br J Psychiatry 177:457–462, 2000

Samuels J, Bienvenu OJ 3rd, Riddle MA, et al: Hoarding in obsessive compulsive disorder: results from a case-control study. Behav Res Ther 40:517–528, 2002

Saxena S: Neuroimaging and the pathophysiology of obsessive-compulsive disorder, in Neuroimaging in Psychiatry. Edited by Fu CH, Senior C, Russell TA, et al. London, Martin Dunitz, 2003, pp 191–224

Saxena S, Rauch SL: Functional neuroimaging and the neuroanatomy of obsessive-compulsive disorder. Psychiatr Clin North Am 23:563–586, 2000

Schneider F, Weiss U, Kessler C, et al: Subcortical correlates of differential classical conditioning of aversive emotional reactions in social phobia. Biol Psychiatry 45:863–871, 1999

Shapiro AK, Shapiro E: Evaluation of the reported association of obsessive-compulsive symptoms or disorder with Tourette's disorder. Compr Psychiatry 33:152–165, 1992

Siever LJ, Buchsbaum MS, New AS, et al: d,l-Fenfluramine response in impulsive personality disorder assessed with [18F]fluorodeoxyglucose positron emission tomography. Neuropsychopharmacology 20:413–423, 1999

Silbersweig DA, Stern E, Frith C, et al: A functional neuroanatomy of hallucinations in schizophrenia. Nature 378:176–179, 1995

Slattery MJ, Dubbert BK, Allen AJ, et al: Prevalence of obsessive-compulsive disorder in patients with systemic lupus erythematosus. J Clin Psychiatry 65:301–306, 2004

Stanley MA, Turner SM, Borden JW: Schizotypal features in obsessive-compulsive disorder. Compr Psychiatry 31:511–518, 1990

Stein DJ: Neurobiology of the obsessive-compulsive spectrum disorders. Biol Psychiatry 47:296–304, 2000

Stein DJ, Newman TK, Savitz J, et al: Warriors versus worriers: the role of COMT gene variants. CNS Spectr 11:745–748, 2006

Stein MB, Goldin PR, Sareen J, et al: Increased amygdala activation to angry and contemptuous faces in generalized social phobia. Arch Gen Psychiatry 59:1027–1034, 2002

Steketee G, Frost R: Compulsive hoarding: current status of the research. Clin Psychol Rev 23:905–927, 2003

Stern E, Silbersweig DA, Chee KY, et al: A functional neuroanatomy of tics in Tourette syndrome. Arch Gen Psychiatry 57:741–748, 2000

Swedo SE, Rapoport JL, Leonard HL, et al: Regional cerebral glucose metabolism of women with trichotillomania. Arch Gen Psychiatry 48:828–833, 1991

Swedo SE, Leonard HL, Garvey M, et al: Pediatric autoimmune neuropsychiatric disorders associated with streptococcal infections: clinical description of the first 50 cases. Am J Psychiatry 155:264–271, 1998

Szechtman H, Sulis W, Eilam D: Quinpirole induces compulsive checking behavior in rats: a potential animal model of obsessive-compulsive disorder (OCD). Behav Neurosci 112:1475–1485, 1998

Thomsen PH, Mikkelsen HU: Development of personality disorders in children and adolescents with obsessive-compulsive disorder: a 6- to 22-year follow-up study. Acta Psychiatr Scand 87:456–462, 1993

Tillfors M, Furmark T, Marteinsdottir I, et al: Cerebral blood flow during anticipation of public speaking in social phobia: a PET study. Biol Psychiatry 52:1113–1119, 2002

Tollefson GD, Rampey AH Jr, Potvin JH, et al: A multicenter investigation of fixed-dose fluoxetine in the treatment of obsessive-compulsive disorder. Arch Gen Psychiatry 51:559–567, 1994

Tracy JI, de Leon J, Qureshi G, et al: Repetitive behaviors in schizophrenia: a single disturbance or discrete symptoms? Schizophr Res 20:221–229, 1996

van den Heuvel OA, Veltman DJ, Groenewegen HJ, et al: Disorder-specific neuroanatomical correlates of attentional bias in obsessive-compulsive disorder, panic disorder, and hypochondriasis. Arch Gen Psychiatry 62:922–933, 2005

van der Wee NJ, Stevens H, Hardeman JA, et al: Enhanced dopamine transporter density in psychotropic-naive patients with obsessive-compulsive disorder shown by [123I]β-CIT SPECT. Am J Psychiatry 161:2201–2206, 2004

Veiel HO: A preliminary profile of neuropsychological deficits associated with major depression. J Clin Exp Neuropsychol 19:587–603, 1997

Vielhaber K, Riemann D, Feige B, et al: Impact of experimentally induced serotonin deficiency by tryptophan depletion on saliva cortisol concentrations. Pharmacopsychiatry 38:87–94, 2005

Volkow ND, Fowler JS: Addiction, a disease of compulsion and drive: involvement of the orbitofrontal cortex. Cereb Cortex 10:318–325, 2000

Volkow ND, Fowler JS, Wang GJ, et al: Decreased dopamine D2 receptor availability is associated with reduced frontal metabolism in cocaine abusers. Synapse 14:169–177, 1993

Volkow ND, Chang L, Wang GJ, et al: Higher cortical and lower subcortical metabolism in detoxified methamphetamine abusers. Am J Psychiatry 158:383–389, 2001

Volkow ND, Fowler JS, Wang GJ, et al: Dopamine in drug abuse and addiction: results from imaging studies and treatment implications. Mol Psychiatry 9:557–569, 2004

Watkins LH, Sahakian BJ, Robertson MM, et al: Executive function in Tourette's syndrome and obsessive-compulsive disorder. Psychol Med 35:571–582, 2005

Wheadon DE, Bushnell W, Steiner M: A fixed dose comparison of 20, 40 or 60mg paroxetine to placebo in the treatment of obsessive compulsive disorder. Poster presented at annual meeting of the American College of Neuropsychopharmacology, Honolulu, HI, December 1993

Whitney KA, Fastenau PS, Evans JD, et al: Comparative neuropsychological function in obsessive-compulsive disorder and schizophrenia with and without obsessive-compulsive symptoms. Schizophr Res 69:75–83, 2004

Wilson JM, Kalasinsky KS, Levey AI, et al: Striatal dopamine nerve terminal markers in human, chronic methamphetamine users. Nat Med 2:699–703, 1996

Wittchen HU, Jacobi F: Size and burden of mental disorders in Europe: a critical review and appraisal of 27 studies. Eur Neuropsychopharmacol 15:357–376, 2005

World Health Organization: International Statistical Classification of Diseases and Related Health Problems, 10th Revision. Geneva, Switzerland, World Health Organization, 1992

Zhang H, Leckman JF, Pauls DL, et al: Genomewide scan of hoarding in sib pairs in which both sibs have Gilles de la Tourette syndrome. Am J Hum Genet 70:896–904, 2002

Zubieta JK, Heitzeg MM, Smith YR, et al: COMT val158met genotype affects mu-opioid neurotransmitter responses to a pain stressor. Science 299:1240–1243, 2003

2

RELATIONSHIP OF BODY DYSMORPHIC DISORDER AND EATING DISORDERS TO OBSESSIVE-COMPULSIVE DISORDER

Katharine A. Phillips, M.D.
Walter H. Kaye, M.D.

Body dysmorphic disorder (BDD) and eating disorders have long been hypothesized to be related to obsessive-compulsive disorder (OCD). More recently, since the advent of the obsessive-compulsive spectrum disorders (OCSDs) concept, they have been considered candidates for inclusion in this grouping of disorders (Abramowitz and Deacon 2005; Brady et al. 1990; Hollander 1993; Jaisoorya et al. 2003; Phillips et al. 1995; Serpell et al. 2002; Simeon et al. 1995; Solyom et al. 1985). Their relationship to OCD has been examined empirically and discussed in the literature and is the focus of this review. It should be noted, however, that BDD has also been hypothesized to be related to other disorders, such as social phobia and major depressive disorder, and eating disorders have been hypoth-

---

This chapter was first published as "The Relationship of Body Dysmorphic Disorder and Eating Disorders to Obsessive-Compulsive Disorder." *CNS Spectrums* 12:347–358, 2007. Copyright 2009. Used with permission.

esized to be related to major depression, anxiety disorders, or substance use disorders (Kleinknecht et al. 1997; Lilenfeld et al. 1998; Phillips 2005a; Phillips and Stout 2006; Phillips et al. 1995; Suzuki et al. 2003).

These possible relationships, however, have received little empirical investigation. Furthermore, BDD and eating disorders themselves seem to have some shared features, such as disturbance in body image. However, their relationship has received very little empirical attention and is not discussed in this chapter. The relationships among all of these disorders have important theoretical and clinical implications and are ripe for empirical study. It is possible that a number of these disorders (e.g., BDD, OCD, and eating disorders) may share some genetic and environmental risk factors as well as pathophysiological mechanisms.

Body Dysmorphic Disorder

Body dysmorphic disorder (BDD) has been considered closely related to OCD for more than a century, and it is widely conceptualized as an OCSD (Abramowitz and Deacon 2005; Brady et al. 1990; Hollander 1993; Jaisoorya et al. 2003; Phillips et al. 1995; Simeon et al. 1995; Solyom et al. 1985; Stekel 1949). BDD's similarities with social phobia have also been noted; the Japanese conceptualization of *taijin kyofusho,* which is similar to social phobia, includes BDD (*shubo-kyofu,* or "the phobia of a deformed body") (Kleinknecht et al. 1997; Suzuki et al. 2003). During the development of DSM-IV (American Psychiatric Association 1994), consideration was given to classifying BDD as an anxiety disorder, but this change was not made because there were insufficient data (Phillips and Hollander 1996). Since then, research on BDD has substantially increased, which includes studies that have directly compared BDD and OCD.

BDD, classified as a somatoform disorder, is defined as a preoccupation with an imagined defect in appearance; if a slight physical anomaly is present, the person's concern is markedly excessive. The preoccupation causes clinically significant distress or impairment in social, occupational, or other important areas of functioning and is not better accounted for by another mental disorder (e.g., dissatisfaction with body shape and size in anorexia nervosa).

Characteristics of Body Dysmorphic Disorder and Its Relationship to Obsessive-Compulsive Disorder

PHENOMENOLOGY OF OBSESSIONS AND COMPULSIONS

Obsessions

BDD preoccupations have many similarities to OCD obsessions (Phillips et al. 1995). They are intrusive, persistent, repetitive, unwanted thoughts that are recognized as one's own (Hardy and Cotterill 1982; Hay 1970; Phillips 2005a; Phillips et al. 1993). Patients usually recognize that the thoughts are excessive, in the sense of realizing that they spend too much time worrying about their appearance. The preoccupations cause significant anxiety and distress, are impairing, and are usually resisted to at least some extent (Phillips et al. 1995, 1998b). In one study (Phillips et al. 1998b, involving 53 subjects with BDD and 53 subjects with OCD, BDD and OCD patients did not significantly differ on any individual obsession item on the Yale-Brown Obsessive Compulsive Scale (Y-BOCS; Phillips et al. 1997). Sometimes, BDD and OCD obsessions have similar content—focusing, for example, on symmetry, "just right" concerns, or a desire for perfection.

BDD obsessions differ from OCD obsessions, however, in their focus on physical appearance. Another difference consistently found in BDD-OCD comparison studies (Eisen et al. 2004; McKay et al. 1997a; Phillips et al. 1998b, 2007) is that BDD obsessions are characterized by poorer insight (greater delusionality) than OCD obsessions. Approximately 2% of OCD patients are currently delusional compared with 27%–39% of BDD patients (Eisen et al. 2004; Phillips et al. 2007). Regarding specific components of delusionality, BDD patients are more convinced than those with OCD that their underlying belief (e.g., "I am ugly and deformed") is accurate, more likely to think others agree with their belief, less willing to consider that their belief is inaccurate, and less likely to recognize that their belief has a psychiatric/psychological cause (Eisen et al. 2004). Thus, OCD criterion C ("the person recognizes that the fear is excessive or unreasonable") often is not characteristic of BDD, if "unreasonable" is interpreted as having good insight.

Another distinction is that core beliefs underlying the obsessions often seem to differ. Although BDD and OCD have not been directly compared in this regard, core beliefs in BDD seem to focus more on unacceptability of the self (e.g., feeling worthless [60%], inadequate [71%], or unlovable [41%], or the fear of ending up isolated and alone [69%]) (Veale et al. 1996a). Unlike OCD, BDD beliefs rarely seem to involve moral repugnance.

Compulsions

Nearly all patients with BDD perform at least one compulsive behavior, such as comparing with others, camouflaging disliked body areas, mirror checking, reassurance seeking, excessive grooming, skin picking, tanning, excessive exercising, touching disliked body areas, clothes changing, seeking dermatological treatment or surgery, and compulsive shopping (e.g., for beauty products) (Phillips et al. 1993, 2005). These behaviors resemble OCD compulsions in that 1) the behaviors are performed intentionally, in response to an obsession; 2) the intent is to reduce anxiety or distress and prevent an unwanted event (e.g., being rejected by others or looking "ugly"); 3) most behaviors are repetitive, time consuming, and excessive; 4) they may be rule bound or done in a rigid manner; and 5) carrying out the act is not pleasurable (Phillips et al. 1993, 1995). Some OCD and BDD compulsions (e.g., checking and reassurance seeking) overlap in content/phenomenology, although their specific focus differs, with a focus on perceived appearance flaws in BDD (Phillips et al. 1995). In one study (Phillips et al. 1998b), BDD and OCD did not significantly differ on any individual Y-BOCS compulsion item.

However, BDD and OCD compulsions differ in their specific content/phenomenology. In addition, some BDD compulsions (e.g., mirror checking) do not seem to follow a simple model of anxiety reduction that occurs in the compulsive checking of OCD (Veale and Riley 2001). Investigation of the functional relationship between anxiety-evoking thoughts (obsessions) and strategies to reduce anxiety (compulsions) is needed to assist in determining the relatedness of BDD and OCD (Abramowitz and Deacon 2005).

ASSOCIATED FEATURES

Anxiety and Depressive Symptoms

One BDD-OCD comparison study (Saxena et al. 2001) found higher state anxiety in BDD, whereas McKay et al. (1997a) found higher state anxiety in OCD on one of two measures. In one study (Saxena et al. 2001), but not the other (McKay et al. 1997a), BDD subjects had more severe depressive symptoms than OCD subjects. In a third study (Phillips et al. 2007), depressive symptoms were more severe for comorbid BDD+OCD subjects than for those with OCD only or BDD only, which was accounted for by more severe BDD symptoms in the comorbid group.

Suicidality

In two of three BDD-OCD comparison studies (Frare et al. 2004; Phillips et al. 1998b, 2007), a higher proportion of BDD subjects reported suicidal ideation. A study that examined lifetime suicide attempts attributed primarily to BDD or OCD found a higher rate among BDD subjects (Phillips et al. 1998b). Another study found a higher lifetime rate of suicide attempts (40%) among subjects with comorbid BDD+OCD than in those with only BDD or only OCD; this appeared accounted for by more severe BDD symptoms in the comorbid group (Phillips et al. 2007).

Functioning and Quality of Life

Functioning and quality of life are similarly very poor in both disorders (Didie et al. 2007). One of three BDD-OCD comparison studies (Frare et al. 2004) found that BDD subjects were more likely to be unemployed and had lower educational attainment. Phillips et al. (2007) found that those with BDD had missed more days of work or school due to their illness.

COMORBIDITY

Three studies (Gunstad and Phillips 2003; Phillips et al. 2005; Zimmerman and Mattia 1998) that used the Structured Clinical Interview for DSM-III-R or for DSM-IV Axis I disorders found that 32%–38% of patients ascertained for BDD had lifetime comorbid OCD. Studies that examined comorbidity in patients ascertained for OCD yielded a broad range (3%–37%) with comorbid BDD (Brawman-Mintzer et al. 1995; Diniz et al. 2004; Hollander et al. 1993; Jaisoorya et al. 2003; Phillips et al. 1998b; Simeon et al. 1995; Wilhelm et al. 1997). Three BDD-OCD comparison studies (Frare et al. 2004; Phillips et al. 1998b, 2007) found no significant differences in lifetime comorbidity for bipolar disorder, psychotic disorders (excluding delusional BDD or delusional OCD), panic disorder, agoraphobia, specific phobia, posttraumatic stress disorder, somatoform disorders, tic disorder, trichotillomania, or eating disorders. One of these studies examined personality disorders, finding no significant difference for 10 of 11 personality disorders (Phillips et al. 2007). However, these studies did find that individuals with BDD were more likely to have paranoid personality disorder (in one study; Phillips et al. 2007) as well as lifetime major depression (in two of three studies; Phillips et al. 1998b, 2007), dysthymia (in one of two studies; Phillips et al. 2007), social phobia (in one of three studies; Phillips et al. 1998b), and substance use disorders (in two of three studies; Frare et al. 2004; Phillips et al. 2007). One study (Frare et al. 2004) found that OCD patients more often had comorbid generalized anxiety disorder. Taken together, these studies suggest that BDD is more often associated with comorbidity than is OCD, although these findings are potentially subject to both type I error (because many comparisons were made) and type II error (because some sample sizes were relatively small).

COURSE OF ILLNESS

Studies indicate that mean age of onset of BDD is 16–17 years of age (Phillips and Diaz 1997; Phillips et al. 2005). Two BDD-OCD comparison studies found no significant difference in age at onset (Phillips et al. 1998b, 2007), although one study found an earlier age at onset for BDD (Frare et al. 2004). The one study (Phillips et al. 2007) that compared onset of subclinical illness found no significant difference between BDD and OCD.

A cross-sectional/retrospective study (Phillips et al. 2007) found that BDD and OCD have a similarly chronic course. In the only prospective study of BDD's course, over 1 year BDD was chronic in 91% of 161 subjects (Phillips et al. 2006c), consistent with studies suggesting that OCD is often chronic. This prospective, naturalistic study also examined longitudinal time-varying associations between BDD and comorbid OCD in 161 subjects (Phillips and Stout 2006). Improvement in comorbid OCD predicted subsequent BDD remission, but improvement in BDD did not predict subsequent remission of comorbid OCD. These mixed findings suggest that BDD and OCD symptoms may be etiologically linked for some subjects (Phillips and Stout 2006). However, full-criteria BDD persisted in about 50% of subjects after their OCD remitted, suggesting that BDD is not simply a symptom of OCD. A stronger longitudinal association was found for BDD and major depression. However, this study was able to detect only larger effects, and relatively few BDD or OCD remissions occurred, which may result in some numerical instability of the results.

DEMOGRAPHIC FEATURES

In nationwide surveys in Germany and the United States (N=2,552 and 2,048), BDD was somewhat more frequent in women (1.9%and 2.5%, respectively) than in men (1.4% and 2.2%, respectively) (Rief et al. 2006; Koran et al. 2008). An epidemiologic study in Italy (N=673) found that BDD was more common in females (1.4% of women vs. 0% of men) (Faravelli et al. 1997), whereas a study in the United States (N=373) found that BDD was slightly more common in males (1.2% vs. 1.0%) (Bienvenu et al. 2000). Some nonepidemiological studies have contained more females than males (Phillips et al. 2006a; Rosen and Reiter 1996; Veale et al. 1996a), others more males than females (Hollander et al. 1993; Perugi et al. 1997), and one an approximately equal proportion of females and males (Phillips and Diaz 1997). In three BDD-OCD comparison studies (Frare et al. 2004; Phillips et al. 1998b, 2007), the gender ratio did not significantly differ.

In two of three studies (Frare et al. 2004; Phillips et al. 1998b, 2007), BDD subjects were significantly younger and less likely to be married than OCD subjects. In one study (Frare et al. 2004), BDD subjects had lower educational attainment. BDD patients have also been found more likely than those with OCD to have an occupation or education in art and design (20% vs. 3%), raising the possibility that an interest in aesthetics may contribute to BDD's development (Veale et al. 2002).

FAMILY HISTORY

A controlled and blinded family study (80 case probands, 73 control probands; Bienvenu et al. 2000) found that BDD occurred significantly more frequently in first-degree relatives of OCD probands than control probands, suggesting that BDD may be a member of the familial OCSDs. In the one BDD-OCD comparison study that examined family history (Phillips et al. 1998b), rates of mood, psychotic, anxiety, and eating disorders were similar in first-degree relatives of BDD and OCD probands. However, first-degree relatives of BDD probands were more likely to have a substance use disorder, which did not appear accounted for by more frequent substance use disorders in BDD probands than in OCD probands.

GENETIC FACTORS AND BRAIN CIRCUITRY

Data on genetic factors and brain circuitry in BDD are limited, with some results but not others supporting a relationship between BDD and OCD. In a preliminary candidate gene study of 57 BDD subjects and 58 healthy control subjects matched for ethnicity and gender (Phillips et al. 2002b), association was demonstrated for $GABA_\alpha$-$\gamma2$ (5q31.1–q33.2) ($P = 0.032$), with the 1(A) allele occurring more frequently in BDD subjects than control subjects. No association was demonstrated for serotonin 5-$HT_{1D-\beta}$ receptor, which has been associated with OCD. Neither was an association demonstrated for other tested candidate genes (*5-HTTLPR,* the 5-HT_{1A} receptor gene, the tryptophan hydroxylase gene, the *VNTR* polymorphism for the serotonin transporter, dopamine receptor genes *DRD4* or *DRD5,* or the dopamine transporter gene).

In a small, preliminary morphometric magnetic resonance imaging study in eight women with BDD versus eight healthy control subjects, the caudate nucleus differed between BDD and control subjects, consistent with conceptualization of BDD as an OCSD (Rauch et al. 2003). However, BDD subjects had a relative leftward shift in caudate nucleus asymmetry, whereas magnetic resonance imaging studies of OCD implicating lateralized abnormalities (Jenike et al. 1996; Peterson et al. 1993; Singer et al. 1993) have suggested a rightward shift in striatal asymmetry. Although some previous OCD studies have shown reduced white matter volume (Breiter et al. 1994; Jenike et al. 1996), BDD subjects had greater total white matter volume (Rauch et al. 2003). A small uncontrolled BDD single photon emission computed tomography study ($N = 6$; Carey et al. 2004) yielded a broad range of discrepant findings that did not support a close relationship between BDD and OCD. One small, preliminary study (Hounie et al. 2004) found that BDD occurred more frequently in patients with rheumatic fever (2 out of 59) than in control subjects (0 out of 39), raising the possibility that BDD and OCD may share some pathophysiological mechanisms involving immune function. In a neuropsychological study ($N = 35$; Deckersbach et al. 2000b), BDD subjects had impaired verbal and nonverbal memory compared with healthy control subjects. This impairment seemed mediated by deficits in organizational encoding strategies, implicating corticostriatal systems. These results are similar to those found for OCD by Deckersbach et al. (2000a). Another BDD study found impaired executive functioning (Hanes 1998).

In an information-processing study (Buhlmann et al. 2002), BDD patients were more likely than healthy control subjects to interpret a range of ambiguous situations (appearance-related, social, and general) as threatening, whereas OCD patients exhibited this negative interpretive bias only in ambiguous general situations. In another study (Buhlmann et al. 2004), BDD patients did not differ from OCD patients or control subjects in terms of general facial-feature discrimination. BDD patients were less accurate than the control group, but not the OCD group, in identifying facial expressions of emotion; this included misinterpreting faces as angry (Buhlmann et al. 2004). Buhlmann et al. (2006) similarly found that BDD patients, relative to control subjects, were less accurate in identifying facial emotional expressions in self-referent scenarios, misinterpreting more neutral expressions as contemptuous and angry (this study did not include OCD patients). These findings are interesting, given that a majority of BDD patients have ideas or delusions of reference (e.g., mistakenly believing that other people are mocking them due to their appearance) (Phillips 2004).

TREATMENT

Pharmacological Dissection/Pharmacotherapy

The treatment of BDD—both pharmacotherapy and cognitive-behavioral therapy— is described in more detail elsewhere, including in a guideline from the United Kingdom's National Institute of Clinical Excellence (National Collaborating Centre for Mental Health 2006) on the treatment of OCD and BDD. In brief, all serotonin reuptake inhibitor (SRI) studies to date (two controlled studies, four open-label trials, and clinical series: Hollander et al. 1999; National Collaborating Centre for Mental Health 2006; Perugi et al. 1996; Phillips 2002, 2006; Phillips and Najjar 2003; Phillips et al. 1998a, 2002a) indicate that these medications are often efficacious for BDD. Furthermore, in a controlled and blinded crossover study (Hollander et al. 1999), the SRI clomipramine was more efficacious than the non-SRI antidepressant desipramine, as in OCD. This latter finding is supported by retrospective data suggesting that SRIs appear more efficacious for BDD than non-SRIs (Phillips 2002). Although somewhat nonspecific, SRI response in BDD (similar to OCD) is usually slow and gradual, appearing over months, and relatively high SRI dosages are often required (although dosage-finding studies have not been done) (Phillips 2002). Unlike OCD, however, in a small, double-blind, randomized trial (Phillips 2005b), pimozide was not more efficacious than placebo as an SRI augmentation agent.

Cognitive-Behavioral Therapy

Like OCD, exposure and response prevention appears efficacious for BDD (National Collaborating Centre for Mental Health 2006; Neziroglu and Khemlani-Patel 2002). However, reports of this technique—without concomitant use of cognitive approaches—are limited to a retrospective study (Gomez Perez 1994) and small case series with up to 10 subjects (Marks and Mishan 1988; McKay et al. 1997b). Most studies (two waiting list controlled studies and case series: Neziroglu and Khemlani-Patel 2002; Rosen et al. 1995; Veale et al. 1996b; Wilhelm et al. 1999) have used both cognitive and behavioral techniques. Cognitive-behavioral therapy strategies for BDD are focused specifically on appearance-related thoughts and behaviors (e.g., appearance concerns and body image, muscle dysmorphia symptoms, pursuit of surgery and dermatological treatment). Clinical experience suggests that (Phillips 2005a), unlike OCD, habit reversal is frequently needed when treating patients with BDD, especially for common BDD symptoms such as skin picking. Clinical experience also suggests that BDD patients' greater delusionality may make them more difficult to engage in treatment and effectively treat. Unanswered questions requiring study are whether the greater delusionality in BDD requires inclusion of a cognitive component to explicitly target poor insight and greater focus on motivation and engagement in therapy.

SUMMARY

More research is needed on BDD and OCD, especially direct comparison studies of the two disorders in all of the domains just described. Studies are also needed that directly compare BDD with other disorders. Research on these disorders' etiology and pathophysiology may be particularly informative (Phillips et al. 2003, 2007). Nonetheless, available data from a variety of domains indicate that BDD and OCD have many similarities but also some differences, suggesting that they are not identical disorders but are probably related. Data on phenomenology, comorbidity, the apparent selective response of BDD to SRIs, and the aforementioned family study (Bienvenu et al. 2000) offer particularly strong support for the conceptualization of BDD as an OCSD.

Body Dysmorphic Disorder's Diagnostic Criteria: Some Issues for DSM-V

Several aspects of BDD's diagnostic criteria need to be considered:

- "Preoccupation" may need to be better operationalized;
- The word "imagined" is problematic and may lead to underdiagnosis of BDD, given that most patients have poor or absent insight and do not realize that their view of their appearance is imagined or distorted;
- A requirement for clinical significance is needed to differentiate BDD from normal appearance concerns; however, it is unclear how to best operationalize this construct (this issue also pertains to other DSM-IV disorders); and
- Careful consideration must be given to insight (delusionality), including its implications for BDD's diagnostic criteria and the classification of delusional and nondelusional variants of BDD. This issue, too, pertains to other disorders in DSM.

Delusionality: A Dimensional Construct?

Whether delusionality is a dimensional construct or both a dimensional and categorical construct is an important classification issue with clinical implications (Phillips 2004; Phillips et al. 2003). A related issue is the relationship between delusional and nondelusional variants of disorders (Phillips 2004; Phillips et al. 2003). DSM-IV-TR (American Psychiatric Association 2000) classifies delusional BDD as a psychotic disorder (delusional disorder, somatic type). Delusional patients may be diagnosed with both delusional disorder and BDD (i.e., double coding is allowed). OCD and hypochondriasis also have delusional variants that DSM-IV-TR classifies as psychotic disorders. In addition, OCD has a poor-insight specifier. OCD patients with and without insight seem generally similar in terms of demographic and clinical characteristics (Eisen and Rasmussen 1993), and studies comparing delusional and nondelusional variants of BDD (Phillips 2004; Phillips et al. 1994, 2006b) suggest that they have many more similarities than differences. Findings such as these raise the question of whether delusional and nondelusional variants of some disorders (Phillips 2004; Phillips et al. 1994, 2006b) constitute the same disorder and whether delusionality is a dimensional construct. If so, how should delusionality be incorporated into DSM-V, and how should delusional and nondelusional variants of disorders optimally be classified? Research is needed on the construct of delusionality and the delusional and nondelusional variants of disorders such as BDD, OCD, hypochondriasis, major depression, and eating disorders (Phillips et al. 2003).

Anorexia Nervosa and Bulimia Nervosa

For at least 50 years, anorexia nervosa has been linked to OCD (Kaye et al. 1997). Earlier reviews of major comorbid symptoms (Rosenberg and Keshavan 1998) showed that OCD symptoms in anorexia were the second most frequently reported after depression. Solyom et al. (1982) found that, even after excluding food- and body-related obsessions, individuals with anorexia nervosa had high trait scores on inventories assessing OCD symptoms that were comparable to scores of patients diagnosed with OCD.

Despite this association between eating disorders and OCD, relatively few studies have directly compared the phenomenology or neurobiology of these disorders. One factor confounding direct comparisons is that anorexia nervosa and bulimia nervosa, a related disorder, are often associated with malnutrition and extremes of eating behaviors, which have substantial effects on behavior and physiology. Thus, the question is often raised as to whether behavioral symptoms are merely state related. In response to this concern, studies (Bulik et al. 1997; Deep et al. 1995; Godart et al. 2002; Kaye et al. 2004a) show that obsessive and anxious symptoms occur premorbidly and persist after recovery but are exaggerated by malnutrition. In addition, recent studies (Anderluh et al. 2003) showed that the majority of individuals with anorexia and bulimia exhibit childhood perfectionism and obsessive-compulsive personality patterns, and these symptoms predate the onset of the eating disorders. Therefore, it can be argued that these are traits that create a vulnerability for developing an eating disorder.

Characteristics of Anorexia Nervosa and Bulimia Nervosa and Their Relationship to Obsessive-Compulsive Disorder

Anorexia nervosa and bulimia nervosa tend to present in adolescence and occur more frequently in females (American Psychiatric Association 2000). They affect an estimated 0.5% and 1.5%–3%, respectively, of females in the general population. These disorders are characterized by restricted and/or binge eating, a relentless pursuit of thinness, and obsessive fears of becoming fat. Although these disorders are often thought to be caused by psychosocial factors, recent studies (Bulik 2005; Kaye et al. 2004b; Treasure and Schmidt 2004) show substantial genetic and neurobiological etiological influences. These are often chronic, disabling conditions.

Anorexia nervosa is divided into two subtypes: restricting and bulimic. In the *restricting subtype,* subnormal body weight and an ongoing malnourished state are maintained by unremitting food avoidance. In the *bulimic subtype,* there is comparable weight loss and malnutrition, yet the course of illness is marked by supervening episodes of binge eating and/or some type of compensatory action, such as self-induced vomiting or laxative abuse. Individuals with bulimia nervosa remain at normal body weight, although many aspire to ideal weights far below the range of normalcy for their age, gender, and height. The core features of bulimia nervosa include repeated episodes of binge eating followed by compensatory self-induced vomiting, laxative abuse, or pathologically extreme exercise or fasting, and excessive concern with weight and shape. Although abnormally low body weight is an exclusion for the diagnosis of bulimia nervosa, some 25%–30% of bulimia patients have a prior history of anorexia. In addition, some individuals with anorexia convert to bulimia. Despite differences in the topography of their feeding behavior, these disorders share equivalent concerns with weight and shape as well as low self-esteem, depression, anxiety, obsessionality, and perfectionism.

PREVALENCE AND PHENOMENOLOGY OF OBSESSIONS AND COMPULSIONS IN ANOREXIA NERVOSA AND BULIMIA NERVOSA

Recently, Godart et al. (2002) reported that the lifetime prevalence of OCD ranged from 9.5% to 62% in restricting-type anorexia nervosa, from 10% to 66% in bulimic-type anorexia nervosa, and from 0% to 42.9% in bulimia nervosa. These studies have tended to use relatively small samples, and methods have varied in terms of rigor. A recent study from the Price Foundation Genetic collaboration (Kaye et al. 2004a) used trained raters and a combination of the Structured Clinical Interview for DSM-IV Axis I Disorders and the Y-BOCS to establish OCD diagnoses in 672 individuals with an eating disorder. The overall rate of OCD was 41%, with no difference in frequency among the three groups.

Several studies have assessed the frequency of specific types of obsessions and compulsions in anorexia nervosa and OCD patients using checklist categories from the Y-BOCS. Two studies found symmetry obsessions to be the most common obsessions in patients with anorexia, occurring in 68.8% of patients in one study (Bastiani et al. 1996) and in 72% in the other study (Matsunaga et al. 1999). These studies found similar rates of ordering and arranging compulsions. The frequency of other types of obsessions and compulsions among the anorexia patients differed in prevalence between these two studies. A third study (Halmi et al. 2003) found that anorexia nervosa subgroups were similar to OCD patients in terms of the frequency of obsessions in the symmetry and somatic categories or in the compulsion categories of ordering and hoarding. In all other categories the subgroups had a significantly lower frequency compared with the OCD patients.

There are several aspects of OCD symptoms in eating disorder patients that should be highlighted. The obsessions and compulsions of anorexia patients are largely ego-syntonic despite interfering significantly in their lives. They feel compelled to perform these rituals and behaviors, even though these behaviors may lead to anxiety. However, the behaviors are not regarded as unwanted. In addition (Mazure et al. 1994), phobic thoughts of food and weight repeatedly enter the mind of these patients, but not necessarily against their will. Although these thoughts or preoccupations may be distressing, they are not regarded as senseless. Similarly, such ego-syntonic acceptance of symmetry and exactness symptoms, unrelated to eating, also occur in anorexia nervosa patients (Bastiani et al. 1996).

There are other reasons why anorexia and bulimia are not often considered to be part of the OCSDs. They are relatively female-gender specific and tend to have a narrow range of onset near in time to puberty. They involve severe and intense body-image distortion, in which emaciated individuals perceive themselves as fat, as well as stereotypic hyperactive motor behavior. Finally, there is often denial of emaciation or illness, lack of insight, and resistance to treatment.

OBSESSIVE-COMPULSIVE PERSONALITY DISORDER SYMPTOMS IN ANOREXIA NERVOSA AND BULIMIA NERVOSA

It has long been recognized that individuals with anorexia or bulimia nervosa commonly have personality disorders. A review (Cassin and von Ranson 2005) of assessments done by raters found that Cluster C disorders are common in restricting-type anorexia nervosa and Cluster B and C disorders are common in bulimia nervosa. Rates of obsessive-compulsive personality disorder (OCPD) were between 2% and 30% for restricting-type anorexia and 3% and 19% for bulimia nervosa. A family study (Lilenfeld et al. 1998) that used blind raters and a control sample found that 46% of restricting-type anorexia subjects had OCPD compared with 4% of bulimia nervosa subjects and 5% of control women. Halmi et al. (2005) found that the frequencies of OCD, OCPD, and OCD/OCPD in a large eating disorder sample were 20%, 13%, and 16%, respectively, with no difference among eating disorder subtypes. Thus, the frequency of OCD and OCPD diagnoses tends to be similar within eating disorder subgroups.

ONSET OF OBSESSIONAL SYMPTOMS IN ANOREXIA NERVOSA AND BULIMIA NERVOSA

Series of studies (Bulik et al. 1997; Deep et al. 1995; Godart et al. 2002; Kaye et al. 2004a) have consistently found that anxiety disorders in anorexia nervosa and bulimia nervosa most commonly appear in childhood, before the onset of either eating disorder. Of the 41% of anorexic and bulimic individuals who had a lifetime diagnosis of OCD (Kaye et al. 2004a), 61% experience the onset of OCD in childhood, prior to the onset of an eating disorder. The mean age of onset of OCD was 14 years, and the mean age of onset of anorexia or bulimia was 17 years. When the entire sample of eating disorder subjects was considered, 23% reported the onset of OCD before the onset of the eating disorder. In addition, individuals also commonly reported (Kaye et al. 2004a) the onset of social phobia, specific phobia, and generalized anxiety disorder in childhood before they developed an eating disorder. People with a history of an eating disorder who were not currently ill and had never been diagnosed with OCD or another anxiety disorder tended to be anxious, perfectionistic, and harm avoidant. The presence of a lifetime anxiety disorder or current anorexia or bulimia nervosa tended to exacerbate anxious, perfectionistic, and harm avoidant symptoms.

ANOREXIA NERVOSA AND BULIMIA NERVOSA IN INDIVIDUALS WITH OBSESSIVE-COMPULSIVE DISORDER

Studies, using a variety of methods, have found increased rates of eating disorder in individuals with OCD. Tamburrino et al. (1994) found that 42% of 31 women with

OCD had a past or current history of an eating disorder (restricting-type anorexia, 26%; bulimia nervosa, 3%; bulimic-type anorexia, 13%). Fahy et al. (1993) found that 11% of 105 women with OCD previously had anorexia nervosa. Rubenstein et al. (1992) found that of 62 OCD patients, 13% met full criteria for anorexia nervosa or bulimia nervosa and another 18% met subthreshold criteria for an eating disorder. Another study (Pigott et al. 1991), which administered the Eating Disorder Inventory, found that scores of female patients with OCD were midway between those of individuals with an eating disorder and healthy comparison women.

FAMILY HISTORY STUDIES

Several studies have found that relatives of individuals with an eating disorder have increased rates of OCD. Lilenfeld et al. (1998) found a 10% rate of OCD in first-degree relatives of individuals with restricting-type anorexia nervosa, which was significantly higher than the 3% rate of OCD in relatives of control subjects. Relatives of patients with bulimia nervosa had a 7% rate of OCD, which was not significantly different than relatives of control subjects. Bellodi et al. (2001) found OCD in 16% of relatives of restricting-type and 15% of relatives of bulimic-type anorexia nervosa subjects and 10% of relatives of bulimia nervosa subjects. Together these were significantly higher than the 1.4% rate of OCD in relatives of control subjects. In comparison, Bienvenu et al. (2000) found no difference in the rates of anorexia and bulimia in first-degree relatives of OCD patients compared with first-degree relatives of control subjects.

Lilenfeld et al. (1998) reported that the first-degree relatives of patients with restricting-type anorexia had a 19% frequency of OCPD, which was significantly higher than the 7% rate in relatives of bulimia nervosa patients and 6% rate in relatives of control women. Rates of OCPD among relatives of anorexia nervosa probands with and without OCPD were virtually identical, suggesting shared familial transmission of anorexia and OCPD. These findings raise the possibility that OCPD and anorexia nervosa represent a continuum of phenotypic expressions of a similar genotype. Alternatively, restricting-type anorexia may occur only in the presence of risk factors for both an eating disorder and OCPD.

Although studies are too few to draw definitive conclusions, these findings raise the possibility of some shared transmission between eating disorders and OCD and/or OCPD. OCD is thought (Mataix-Cols et al. 2005) to be a heterogeneous condition. Perhaps anorexia nervosa and bulimia nervosa share transmission with the cluster of OCD patients with symmetry and exactness symptoms, or with some dimension of OCPD.

NEUROBIOLOGY AND GENETICS

Considerable physiological studies have shown that individuals with anorexia nervosa and bulimia nervosa have disturbances of serotonin activity (Kaye et al. 2004b). These disturbances occur when individuals are ill and persist after recovery. A disturbance of serotonin function has also been implicated in OCD (Saxena 2003). Whether people with an eating disorder and OCD share identical disturbances of serotonin function is less clear. As noted earlier, malnutrition and pathological eating influence serotonin function, making direct comparisons problematic. One potential means of answering such questions is to assess 5-HT genes. In fact, there are indications that individuals with an eating disorder and OCD may have alterations in the 5-HT_{2A} receptor and 5-HT transporter genes (Hemmings and Stein 2006; Klump and Gobrogge 2005). However, these studies tend to be small, with many inconsistent findings. Confirmation of such findings will need to rely on much larger samples and contemporary assessment of haplotypes as well as an understanding of the many genes that contribute to serotonin and related neuronal circuit function.

BRAIN IMAGING

Considerable studies have used brain imaging to study OCD. A review by Saxena (2003) reported that studies of OCD patients have consistently found altered activity in the orbitofrontal cortex, with less consistent abnormalities in the caudate nuclei, thalamus, and anterior cingulate, which also show neurochemical alterations suggestive of neuronal dysfunction. Many fewer brain imaging studies have been done in anorexia nervosa and bulimia nervosa (Kaye et al. 2006), and no studies to our knowledge have directly compared eating disorders with OCD. It is well known that malnourishment in both anorexia and bulimia is associated with shrinkage of brain tissue as well as metabolic alterations. Thus, comparing studies in ill, symptomatic eating disorder subjects with those of OCD subjects may be problematic, because it is not certain how brain imaging findings in eating disorders are influenced by malnutrition. Another approach is to study eating disorder subjects after recovery, when there is normalization of eating, nutrition, and weight. Many temperament characteristics, including obsessionality, persist in the recovered state, but there is normalization of brain mass (Wagner et al. 2006). Thus, any persisting alterations are likely to be traits, but they may also reflect a "scar" caused by chronic malnutrition. Still, brain imaging studies in eating disorder subjects (Kaye et al. 2006) have tended to find alterations in limbic regions. These findings are consistent with dysfunction of affect regulation, executive function, and impulse control. However, the question of whether eating disorders and OCD involve similar regions/circuits remains uncertain and will likely require direct comparisons of matched eating disorder and OCD subjects. It should also be noted that several studies have found relationships between body image distortion and changes in the left parietal lobe in anorexia nervosa (Kaye et al. 2006). It has long been recognized that the parietal cortex mediates perceptions of the body. In summary, neuroimaging data suggest some shared brain circuitry between eating disorders and OCD, but state and methodological differences confound comparisons.

TREATMENT

Several consensus publications have recently reviewed treatment options for anorexia nervosa and bulimia nervosa. These include guidelines from the American Psychiatric Association (2006) and the National Institute of Clinical Excellence (2004). These publications should be consulted for more specific details about therapy. In addition, Web sites such as the National Eating Disorders Association (www.nationaleatingdisorders.org) can be accessed for more information and treatment referrals.

In brief, controlled trials have provided convincing evidence for the efficacy of both psychological and antidepressant treatments for bulimia nervosa. Still, although most subjects show a decrease in the frequency of binge eating and purging episodes, relatively few develop complete abstinence. In contrast, relatively few controlled trials have been done in anorexia nervosa. Individuals with anorexia are often resistant to treatment because they tend to have ego-syntonic symptoms or may deny being underweight or in need of treatment. Few controlled trials of any therapy have been performed, in part because it has been difficult to enlist cooperation of individuals with anorexia and in part because psychological and pharmacological strategies that have been successful in other disorders appear to be less effective in this illness. For severely emaciated patients, hospitalization for supportive medical care and weight restoration may be useful or necessary. Still, relapse is common after discharge. More recent controlled trials (Lock and le Grange 2005) have suggested that the Maudsley Family Therapy techniques seem to be particularly helpful in younger patients with anorexia nervosa. Follow-up studies (Lock and le Grange 2005) suggest that these interventions may also help prevent relapse in patients who achieve weight restoration. Recent studies (Pike et al. 2003) have begun more systematic evaluation of the potential benefits of manualized cognitive-behavioral and family therapies for this disorder. A range of medications, including SRIs and neuroleptics, have been tried in anorexia nervosa, but there have been few controlled trials in ill, malnourished patients. Some data (Kaye et al. 2001; Walsh et al. 2006) raised the possibility that fluoxetine may be useful in reducing relapse after weight restoration, particularly in those with restricting-type compared with bulimic-type anorexia.

SUMMARY

There is compelling evidence that eating disorders and OCD are related. Individuals with eating disorders often have comorbid OCD, and eating disorders occur in some subjects who present with OCD. Moreover, OCD symptoms first present in childhood in about one-quarter of individuals who later develop anorexia nervosa or bulimia nervosa. Finally, a diagnosis of OCD occurs in family members of people with eating disorders. There are clear differences between the disorders, however. Anorexia and bulimia are gender specific and accompanied by eating and body-image symptoms. Anorexia in particular is associated with OCPD; perfectionism; and inflexible, ascetic personalities, and these symptoms are common in family members. In addition, anorexic individuals, particularly in the ill state, have ego-syntonic symptoms, are resistant to treatment, and lack insight. It has been proposed (Mataix-Cols et al. 2005) that OCD is a heterogeneous condition. Perhaps anorexia and bulimia have more in common with OCD patients with symmetry and exactness dimensions or with OCD patients with OCPD and/or overvalued ideation. These questions are unlikely to be answered until direct comparisons of phenomenology, genetics, and brain imaging are conducted in eating disorder and OCD patients.

Some Issues for DSM-V

DSM-V should consider including as part of the diagnostic criteria or as an associated descriptive feature a description of common premorbid vulnerabilities to eating disorders, such as obsessionality, anxiety, harm avoidance, and perfectionism. These traits also often persist after people recover from anorexia nervosa and bulimia nervosa. More recently it has become clear that certain neurocognitive patterns occur in anorexia that persist after recovery, such as delayed set-shifting. Together these appear to be traits that contribute toward a vulnerability of developing anorexia and bulimia.

Although many malnourished individuals with anorexia nervosa have normal laboratory examinations, there is considerable evidence that they have abnormal brain neurotransmitter function, which contributes to symptoms and perhaps resistance to treatment. The optimal way to reflect this in the DSM-V is unclear; however, information on neurobiology as well as genetic contributions to the development of eating disorders should be included.

Anorexia nervosa is associated with a cluster of common symptoms, such as overexercise, denial, and resistance to treatment. These clinical features should be included in DSM-V because they are key elements that make it difficult to treat this disorder.

Conclusion

Views of the relationship between OCD, BDD, and eating disorders have tended to be based largely on observations of phenomenology. Although such observations are of critical importance, it is necessary to also increase understanding of these disorders' etiology and pathophysiology, including how behavior is coded in the brain. It has been difficult to correlate brain function and behavior in living human beings because our technology has been indirect and relatively imprecise. Now, a revolution is taking place in understanding the brain and behavior. Considerable basic science studies have produced a wealth of information about the function of brain pathways and neurotransmitters. Moreover, substantial advances have occurred in technologies, such as brain imaging and genetics, that make it possible to apply this new knowledge to studies in living people. Increased understanding of environmental determinants of illness, and their effects on the brain, is also occurring. The shared symptoms of BDD, eating disorders, and OCD suggest that they may involve the same brain pathways. However, each may be a syndrome consisting of one, or likely many, different patterns of molecular disturbances. A definitive answer to questions about the relationship between these syndromes may not be possible until we have the tools necessary to understand the genetic and environmental bases of these disorders and to better define brain pathway function and behavior.

References

Abramowitz JS, Deacon BJ: Obsessive-compulsive disorders: essential phenomenology and overlap with other anxiety disorders, in Concepts and Controversies in Obsessive-Compulsive Disorder. Edited by Abramowitz JS, Houts AC. New York, Springer, 2005, pp 119–135

American Psychiatric Association: Diagnostic and Statistical Manual of Mental Disorders, 4th Edition. Washington, DC, American Psychiatric Association, 1994

American Psychiatric Association: Diagnostic and Statistical Manual of Mental Disorders, 4th Edition, Text Revision. Washington, DC, American Psychiatric Association, 2000

American Psychiatric Association: Practice Guideline for the Treatment of Patients with Eating Disorders, 3rd Edition. Washington, DC, American Psychiatric Association, 2006

Anderluh MB, Tchanturia K, Rabe-Hesketh S, et al: Childhood obsessive-compulsive personality traits in adult women with eating disorders: defining a broader eating disorder phenotype. Am J Psychiatry 160:242–247, 2003

Bastiani AM, Altemus M, Pigott TA, et al: Comparison of obsessions and compulsions in patients with anorexia nervosa and obsessive compulsive disorder. Biol Psychiatry 39:966–969, 1996

Bellodi L, Cavallini MC, Bertelli S, et al: Morbidity risk for obsessive-compulsive spectrum disorders in first-degree relatives of patients with eating disorders. Am J Psychiatry 158:563–569, 2001

Bienvenu OJ, Samuels JF, Riddle MA, et al: The relationship of obsessive-compulsive disorder to possible spectrum disorders: results from a family study. Biol Psychiatry 48:287–293, 2000

Brady KT, Austin L, Lydiard RB: Body dysmorphic disorder: the relationship to obsessive-compulsive disorder. J Nerv Ment Dis 178:538–540, 1990

Brawman-Mintzer O, Lydiard RB, Phillips KA, et al: Body dysmorphic disorder in patients with anxiety disorders and major depression: a comorbidity study. Am J Psychiatry 152:1665–1667, 1995

Breiter HC, Filipek PA, Kennedy DN, et al. Retrocallosal white matter abnormalities in patients with obsessive-compulsive disorder. Arch Gen Psychiatry 51:663–664, 1994

Buhlmann U, Wilhelm S, McNally RJ, et al: Interpretive biases for ambiguous information in body dysmorphic disorder. CNS Spectr 7:435–443, 2002

Buhlmann U, McNally RJ, Etcoff NL, et al: Emotion recognition deficits in body dysmorphic disorder. J Psychiatr Res 38:201–206, 2004

Buhlmann U, Etcoff NL, Wilhelm S: Emotion recognition bias for contempt and anger in body dysmorphic disorder. J Psychiatr Res 40:105–111, 2006

Bulik CM: Exploring the gene-environment nexus in eating disorders. J Psychiatry Neurosci 30:335–339, 2005

Bulik CM, Sullivan PF, Fear JL, et al: Eating disorders and antecedent anxiety disorders: a controlled study. Acta Psychiatr Scand 96:101–107, 1997

Carey P, Seedat S, Warwick J, et al: SPECT imaging of body dysmorphic disorder. J Neuropsychiatry Clin Neurosci 16:357–359, 2004

Cassin S, von Ranson K: Personality and eating disorders: a decade in review. Clin Psychol Rev 25:895–916, 2005

Deckersbach T, Otto MW, Savage CR, et al: The relationship between semantic organization and memory in obsessive-compulsive disorder. Psychother Psychosom 69:101–107, 2000a

Deckersbach T, Savage CR, Phillips KA, et al: Characteristics of memory dysfunction in body dysmorphic disorder. J Int Neuropsychol Soc 6:673–681, 2000b

Deep AL, Nagy LM, Weltzin TE, et al: Premorbid onset of psychopathology in long-term recovered anorexia nervosa. Int J Eat Disord 17:291–297, 1995

Didie ER, Walters MM, Pinto A, et al: Comparison of quality of life and psychosocial functioning in obsessive-compulsive disorder and body dysmorphic disorder. Ann Clin Psychiatry 19:181–186, 2007

Diniz JB, Rosario-Campos MC, Shavitt RG, et al: Impact of age at onset and duration of illness on the expression of comorbidities in obsessive-compulsive disorder. J Clin Psychiatry 65:22–27, 2004

Eisen JL, Rasmussen SA: Obsessive compulsive disorder with psychotic features. J Clin Psychiatry 54:373–379, 1993

Eisen JL, Phillips KA, Coles ME, et al: Insight in obsessive compulsive disorder and body dysmorphic disorder. Compr Psychiatry 45:10–15, 2004

Fahy TA, Osacar A, Marks I: History of eating disorders in female patients with obsessive-compulsive disorder. Int J Eat Disord 14:439–443, 1993

Faravelli C, Salvatori S, Galassi F, et al: Epidemiology of somatoform disorders: a community survey in Florence. Soc Psychiatry Psychiatr Epidemiol 32:24–29, 1997

Frare F, Perugi G, Ruffolo G, et al: Obsessive-compulsive disorder and body dysmorphic disorder: a comparison of clinical features. Eur Psychiatry 19:292–298, 2004

Godart NT, Flament MF, Perdereau F, et al: Comorbidity between eating disorders and anxiety disorders: a review. Int J Eat Disord 32:253–270, 2002

Gomez Perez JC: Dysmorphophobia: clinical features and outcome with behavior therapy. Eur Psychiatry 9:229–235, 1994

Gunstad J, Phillips KA: Axis I comorbidity in body dysmorphic disorder. Compr Psychiatry 44:270–276, 2003

Halmi KA, Sunday S, Klump KL, et al: Obsessions and compulsions in anorexia nervosa subtypes. Int J Eat Disord 33:308–319, 2003

Halmi K, Tozzi F, Thornton L, et al: The relation among perfectionism, obsessive-compulsive personality disorder and obsessive-compulsive disorder in individuals with eating disorders. Int J Eat Disord 38:371–374, 2005

Hanes KR: Neuropsychological performance in body dysmorphic disorder. J Int Neuropsychol Soc 4:167–171, 1998

Hardy GE, Cotterill JA: A study of depression and obsessionality in dysmorphophobic and psoriatic patients. Br J Psychiatry 140:19–22, 1982

Hay GG: Dysmorphophobia. Br J Psychiatry 116:399–406, 1970

Hemmings S, Stein D: The current status of association studies in obsessive-compulsive disorder. Psychiatr Clin North Am 29:411–444, 2006

Hollander E: Introduction, in Obsessive-Compulsive Related Disorders. Edited by Hollander E. Washington, DC, American Psychiatric Press, 1993, pp 17–48

Hollander E, Cohen LS, Simeon D: Body dysmorphic disorder. Psychiatr Ann 23:359–364, 1993

Hollander E, Allen A, Kwon J, et al: Clomipramine vs desipramine crossover trial in body dysmorphic disorder: selective efficacy of a serotonin reuptake inhibitor in imagined ugliness. Arch Gen Psychiatry 56:1033–1039, 1999

Hounie AG, Pauls DL, Mercadante MT, et al. Obsessive-compulsive spectrum disorders in rheumatic fever with and without Sydenham's chorea. J Clin Psychiatry 65:994–999, 2004

Jaisoorya TS, Reddy YC, Srinath S: The relationship of obsessive-compulsive disorder to putative spectrum disorders: results from an Indian study. Compr Psychiatry 44:317–323, 2003

Jenike MA, Breiter HC, Baer L, et al: Cerebral structural abnormalities in obsessive-compulsive disorder: a quantitative morphometric magnetic resonance imaging study. Arch Gen Psychiatry 53:625–632, 1996

Kaye WH, Weltzin TE, Hsu L: Relationship between anorexia nervosa and obsessive and compulsive behaviors. Psychiatr Ann 23:365–373, 1997

Kaye WH, Nagata T, Weltzin TE, et al: Double-blind placebo-controlled administration of fluoxetine in restricting and restricting-purging type anorexia nervosa. Biol Psychiatry 49:644–652, 2001

Kaye W, Bulik C, Thornton L, et al: Comorbidity of anxiety disorders with anorexia and bulimia nervosa. Am J Psychiatry 161:2215–2221, 2004a

Kaye W, Strober M, Jimerson D: The neurobiology of eating disorders, in The Neurobiology of Mental Illness. Edited by Charney DS, Nestler EJ. New York, Oxford Press, 2004b, pp 1112–1128

Kaye W, Wagner A, Frank G, et al: Review of brain imaging in anorexia and bulimia nervosa, in AED Annual Review of Eating Disorders, Pt 2. Edited by Mitchell J, Wonderlich S, Steiger H, et al. Abingdon, United Kingdom, Radcliffe Publishing Ltd, 2006, pp 113–130

Kleinknecht RA, Dinnel DL, Kleinknecht EE: Cultural factors in social anxiety: a comparison of social phobia symptoms and taijin kyofusho. J Anxiety Disord 11:157–177, 1997

Klump K, Gobrogge K: A review and primer of molecular genetic studies of anorexia nervosa. Int J Eat Disord 37(suppl):S43–S48; discussion S87–S89, 2005

Lilenfeld LR, Kaye WH, Greeno CG, et al: A controlled family study of anorexia nervosa and bulimia nervosa: psychiatric disorders in first-degree relatives and effects of proband comorbidity. Arch Gen Psychiatry 55:603–610, 1998

Lock J, le Grange D: Family based treatment of eating disorders. Int J Eat Disord 37(suppl): S64–S67, discussion S87–S89, 2005

Marks I, Mishan J: Dysmorphophobic avoidance with disturbed bodily perception: a pilot study of exposure therapy. Br J Psychiatry 152:674–678, 1988

Mataix-Cols D, Rosario-Campos M, Leckman J: A multidimensional model of obsessive-compulsive disorder. Am J Psychiatry 162:228–238, 2005

Matsunaga H, Miyaga A, Iwasaki H, et al: A comparison of clinical features among Japanese eating-disordered women with obsessive-compulsive disorder. Compr Psychiatry 40:337–342, 1999

Mazure CM, Halmi KA, Sunday SR, et al: The Yale-Brown-Cornell Eating Disorder Scale: development, use, reliability and validity. J Psychiatr Res 28:425–445, 1994

McKay D, Neziroglu F, Yaryura-Tobias JA: Comparison of clinical characteristics in obsessive-compulsive disorder and body dysmorphic disorder. J Anxiety Disord 11:447–454, 1997a

McKay D, Todaro J, Neziroglu F, et al: Body dysmorphic disorder: a preliminary evaluation of treatment and maintenance using exposure with response prevention. Behav Res Ther 35:67–70, 1997b

National Collaborating Centre for Mental Health: Core Interventions in the Treatment of Obsessive-Compulsive Disorder and Body Dysmorphic Disorder (A Guideline From the National Institute for Health and Clinical Excellence, National Health Service). London, England, British Psychiatric Society and Royal College of Psychiatrists, 2006. Available online at http://www.nice.org.uk/page.aspx?o=289817.

National Institute for Clinical Excellence: Core Interventions in the Treatment and Management of Anorexia Nervosa, Bulimia Nervosa and Related Eating Disorders. London, England, The British Psychological Society, 2004

Neziroglu F, Khemlani-Patel S: A review of cognitive and behavioral treatment for body dysmorphic disorder. CNS Spectr 7:464–471, 2002

Perugi G, Giannotti D, Di Vaio S, et al: Fluvoxamine in the treatment of body dysmorphic disorder (dysmorphophobia). Int Clin Psychopharmacol 11:247–254, 1996

Perugi G, Akiskal HS, Giannotti D, et al: Gender-related differences in body dysmorphic disorder (dysmorphophobia). J Nerv Ment Dis 185:578–582, 1997

Peterson B, Riddle MA, Cohen DJ, et al: Reduced basal ganglia volumes in Tourette's syndrome using three-dimensional reconstruction techniques from magnetic resonance images. Neurology 43:941–949, 1993

Phillips KA: Pharmacologic treatment of body dysmorphic disorder: review of the evidence and a recommended treatment approach. CNS Spectr 7:453–463, 2002

Phillips KA: Psychosis in body dysmorphic disorder. J Psychiatr Res 38:63–72, 2004

Phillips KA: The Broken Mirror: Understanding and Treating Body Dysmorphic Disorder, Revised and Expanded Edition. New York, Oxford University Press, 2005a

Phillips KA: Placebo-controlled study of pimozide augmentation of fluoxetine in body dysmorphic disorder. Am J Psychiatry 162:377–379, 2005b

Phillips KA: An open-label study of escitalopram in body dysmorphic disorder. Int Clin Psychopharmacol 21:177–179, 2006

Phillips KA, Diaz S: Gender differences in body dysmorphic disorder. J Nerv Ment Dis 185:570–577, 1997

Phillips KA, Hollander E: Body dysmorphic disorder, in DSM-IV Sourcebook, Vol 2. Edited by Widiger TA, Frances AJ, Pincus HA, et al. Washington, DC: American Psychiatric Association, 1996, pp 949–960

Phillips KA, Najjar F: An open-label study of citalopram in body dysmorphic disorder. J Clin Psychiatry 64:715–720, 2003

Phillips KA, Stout RL: Associations in the longitudinal course of body dysmorphic disorder with major depression, obsessive compulsive disorder, and social phobia. J Psychiatr Res 40:360–369, 2006

Phillips KA, McElroy SL, Keck PE Jr, et al: Body dysmorphic disorder: 30 cases of imagined ugliness. Am J Psychiatry 150:302–308, 1993

Phillips KA, McElroy SL, Keck PE Jr, et al: A comparison of delusional and nondelusional body dysmorphic disorder in 100 cases. Psychopharmacol Bull 30:179–186, 1994

Phillips KA, McElroy SL, Hudson JI, et al: Body dysmorphic disorder: an obsessive compulsive spectrum disorder, a form of affective spectrum disorder, or both? J Clin Psychiatry 56(suppl):S41–S52, 1995

Phillips KA, Hollander E, Rasmussen SA, et al: A severity rating scale for body dysmorphic disorder: development, reliability, and validity of a modified version of the Yale-Brown Obsessive Compulsive Scale. Psychopharmacol Bull 33:17–22, 1997

Phillips KA, Dwight MM, McElroy SL: Efficacy and safety of fluvoxamine in body dysmorphic disorder. J Clin Psychiatry 59:165–171, 1998a

Phillips KA, Gunderson CG, Mallya G, et al: A comparison study of body dysmorphic disorder and obsessive compulsive disorder. J Clin Psychiatry 59:568–575, 1998b

Phillips KA, Albertini RS, Rasmussen SA: A randomized placebo-controlled trial of fluoxetine in body dysmorphic disorder. Arch Gen Psychiatry 59:381–388, 2002a

Phillips KA, Richter MA, Tharmalingam S, et al: A preliminary candidate gene study of body dysmorphic disorder. Presented at the American College of Neuropsychopharmacology 42nd Annual Meeting, San Juan, Puerto Rico, December 2002b

Phillips KA, Price LH, Greenberg BD, et al: Should DSM's diagnostic groupings be changed?, in Advancing DSM: Dilemmas in Psychiatric Diagnosis. Edited by Phillips KA, First MB, Pincus H. Washington, DC, American Psychiatric Publishing, 2003, pp 57–84

Phillips KA, Menard W, Fay C, et al: Demographic characteristics, phenomenology, comorbidity, and family history in 200 individuals with body dysmorphic disorder. Psychosomatics 46:317–325, 2005

Phillips KA, Menard W, Fay C: Gender similarities and differences in 200 individuals with body dysmorphic disorder. Compr Psychiatry 47:77–87, 2006a

Phillips KA, Menard W, Pagano M, et al: Delusional versus nondelusional body dysmorphic disorder: clinical features and course of illness. J Psychiatr Res 40:95–104, 2006b

Phillips KA, Pagano ME, Menard W, et al: A 12-month follow-up study of the course of body disorder. Am J Psychiatry 163:907–912, 2006c

Phillips KA, Pinto A, Menard W, et al: Obsessive-compulsive disorder versus body dysmorphic disorder: a comparison study of two possibly related disorders. Depress Anxiety 24:399–409, 2007

Pigott TA, Altemus M, Rubeinstein C, et al: Symptoms of eating disorders in patients with obsessive-compulsive disorder. Am J Psychiatry 148:1552–1557, 1991

Pike KM, Walsh BT, Vitousek K, et al: Cognitive behavior therapy in the posthospitalization treatment of anorexia nervosa. Am J Psychiatry 160:2046–2049, 2003

Rauch SL, Phillips KA, Segal E, et al: A preliminary morphometric magnetic resonance imaging study of regional brain volumes in body dysmorphic disorder. Psychiatry Res 122:13–19, 2003

Rief W, Buhlmann U, Wilhelm S, et al: The prevalence of body dysmorphic disorder: a population-based survey. Psychol Med 36:877–885, 2006

Rosen JC, Reiter J: Development of the Body Dysmorphic Disorder Examination. Behav Res Ther 34:755–766, 1996

Rosen JC, Reiter J, Orosan P: Cognitive-behavioral body image therapy for body dysmorphic disorder. J Consult Clin Psychol 63:263–269, 1995

Rosenberg DR, Keshavan MS: A.E. Bennett Research Award: toward a neurodevelopmental model of obsessive-compulsive disorder. Biol Psychiatry 43:623–640, 1998

Rubenstein C, Pigott T, L'Heureux F, et al: A preliminary investigation of the lifetime prevalence of anorexia and bulimia nervosa in patients with obsessive compulsive disorder. J Clin Psychiatry 53:309–314, 1992

Saxena S: Neuroimaging and the pathophysiology of obsessive-compulsive disorder, in Neuroimaging in Psychiatry. Edited by Fu C, Senior C, Russell T, et al. London, England, Martin Dunitz, 2003, pp 191–224

Saxena S, Winograd A, Dunkin JJ, et al: A retrospective review of clinical characteristics and treatment response in body dysmorphic disorder versus obsessive-compulsive disorder. J Clin Psychiatry 62:67–72, 2001

Serpell L, Livingstone A, Neiderman M, et al: Anorexia nervosa: obsessive-compulsive disorder, obsessive-compulsive personality disorder, or neither? Clin Psychol Rev 22:647–669, 2002

Simeon D, Hollander E, Stein DJ, et al: Body dysmorphic disorder in the DSM-IV field trial for obsessive-compulsive disorder. Am J Psychiatry 152:1207–1209, 1995

Singer HS, Reiss AL, Brown JE, et al: Volumetric MRI changes in basal ganglia of children with Tourette's syndrome. Neurology 43:950–956, 1993

Solyom L, Freeman RJ, Miles JE: A comparative psychometric study of anorexia nervosa and obsessive neurosis. Can J Psychiatry 27:282–286, 1982

Solyom L, DiNicola VF, Phil M, et al: Is there an obsessive psychosis? Aetiological and prognostic factors of an atypical form of obsessive-compulsive neurosis. Can J Psychiatry 30:372–380, 1985

Stekel W: Compulsion and Doubt. Translated by Gutheil EA. New York, Liveright, 1949

Suzuki K, Takei N, Kawai M, et al: Is taijin kyofusho a culture-bound syndrome? Am J Psychiatry 160:1358, 2003

Tamburrino M, Kaufman R, Hertzer J: Eating disorder history in women with obsessive compulsive disorder. J Am Med Womens Assoc 49:24–26, 1994

Treasure J, Schmidt U: Anorexia nervosa. Clin Evid 11:1192–1203, 2004

Veale D, Riley S: Mirror, mirror on the wall, who is the ugliest of them all? The psychopathology of mirror gazing in body dysmorphic disorder. Behav Res Ther 39:1381–1393, 2001

Veale D, Boocock A, Gournay K, et al: Body dysmorphic disorder: a survey of fifty cases. Br J Psychiatry 169:196–201, 1996a

Veale D, Gournay K, Dryden W, et al: Body dysmorphic disorder: a cognitive behavioural model and pilot randomised controlled trial. Behav Res Ther 34:717–729, 1996b

Veale D, Ennis M, Lambrou C: Possible association of body dysmorphic disorder with an occupation or education in art and design. Am J Psychiatry 159:1788–1790, 2002

Wagner A, Greer P, Bailer UF, et al: Normal brain tissue volumes after long-term recovery in anorexia and bulimia nervosa. Biol Psychiatry 59:291–293, 2006

Walsh BT, Kaplan AS, Attia E, et al: Fluoxetine after weight restoration in anorexia nervosa: a randomized controlled trial. JAMA 295:2605–2612, 2006

Wilhelm S, Otto MW, Zucker BG, et al: Prevalence of body dysmorphic disorder in patients with anxiety disorders. J Anxiety Disord 11:499–502, 1997

Wilhelm S, Otto MW, Lohr B: Cognitive behavior group therapy for body dysmorphic disorder: a case series. Behav Res Ther 37:71–75, 1999

Zimmerman M, Mattia JI: Body dysmorphic disorder in psychiatric outpatients: recognition, prevalence, comorbidity, demographic, and clinical correlates. Compr Psychiatry 39:265–270, 1998

3

TOURETTE'S SYNDROME, TRICHOTILLOMANIA, AND OBSESSIVE-COMPULSIVE DISORDER

How Closely Are They Related?

Ygor Arzeno Ferrão, M.D., Ph.D.
Euripedes Constantino Miguel, M.D., Ph.D.
Dan J. Stein, M.D., Ph.D.

The question of whether Tourette's syndrome and trichotillomania are best conceptualized as obsessive-compulsive spectrum disorders (OCSDs) has been raised by family studies on the close relationship between Tourette's syndrome and obsessive-compulsive disorder (OCD) (Pauls et al. 1986; Rosario-Campos et al. 2005) and by psychopharmacological research indicating that both trichotillomania and OCD respond more robustly to clomipramine than to desipramine (Swedo et al. 1989; Zohar and Insel 1987). A range of studies have subsequently allowed comparison of the phenomenology, psychobiology, and management of Tourette's syn-

This chapter was first published as "Tourette's Syndrome, Trichotillomania, and Obsessive-Compulsive Disorder: How Closely Are They Related?" *Psychiatry Research* 170:32–42, 2009. Copyright 2009. Used with permission.

drome and trichotillomania with those of OCD. These disorders are characterized by repetitive behaviors and may have a number of phenomenological intersections as depicted in Figure 3–1 (Chamberlain et al. 2006; Ferrão et al. 2006; Lochner et al. 2005). Thus, some kinds of hair-pulling resemble tic-like behaviors or compulsions insofar as they are preceded by an urge to pull and followed by a sense of relief (Figure 3–1, area A) or are preceded by obsessive thoughts (Figure 3–1, area B); tics and compulsions can overlap insofar as some compulsions are preceded by sensory phenomena and some tics are in response to obsessions (Figure 3–1, area B); and some patients have hair-pulling, tics, and compulsions (Figure 3–1, area D).

In this chapter we briefly review the current literature on the relationship of these disorders with OCD, beginning with Tourette's syndrome and moving on to trichotillomania.

Tourette's Syndrome and Obsessive-Compulsive Disorder

PHENOMENOLOGY

The main phenomenological differences between Tourette's syndrome and OCD are presented in Table 3–1. In OCD, compulsions are typically performed in response to obsessive thoughts, images, or impulses. In contrast, in Tourette's syndrome tics are not commonly preceded by obsessions. In addition, tics are sometimes performed involuntarily, whereas compulsions are always performed intentionally. Tics that are performed voluntarily and compulsions not preceded by obsessions represent an area of overlap between OCD and Tourette's syndrome.

Repetitive Behaviors Instead of Compulsions or Tics

The Tourette Syndrome Classification Study Group (1993) described *tics* as an "involuntary" (i.e., completely unintentional) response to either an urge or an unpleasant sensation (i.e., sensory phenomena) perceived as "voluntary." Nevertheless, as indicated earlier, there are areas of overlap between complex motor tics and compulsions. For instance, repetitive behaviors such as touching or eye blinking may result from a need to relieve an urge or an unpleasant sensation or to neutralize a superstitious fear. Thus, depending on the nature of the subjective experience, the same repetitive behavior is labeled differently in our current nosology (Miguel et al. 1995).

The term *intentional repetitive behavior* may have the advantage of encompassing various presentations of stereotyped repetitive behaviors reported in Tourette's syndrome and OCD patients (as well as a number of other disorders, such as trichotillomania and stereotypic movement disorder) while at the same time allowing a clear differentiation from unintentional or involuntary tic phenomena (e.g., simple tics) (Miguel et al. 1995). The intentional repetitive behaviors of both Tou-

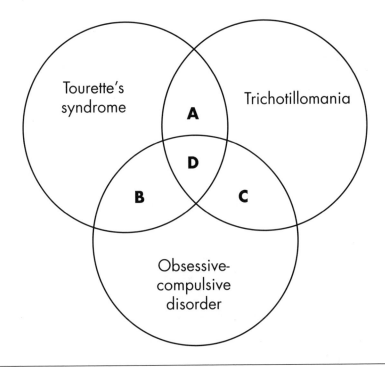

FIGURE 3–1. Obsessive-compulsive disorder, Tourette's syndrome, and trichotillomania.

A, automatic trichotillomania; **B,** tic-like compulsion, complex tic ("compulsion-like" tic) and sensory phenomena; **C,** focused trichotillomania or hair-focused obsessions or compulsions ("grooming-like" obsessive-compulsive symptoms) and sensory phenomena; **D,** complex repetitive behavior disorder.

rette's syndrome and OCD can be conceptualized as responses to unpleasant internal cues.

Obsessive-Compulsive Disorder With Tics

On a theoretical continuum of tics and compulsions, it can be hypothesized that a nodal point exists where the shift from "unintentional" to "intentional" repetitive behaviors takes place. Subjective experiences that precede these behaviors may be helpful in defining this demarcation (Miguel et al. 1995) and may be particularly useful to investigate in the subgroup of OCD with tics. OCD patients with tics often report compulsions not preceded by obsessions, and instead usually perform their repetitive behaviors to relieve sensory phenomena (i.e., bodily sensations, general feelings) or to reach a specific sensation or feeling "just right" (Leckman et al. 1994; Miguel et al. 1995, 1997, 2000).

TABLE 3–1. Phenomenological features of Tourette's syndrome, trichotillomania, and obsessive-compulsive disorder

	Tourette's syndrome	Trichotillomania	Obsessive-compulsive disorder
Cognitive process	More frequently report obsessions of symmetry and exactness, and aggressive obsessions.	Obsessions are rarely present.	Obsessions are common and can be frequent. All types of obsessions are present.
Repetitive behaviors	Repetitive behaviors (motor and vocal tics) can be performed unintentionally, although, in most cases, at least one repetitive behavior is performed intentionally. Unintentional repetitive behaviors are experienced as irresistible, but can be suppressed for varying lengths of time. They are usually sudden, rapid, recurrent, nonrhythmic, and stereotypical.	Repetitive behaviors are performed unintentionally or intentionally (i.e., automatic vs. focused). They are experienced as irresistible but can be suppressed for varying lengths of time. They are usually planned, recurrent, and stereotypical.	Performed intentionally (conscious behavior)
	Intentional repetitive behaviors are usually not preceded by obsessions but by subjective experiences such as sensory phenomena (i.e., general, uncomfortable feelings or perceptions or bodily sensations).	Can be preceded by sensory phenomena.	Performed in response to obsessions or according to rigid rules. Occasionally performed in response to "bodily sensations."

TABLE 3–1. Phenomenological features of Tourette's syndrome, trichotillomania, and obsessive-compulsive disorder *(continued)*

	Tourette's syndrome	Trichotillomania	Obsessive-compulsive disorder
Repetitive behaviors *(continued)*	Occasionally performed in response to or to relieve physical anxiety (autonomic anxiety).	Occasionally performed in response to or to relieve physical anxiety (autonomic anxiety).	Occasionally performed in response or to relieve physical anxiety (autonomic anxiety).
	Associated with relief rather than pleasure.	May be associated with relief and/or pleasure.	Associated with relief rather than pleasure.
	Distressing or socially disabling.	Distressing or socially disabling.	Distressing or socially disabling.
	Repetitive but can be of short duration.	Repetitive but frequently less durable.	Repetitive (until the goal is achieved).
	Frequently less rigid.	Can be less rigid.	Often rule-bound or performed in a rigid manner.

In terms of type of obsessive-compulsive symptoms, patients with OCD plus tics more frequently report intrusive violent, sexual, or religious images/thoughts; somatic obsessions; counting rituals; tic-like compulsions; and hoarding (Diniz et al. 2005; Eapen et al. 1997; George et al. 1993; Holzer et al. 1994; Petter et al. 1998; Swerdlow et al. 1999). When symptoms are measured based on dimensions, the aggressive/sexual/religious factor and the symmetry/ordering/arranging factor are also more frequently associated with the OCD plus tics subtype (Hasler et al. 2005; Leckman et al. 1997).

Compared with patients with OCD alone, OCD patients with tics usually present with an earlier age of onset (Diniz et al. 2004, 2005; Leckman et al. 1995; Miguel et al. 1997; Rosario-Campos et al. 2001) and are more frequently males (Holzer et al. 1994; Leckman et al. 1995). Diniz et al. (2005) found that OCD patients with chronic motor or vocal tics were similar to OCD patients with Tourette's syndrome regarding the frequency of intrusive sounds, repeating behaviors, counting, and tic-like compulsions, but these symptoms were more frequent in those groups than in OCD patients without tics. For age at obsessive-compulsive symptom onset, sensory phenomena score, number of comorbidities, frequency of somatic obsessions, bodily sensations and just-right perceptions, OCD patients with chronic motor or vocal tics tended to be in between the other two groups. From a phenomenological point of view, these results provide further evidence of a possible continuum between OCD and Tourette's syndrome in which patients with OCD plus tics have intermediate phenotypic features (Diniz et al. 2005).

Comorbidity

Studies have reported that patients with tic-related OCD present higher rates of trichotillomania, body dysmorphic disorder (BDD), mood disorders, social phobia, other anxiety disorders, and attention-deficit/hyperactivity disorder when compared with patients with non-tic-related OCD (Coffey et al. 1998; Diniz et al. 2005; Petter et al. 1998). Comorbid bipolar disorder in OCD and Tourette's syndrome has also been associated with a higher prevalence when OCD and Tourette's syndrome are combined (Berthier et al. 1998; Coffey et al. 1998; Kerbeshian et al. 1995). More detailed studies are necessary to determine whether comorbid tics in OCD are merely a marker of increased severity and increased comorbidity or whether the combination of symptoms points to a specific set of underlying psychobiological variations.

The main Tourette's syndrome and OCD psychiatric comorbidities are presented in Table 3–2.

Course of the Illness

Tourette's syndrome usually starts with motor tics between the ages of 3 and 8 years, with transient periods of intense eye blinking or some other facial tic. Phonic tics such as throat clearing typically follow the onset of motor tics by several years. Motor and phonic tic severity peaks early in the second decade (Leckman et al. 2003). In OCD plus Tourette's syndrome patients, the worst-ever OCD symptoms occurred approximately 2 years later than worst-ever tic symptoms, and the OCD symptoms were more likely to persist than tic symptoms (Bloch et al. 2006b).

OCD and Tourette's syndrome are usually characterized by waxing and waning courses. Early-onset OCD (which is more associated with tic disorders) more frequently has a waxing and waning course, whereas late forms of OCD may have an episodic course (Ravizza et al. 1997).

The main Tourette's syndrome and OCD course features are presented in Table 3–3.

PSYCHOBIOLOGY

Genetic Data

Family and twin studies.   Genetic family studies have shown not only higher rates of obsessive-compulsive symptoms and OCD in relatives of Tourette's syndrome patients (Comings and Comings 1987; Eapen et al. 1993; Pauls and Leckman 1986; Pauls et al. 1986, 1991; Robertson et al. 1988) but also higher rates of tics or Tourette's syndrome in first-degree relatives of OCD patients (Grados et al. 2001; Hanna et al. 2005; Leonard et al. 1992; Pauls et al. 1995; Rosario-Campos et al. 2005) when compared with control subjects. Some studies do not support a relationship between Tourette's syndrome and OCD (Reddy et al. 2001), suggesting that larger community samples will better explain the hypotheses of OCD familial transmission and comorbidity with tic disorders.

Twin studies (Hyde et al. 1992; Price et al. 1985; Zhang et al. 2002) have shown concordance rates for Tourette's syndrome in monozygotic twins to range between 60% and 80%, compared with less than 20% in dizygotic twins (Hyde et al. 1992; Price et al. 1985). When the phenotype assessed is the presence of all kinds of chronic tics, the concordance rates increase to almost 100% in monozygotic twins (Walkup et al. 1988). The concordance rates for OCD in monozygotic twins, although smaller than in Tourette's syndrome (27%–47%), also reinforce the notion that OCD is genetically mediated (van Grootheest et al. 2005).

Segregation analyses.   Results from early segregation analyses suggest that the pattern of transmission within Tourette's syndrome families is consistent with autosomal transmission (Leckman et al. 2003; Pauls et al. 1986, 1990). However, more recent segregation analyses are not always entirely consistent (Cuker et al. 2004; Hasstedt et al. 1995; Kurlan et al. 1994; McMahon et al. 1996; Seuchter et al. 2000; Walkup et al. 1996).

TABLE 3–2. Comorbidity in Tourette's syndrome, trichotillomania, and obsessive-compulsive disorder

Disorders	Tourette's syndrome	Trichotillomania	Obsessive-compulsive disorder
Major depression	Higher Associated with tic severity Less prevalent than in OCD patients	Higher	Higher Associated with longer duration of the OCD
Tic disorders, including Tourette's syndrome		Higher	Higher Associated with early age at OCD onset
Panic disorder	Higher in patients with TS with additional comorbidity such as bipolar disorder or OCD	Associated with other anxiety disorders such as OCD	Higher Associated with other anxiety disorders
Generalized anxiety disorder	Associated with major depressive disorder	Higher	Higher Associated with major depressive disorder
Social phobia	Associated with OCD in TS patients	Higher	Associated with longer duration of the OCD, early age at OCD onset, and bipolar disorder
Body dysmorphic disorder	Higher Associated with the TS-OCD combination	Higher	Higher Associated with early age at OCD onset, OCD+tics, and familial aggregation

TABLE 3–2. Comorbidity in Tourette's syndrome, trichotillomania, and obsessive-compulsive disorder *(continued)*

Disorders	Tourette's syndrome	Trichotillomania	Obsessive-compulsive disorder
Trichotillomania	Higher Associated with the TS-OCD combination		Higher Associated with early age at OCD onset, OCD+tics, and familial aggregation
Bipolar disorder	Higher Associated with high frequency of additional psychopathology	No strong evidence (case reports only)	Higher Associated with tics, symmetry obsessions, ordering rituals, and early age at OCD onset Associated with lower quality of life
Eating disorders (females and possibly males)	No known association with TS	Higher	Higher Associated with familial aggregation of symptoms and with obsessive-compulsive personality disorder
Attention-deficit disorder (children)	Higher Associated with behavioral disorders	Higher	Associated with OCD+tics Associated with children with OCD

TABLE 3–2. Comorbidity in Tourette's syndrome, trichotillomania, and obsessive-compulsive disorder *(continued)*

Disorders	Tourette's syndrome	Trichotillomania	Obsessive-compulsive disorder
Oppositional defiant disorder (children)	Higher Associated with behavioral disorders	No known association	No known association
Alcohol abuse/dependence	Higher Higher in first-degree relatives of probands with tics and/or ADHD	Higher	Higher in community samples
Obsessive-compulsive personality disorder	Not associated with tic disorders	Higher	Higher Associated with hoarding symptoms in OCD patients
Posttraumatic stress disorder or traumatic experiences	No evidence	Higher	Higher
Schizotypal personality disorder	Not associated with tic disorders	Not associated	Associated with worse treatment response
Other impulse-control disorders	No known association	Higher, especially with kleptomania, omniomania, and skin picking	Higher, especially with omniomania, trichotillomania, and skin picking

Note. Disorders with increased prevalence compared with that seen in the general population.
ADHD=attention-deficit/hyperactivity disorder; OCD=obsessive-compulsive disorder; TS=Tourette's syndrome.

TABLE 3–3. Course of illness (clinical samples) in Tourette's syndrome, trichotillomania, and obsessive-compulsive disorder

Features	Tourette's syndrome	Trichotillomania	Obsessive-compulsive disorder
Age at onset	Onset before 10 years of age in most patients (mean ~7 years)	Onset often around puberty; childhood onset transitory	Onset by age 15 in ~30% of cases and by age 10 in ~20%; ~50% by age 10 in tertiary-care facilities
Female/male ratio	Female/male ratio <1 (~1:4)	Among adults, 75%–90% are female; among children, female/male ratio is near 1	Female/male ratio slightly >1 in adult samples; female/male ratio slightly <1 in cases of early age at onset of obsessive-compulsive disorder
Chronic course	Usually chronic with waxing and waning (80%), impairment because of tics persists in only 14%; symptoms usually improve with age	Usually chronic (~60%), severity varying according to environmental stressors	Usually chronic, waxing and waning in 50%–80%; symptoms typically worsen with age
Episodic course	Rarely episodic	Rarely episodic in adults but can be transitory in children	May be episodic (≥6 months symptom free) in ~25%
Remission	Reduction or remission of tic symptoms in early adulthood is common (~85%)	Remission can occur but is not common	Remission (no symptoms for ≥5 years) occurs in ~20%

Similarly, in OCD, some studies are consistent with a simple Mendelian mode of transmission, whereas others suggest a more complex pattern of transmission with multifactorial components. (Alsobrook et al. 1999; Cavallini et al. 1999; Nestadt et al. 2000; Nicolini et al. 1991). Despite the differences in findings, methodologies, and proposed models of inheritance, the bulk of family and segregation analyses studies support the idea that genes play a major role in the etiology of both Tourette's syndrome and OCD.

Molecular genetic findings.   The candidate genes that have been examined in association studies with Tourette's syndrome patients and control subjects include various serotonergic genes *(5-HTT)*, dopamine receptor genes *(DRD1, DRD2, DRD4,* and *DRD5)*, the dopamine transporter gene, and various noradrenergic genes *(ADRA2a, ADRA2C,* and *DBH)* (Leckman 2002). More recently, functional variants at the *SLITRK1* locus were associated with Tourette's syndrome (Abelson et al. 2005). In OCD, there have been positive associations with polymorphisms of the genes for the serotonin transporter *(5-HTTLPR)* (Kim et al. 2005), serotonin receptors *(5HT1B)*, dopamine receptors *(DRD2, DRD4)*, COMT, monoamine oxidase A (Denys et al. 2004, 2006; Karayiorgou et al. 1999), and glutamate receptors *(GRIN2B, GRIK2)* (Arnold et al. 2006). More recent findings implicate the genetic locus on chromosome 9p24 that codes for a high-affinity neuronal/epithelial excitatory amino-acid transporter (ECCA-1) known as *SLC1A1* (Leckman and Kim 2006). OCD plus tic disorders (including Tourette's syndrome) has been associated with variants in the serotonin transporter gene, dopamine receptor genes *(DRD4, DRD4)*, and mu opioid receptor gene. In conclusion, there is some evidence that common genes confer vulnerability for both disorders, with both OCD and tic disorders rarely being associated with single genetic variants (Abelson et al. 2005), but possibly more commonly the result of the action of multiple genes interacting with each other and with environmental factors.

Neural Circuitry

Volumetric magnetic resonance imaging (MRI) studies of Tourette's syndrome subjects have shown abnormal volumes and asymmetry in striatum and globus pallidus, corpus callosum, and prefrontal, premotor, and orbitofrontal cortices (Baumgardner et al. 1996; Mostofsky et al. 1999; Peterson et al. 1993, 2003) and shape deformity of the corpus striatum, especially the caudate nucleus (Choi et al. 2007). In a recent prospective study, smaller childhood caudate volumes correlated significantly and inversely with the severity of tics and obsessive-compulsive symptoms in early adulthood but did not correlate with the severity of symptoms at the time of the MRI scan, suggesting that morphologic disturbances of the caudate nucleus within cortico-striatal-thalamo-cortical circuits are central to the persistence of both tics and obsessive-compulsive symptoms into adulthood (Bloch et al. 2005).

Functional studies with positron emission tomography (PET) and single photon emission computed tomography (SPECT) have shown that the occurrence of tics in Tourette's syndrome patients is correlated with decreased activity in the caudate and thalamus, together with increased activity of the lateral and medial premotor cortex, supplementary motor areas, anterior cingulate gyrus, dorsolateral-rostral prefrontal cortex, inferior parietal cortex, putamen, caudate, primary motor cortex, Broca's area, superior temporal gyrus, insula, and claustrum (Stern et al. 2000). Vocal tics, including coprolalia, seem to activate prerolandic and postrolandic language regions, insula, caudate, thalamus and cerebellum, whereas motor tics seem associated with activity in sensorimotor cortex (Bohlhalter et al. 2006; Stern et al. 2000; Temel et al. 2004).

Structural and functional studies in OCD studies have consistently shown abnormalities in the orbitofrontal cortex, anterior cingulate gyrus, caudate nucleus, and thalamus in groups of OCD patients relative to healthy control subjects (Rauch 2000; Whiteside et al. 2004). Thus, the pathophysiology of both OCD and Tourette's syndrome seems to involve cortico-striatal-thalamic-cortical circuits. It is has been suggested that imaging findings in particular cases of Tourette's syndrome may reflect a proband's family history (of Tourette's syndrome or OCD) (Moriarty et al. 1997). However, compared with OCD, abnormalities in Tourette's syndrome are generally found in other cortical regions, including motor and sensory cortical areas and their projections to dorsolateral striatal regions (Rauch 2000; Whiteside et al. 2004).

PET and SPECT studies in Tourette's syndrome suggest an increased density of presynaptic dopamine transporters and postsynaptic dopamine D_2 receptors as well as a greater dopamine release in the putamen when compared with healthy control subjects (Singer 2005). Similarly, OCD studies have demonstrated abnormalities in DAT and D_2 receptor density, whereas findings with serotonergic ligands are less consistent to date. These data again reinforce the idea that OCD and tics might be part of a spectrum and are consistent with the efficacy of dopamine antagonists in association with reuptake serotonin inhibitors for the treatment of OCD with tics. Whiteside et al. (2006), using single voxel magnetic resonance spectroscopy (MRS), compared adult patients with OCD and a control group. They found that patients with OCD had increased levels of a combined measure of glutamate, glutamine, and *N*-acetyl-L-aspartic acid relative to creatine in the right orbitofrontal white matter (and that it was positively correlated to OCD symptoms) and reduced levels of myo-inositol relative to creatine in the head of the caudate nucleus bilaterally (and that it was related to trait and/or state anxiety) (Whiteside et al. 2006). Patients with Tourette's disorder demonstrated a reduction in *N*-acetyl-aspartate and choline in the left putamen, along with reduced levels of creatine bilaterally in the putamen. In the frontal cortex, patients had significantly lower concentrations of *N*-acetyl-aspartate bilaterally, lower levels of creatine on the right side, and reduced myoinositol on the left side (DeVito et al. 2005).

Immune Function

Seminal research has described a subgroup of childhood-onset OCD or tic disorder patients with onset and subsequent exacerbations of their symptoms following infections with group A β-hemolytic *Streptococcus*. This subgroup was designated by the acronym PANDAS: pediatric autoimmune neuropsychiatric disorders associated with streptococcal infections (Swedo et al. 1997). It is hypothesized that PANDAS may arise when antibodies directed against invading bacteria cross-react with basal ganglia structures, resulting in exacerbations of OCD or tic disorders (Mell et al. 2005; Swedo 1993).

Additional studies have reported high frequencies of obsessive-compulsive symptoms, OCD, and tic disorders in rheumatic fever with and without Sydenham's chorea. These psychopathological manifestations have been described in acute and chronic phase rheumatic fever patients (Alvarenga et al. 2006; Mercadante et al. 2000, 2005).

More recently, Hounie et al. (2007) undertook a case-control family study to estimate the frequency of OCSD in first-degree relatives of rheumatic fever patients and control subjects. In this study OCSD encompassed Tourette's syndrome, trichotillomania, and body dysmorphic disorder in addition to OCD. The authors found that the rate of OCSDs was significantly higher among first-degree relatives of rheumatic fever probands than among those of control subjects, which is consistent with the hypothesis that a familial relationship exists between OCSD and rheumatic fever. However, a study failed to provide support of D8/17 as an immunological marker associated with rheumatic fever as a predictor of childhood psychiatric disorders in a community sample (Inoff-Germain et al. 2003).

In conclusion, some early onset forms of Tourette's syndrome and OCD may be causally related to streptococcal infections and immune abnormalities, raising the possibility of another common etiological factor for both disorders.

TREATMENT

Table 3–4 summarizes treatment options in Tourette's syndrome and OCD.

Pharmacology

Despite the evidence suggesting an association between OCD and Tourette's syndrome, when it comes to treatment these disorders are managed differently. The first-choice pharmacological treatment for Tourette's syndrome includes antipsychotics, whereas that for OCD comprises the selective serotonin reuptake inhibitors (SSRIs) (Scahill et al. 2006). However, some augmentation strategies, such as the addition of haloperidol to an SSRI, are especially effective for OCD patients with comorbid tic disorders resistant to fluvoxamine (McDougle et al. 1994). Augmentation with atypical antipsychotics that have mixed effects on dopamine and sero-

TABLE 3–4. Interventional treatment options in Tourette's syndrome (TS), trichotillomania, and obsessive-compulsive disorder (OCD)

Intervention	Tourette's syndrome	Trichotillomania	Obsessive-compulsive disorder
Serotonin reuptake inhibitor (SRI) or selective serotonin reuptake inhibitor (SSRI)	Does not alter tic severity	SRIs and SSRIs, including clomipramine (serotonergic), can be effective	SRIs and SSRIs, including clomipramine (serotonergic), are effective
Dose response	Most compounds used in low dosages	No evidence of dose-response association	Dose response relationship for most compounds
Antipsychotics	First- and second-generation antipsychotics effective, regardless of other drugs used in combination	May be effective	First- and second-generation antipsychotics effective for SRI-resistant cases when combined with an SRI
Neurosurgery	Few case reports suggesting efficacy, except with reversible techniques	No evidence	Ablative and reversible neurosurgical procedures effective
Repetitive transcranial magnetic stimulation	No evidence of efficacy	No evidence	Perhaps effect only transient; possibly not effective with available techniques
Electroconvulsive therapy	Not clearly effective	No evidence	Not clearly effective

tonin has also been proved effective in treatment-resistant OCD cases, irrespective of the presence or absence of tics (Ipser et al. 2006; Miguel et al. 2003). In contrast, in one study (Saxena et al. 1996), comorbid tics were associated with poor response to risperidone augmentation. In another study, clomipramine alone was effective in patients with OCD independently of the presence of tics (Shavitt et al. 2006). Nevertheless, a recent systematic review (Bloch et al. 2006a), which evaluated clinical trials of the augmentation of serotonin reuptake inhibitors with antipsychotics, reported that the presence of tics was associated with better treatment response in OCD. These data may be suggestive, from a pharmacological perspective, of a continuum between OCD and Tourette's syndrome.

Psychotherapy

Exposure and response prevention and cognitive treatment approaches, which are the first choice in the treatment of mild and moderate OCD, have not been used for Tourette's syndrome and are probably not effective. The most effective psychological approach for tics in Tourette's syndrome is habit reversal (Wagaman et al. 1995; Wilhelm et al. 2003; Woods et al. 1996). The presence of tics has been suggested not to influence the cognitive-behavior therapy for OCD (Himle et al. 2003), but further work is needed to confirm this.

Other Interventions

Electroconvulsive therapy.   The few cases in which obsessive-compulsive symptoms and tics improved with electroconvulsive therapy (ECT) probably reflected the effects of ECT on comorbid conditions rather than reduction of OCD or tics per se (Strassing et al. 2004). The clinical efficacy of ECT in OCD and Tourette's syndrome has not yet been studied in rigorously designed trials (Karadenizli et al. 2005; Rapoport et al. 1998).

Neurosurgery.   Classical neurosurgical interventions (such as stereotactic anterior capsulotomy, limbic leucotomy, or cingulotomy), which may be effective in 50% or more cases of refractory OCD (Lopes et al. 2004), have also been conducted in Tourette's syndrome patients. In contrast, such interventions have not been associated with symptom improvement in Tourette's syndrome (Kurlan et al. 1988, 1990; Rauch et al. 1995; Robertson et al. 1990). Severe side effects were described in Tourette's syndrome when infrathalamic and cingulotomy lesions were combined (Leckman et al. 1993; Rauch et al. 1995).

Techniques not used in OCD have been employed for the treatment of Tourette's syndrome (e.g., chemothalamectomy of the ventrolateral nucleus, dentatotomy, and bilateral campotomy) with no adequate assessment of improvement measures (Baker 1962; Beckers 1973; Cooper 1962; Nadvornik et al. 1972; Stevens 1964). Symptom improvements have ranged from 50% (with lesions in the intralaminar and medial thalamic nuclei and in the ventro-oralis internus nucleus) to 70%–100% (lesioning ventrolateral nuclei/lamella medialis of thalamus). On the other hand, important side effects such as cerebellar signs, dystonia, dysarthria, and hemiballism were reported (Babel et al. 2001; Temel and Visser-Vandewalle 2004). None of these interventions have been tested in randomized, controlled trials.

Deep brain stimulation.   Several case reports of deep brain stimulation in Tourette's syndrome have described successful results with placement of electrodes in various sites, mainly in the anterior internal capsule, in the medial thalamus, and in the globus pallidus internus (Ackermans et al. 2006; Dell'Osso et al. 2005; Diederich et al. 2005; Flaherty et al. 2005; Houeto et al. 2005; Vandewalle et al. 1999). Different brain areas have been targeted in OCD, with effective results after the stimulation of areas such the anterior limb of the internal capsule (Greenberg et al. 2006).

Repetitive transcranial magnetic stimulation.   Repetitive transcranial magnetic stimulation (rTMS) does not currently appear effective in either Tourette's syndrome or OCD (Chae et al. 2004; Gilbert 2006; Munchau et al. 2002; Orth et al. 2005). Given advances in rTMS methods, further work is needed, and possibly new approaches using this technique may turn out to be effective.

Immunological interventions.   Additional treatments, such as antibiotic prophylaxis, have been investigated in the subgroup of OCD and/or Tourette's syndrome with an abrupt onset and symptom exacerbation associated with streptococcal infections. Garvey et al. (1999) found no effectiveness of prophylaxis with oral penicillin, but Snider et al. (2005) found that both azithromycin and penicillin were effective in preventing exacerbation of neuropsychiatric symptoms in children with PANDAS. Plasma exchange and intravenous immunoglobulin were both effective in ameliorating symptoms in children with infection-triggered OCD and tic disorders. (Perlmutter et al. 1999). Additional work is needed to replicate and extend these findings.

Trichotillomania

The question of whether trichotillomania is best conceptualized as an OCSD was raised when clomipramine was reported to be more effective than desipramine for patients with chronic hair-pulling (Swedo et al. 1989). This thought-provoking study replicated findings that serotonin reuptake inhibitors were more robust than noradrenaline reuptake inhibitors in the treatment of OCD (Zohar and Insel 1987). A range of studies have subsequently compared the phenomenology, neurobiology, neuropsychology, and management of trichotillomania and OCD (Bohne et al. 2005a, 2005b; Carpenter et al. 2002; Chamberlain et al. 2006; Coetzer and Stein 1999; Lochner et al. 2002, 2004, 2005; Niehaus et al. 1999; Stanley et al. 1992; Stein et al. 1997b; Swedo 1993; Tukel et al. 2001).

PHENOMENOLOGY

Repetitive Behaviors

As mentioned earlier, OCD is typically characterized by the presence of both obsessions and compulsions, and often these cover a number of different areas (e.g., checking, washing). In contrast, trichotillomania is typically characterized by a focus solely on hair-pulling. However, there may be some overlap with the phenomenology of OCD; hair-pulling may be triggered by concerns about symmetry; hair-pulling is often performed in a repetitive and ritualistic fashion; and hair-pulling may be preceded by an increase in anxiety and followed by a decrease in anxiety (Table 3–1).

On the other hand, functional analysis of hair-pulling, compulsions, and tics often indicates important differences between these symptoms. Tics frequently involve abrupt movements of one or more muscle groups and occur in response to a sensory urge, whereas hair-pulling always involves many muscle groups, resulting in a series of complex movements, with a very specific "grooming" purpose. Similarly, the cognitive mechanisms, such as thought–action fusion, inflated sense of responsibility, and the need for control over thoughts that operate in OCD are not particularly characteristic of either Tourette's syndrome or trichotillomania.

One hypothesis has been that hair-pulling occurs in two different forms— focused and automatic. The focused form is redolent of OCD insofar as it is preceded by anxiety and results in a decrease in anxiety. However, the automatic form of hair-pulling is rather different; it is somewhat reminiscent of a trance state in that patients are only minimally aware of their behavior at the time that they are doing it, and it may be associated with dissociative symptoms. Nevertheless, there has been only some clinical or psychobiological validation of this distinction to date (Woods et al. 2005).

It is notable that a number of other conditions characterized by repetitive non-functional behavior, for example, skin picking, are not well defined in our current nosology. The category of stereotypic movement disorder specifically excludes patients with tics and hair-pulling and is typically used for patients with intellectual disability. Nevertheless, these behaviors would seem to fit the definition of a clinical stereotypy as a repetitive nonfunctional motor behavior (Table 3–1). Furthermore, there is increasing recognition of the high prevalence of stereotypic behaviors in subjects with normal intelligence and of a significant overlap in their phenomenology with hair-pulling (Lochner et al. 2005). Given these data, as well as available methods for assessment and treatment (Castellanos et al. 1996; Keuthen et al. 2001), this is a significant omission in DSM-IV-TR (American Psychiatric Association 2000).

Disability

It is appropriate to think of OCD as a highly disabling disorder. However, clinicians sometimes err on the side of underestimating the disability associated with trichotillomania. One of the first systematic reports of hair-pulling was a surgical series that documented literally hundreds of cases of trichobezoar patients (De-Bakey and Ochsner 1939). There is increasing appreciation of the distress associated with hair-pulling and of the significant disability associated with this condition (Diefenbach et al. 2005; Seedat and Stein 1998; Soriano et al. 1996; Woods et al. 2006a). There is also growing awareness of the distress and disability associated with other stereotypic behaviors such as skin picking (Arnold et al. 2001; Keuthen et al. 2001).

Comorbidity

A number of studies have compared comorbid disorders in patients with trichotillomania and OCD. It is notable that there is high comorbidity of mood, anxiety, eating, and substance abuse disorders in both groups. Although small, the relevant studies indicate that comorbidity is somewhat greater in OCD than in trichotillomania (Bienvenu et al. 2000; Stanley et al. 1992; Tukel et al. 2001). Furthermore, these particular sets of comorbidity are arguably fairly nonspecific; they are found in a range of mood and anxiety disorders.

Comorbidity of OCD and tics in patients with trichotillomania would provide stronger evidence, perhaps, that trichotillomania is an OCSD. The data do suggest a higher incidence of OCD in trichotillomania than might be expected in the general population (Jaisoorya et al. 2003). Furthermore, Coffey et al. (1998) found that patients with Tourette's syndrome alone or OCD plus Tourette's syndrome had higher rates of trichotillomania than patients with OCD alone.

It is notable, however, that patients with trichotillomania have a high incidence of other habits, including skin picking (Christenson et al. 1991; see Table 3–2). High comorbidity of different clinical stereotypies, including hair-pulling, suggests that there may be clinical utility in categorizing these conditions in the same section of DSM-V.

PSYCHOBIOLOGY

Neurocircuitry/Neuroimmunology/Neuropsychology

There is strong evidence that OCD is mediated by corticostriatal circuitry (Whiteside et al. 2004). The database of neurological lesion studies (Ferrão and Scheidt 2003; Managoli and Vilhekar 2003) and of structural and functional imaging studies of trichotillomania is much smaller, so conclusions must be more tentative.

There is some evidence that trichotillomania is characterized by reduced putamen volume (O'Sullivan et al. 1997), although not all studies have been consistent (Stein et al. 1997b). There is also evidence of cerebellar involvement in trichotillomania (Keuthen et al. 2007; O'Sullivan et al. 1997). Functional imaging studies have indicated some overlap with OCD, but probably insufficient overlap to argue that the two disorders are mediated by similar neurocircuitry (Stein et al. 2002; Swedo et al. 1991). However, decreased frontal activity may predict response to serotonin reuptake inhibitors in both disorders (Stein et al. 2002; Swedo et al. 1991).

It has been postulated that corticostriatal dysfunction in OCD may be mediated by autoantibodies after streptococcal infection. There have been reports linking hair-pulling to autoimmune dysfunction, but these are very preliminary in nature (Mercadante et al. 2005), and other studies (e.g., Carpenter et al. 2002) fail to support speculation that ongoing immune activation may be causally involved in the pathogenesis of OCD or trichotillomania.

A series of studies have compared neuropsychological tasks in trichotillomania and OCD (Bohne et al. 2005b; Chamberlain et al. 2006; Coetzer and Stein 1999). For example, Bohne et al. (2005b) compared 23 individuals with trichotillomania, 21 individuals with OCD, and 26 healthy control subjects in terms of their ability to perform neuropsychological tasks. Neither the trichotillomania group nor the OCD group had generalized neuropsychological deficits compared with the control group. The individuals in the trichotillomania group presented increased perseveration on the Object Alternation Task, suggesting difficulties in response flexibility. Those in the OCD group presented impaired ability to learn from feedback on the Wisconsin Card Sorting Test. Chamberlain et al. (2006) compared 20 patients with OCD, 20 patients with trichotillomania, and 20 matched control subjects (groups were matched for age, education, verbal IQ, and gender). The OCD and trichotillomania groups presented impaired spatial working memory. The individuals in the OCD group presented additional impairments (in executive planning and visual pattern recognition memory) and missed more responses to sad target words than did those in the other groups on an affective go/no-go task. In addition, OCD patients failed to modulate their behavior between conditions on the reflection-impulsivity test, which is suggestive of cognitive inflexibility. Both clinical groups presented intact decision-making and probabilistic reversal learning. Again, although there is some overlap, there appear to be important differences between the two disorders.

Neurochemistry/Neurogenetics/Animal Models

Glutamate, serotonin, and dopamine play an important role in modulating the corticostriatal circuits that underpin OCD. Given the suggestion that both trichotillomania and OCD respond selectively to serotonin reuptake inhibitors, there has been interest in studying the serotonin system in trichotillomania. There have, however, been relatively few studies to date, and there are no studies of trichotillomania with the more sophisticated molecular imaging techniques currently available. It is noteworthy, however, that dopamine agonists have been reported to exacerbate hair-pulling and that dopamine blockers may play a role in pharmacotherapy (George and Moselhy 2005; Senturk and Tanriverdi 2002; Stein and Hollander 1992; Stein et al. 1997a; Stewart and Nejtek 2003).

Family studies have indicated that both trichotillomania and OCD are more common in family members of trichotillomania probands (Christenson et al. 1992; Lenane et al. 1992). Furthermore, family studies show that pathological grooming symptoms (e.g., nail biting, skin picking, hair-pulling) occur more commonly in relatives of OCD probands than expected (Nestadt et al. 2003). Similarly, these conditions are more common in familial than in spontaneous early onset OCD (Hanna et al. 2005).

There are currently few data on the genetic variants in association with trichotillomania, but a preliminary study points to the involvement of a variant in *5HT2A* (Hemmings et al. 2004), a gene that has been associated with impulsive disorders. Candidate genes that seem worth pursuing include *hoxB8* (which may play a role in grooming in animal models; Greer and Capecchi 2002) and *SLITRK1* (variants of which have been associated with trichotillomania) (Abelson et al. 2005; Zuchner et al. 2006).

It is possible that animal models will ultimately shed light on the neurobiology of trichotillomania. An interesting model is barbering (fur and whisker trimming) in mice (Garner et al. 2004). However, the underlying biology of this behavior remains to be fully understood. An understanding of the neurobiology of stereotypies and habits may be relevant to trichotillomania; such work currently emphasizes the role of striatal dopamine (Marsh et al. 2004).

TREATMENT

Like the psychobiological literature, the treatment literature on trichotillomania is sparse compared with that on OCD (see Table 3–4). So once again, conclusions on similarities and differences between the disorders must be somewhat tentative.

Studies of the pharmacotherapy of trichotillomania have been relatively disappointing. SSRIs are frequently effective in open-label studies but have not proved clearly effective in controlled studies (Woods et al. 2006b). Furthermore, short-term response may be lost during maintenance therapy. There has been interest in antipsychotic agents for the augmentation of serotonin reuptake inhibitors in trichotillomania, and a recent controlled study of olanzapine has yielded promising data (Stewart and Nejtek 2003).

Habit reversal therapy appears effective in trichotillomania. The principles of this treatment are, however, different from those of exposure and response prevention. Instead, habit reversal conceptualizes hair-pulling as one of a range of differ-

ent stereotypes (e.g., skin picking) that people may experience. In this view, negative reinforcement is important in OCD, whereas positive reinforcement is key
in trichotillomania and stereotypies (Azrin and Nunn 1973; Miltenberger et al.
1998).

Conclusion

How similar are Tourette's syndrome and trichotillomania to OCD? It seems clear
from data on phenomenology, psychobiology, and treatment that Tourette's syndrome
and trichotillomania are not simply variants of OCD. Nevertheless, some genetic
(Pauls et al. 1986) and imaging (Moriarty et al. 1997) data indicate that Tourette's
syndrome and OCD may have significant overlap in their underlying mechanisms,
and Tourette's syndrome is arguably the disorder most closely related to OCD. In
the case of trichotillomania, there is less information available on underlying psychobiological mechanisms, but there are some data to support an argument that hair-
pulling can be conceptualized primarily as a stereotypic disorder, along with conditions such as repetitive skin picking, which are currently neglected in DSM-IV-TR.
Any discussion of the psychobiological validation of a spectrum between Tourette's
syndrome, trichotillomania, and OCD must, however, be tempered by the admis-
sion that our knowledge of the psychobiology of any one of these disorders is currently only partial.

Even in the absence of a full understanding of psychobiology, is there a rationale for conceptualizing OCD, Tourette's syndrome, and stereotypic disorders as
lying on a spectrum? We would argue that with respect to trichotillomania and stereotypic disorders, the obsessive-compulsive spectrum concept has significant conceptual and clinical utility. At a conceptual level, the idea of a spectrum provides a
useful framework for integrating data on overlaps as well as differences in the phenomenology, psychobiology, and treatment across these disorders. Thus, for example, work on cortico-striatal-thalamic-cortical circuitry in Tourette's syndrome and
OCD may shed light on why both disorders are characterized by impulse dyscon-
trol as well as why Tourette's syndrome is characterized predominantly by motoric
symptoms. From a clinical perspective there may be significant utility in empha-
sizing the different relationships between Tourette's syndrome, trichotillomania, and
OCD: this reminds clinicians to screen for these otherwise neglected disorders (e.g.
stereotypies are typically omitted in screening for common mental disorders), to
evaluate important comorbidities (e.g., determining the presence of tics in OCD),
and to consider particular treatment options (e.g., although antipsychotics are one
of the first-line treatments of Tourette's syndrome, they may be useful in the augmentation therapy of OCD and trichotillomania). Nevertheless, we are also mind-
ful of the possibility that such an approach may be disadvantageous insofar as
Tourette's syndrome, trichotillomania, and OCD each require a unique conceptual

and clinical framework involving nonoverlapping assessment measures and treatment options.

Acknowledgments

The authors thank Albina Torres, Alice de Mathis, Marcos Mercadante, Marcelo Hoexter, Juliana Diniz, Cristina Belloto, Antonio Carlos Lopes, Roseli Gedanke Shavitt, Ana G. Hounie, and Maria Conceição Rosário, members of The Brazilian Obsessive-Compulsive Research Consortium, for their invaluable contribution to this article. The work was also supported by grants from the Fundação de Amparo à Pesquisa do Estado de São Paulo (FAPESP, Foundation for the Support of Research in the state of São Paulo): to Dr. Miguel (#2005/55628–08). Additional support was provided by the Conselho Nacional de Desenvolvimento Científico e Tecnológico (CNPQ, Brazilian Council for Scientific and Technological Development) grant to Dr. Miguel (grant #521369/96–7). Dr. Ygor is supported by the Research Council of Porto Alegre Institute (grant # 660018). Dr. Stein is supported by the Medical Research Council of South Africa.

References

Abelson JF, Kwan KY, O'Roak BJ, et al: Sequence variants in SLITRK1 are associated with Tourette's syndrome. Science 310:317–320, 2005

Ackermans L, Temel Y, Cath D, et al: Deep brain stimulation in Tourette's syndrome: two targets? Move Disord 21:709–713, 2006

Alsobrook JP, Leckman JF, Goodman WK, et al: Segregation analysis of obsessive-compulsive disorder using symptom-based factor scores. Am J Med Genet 88:669–675, 1999

Alvarenga PG, Hounie AG, Mercadante MT, et al: Obsessive-compulsive symptoms in heart disease patients with and without history of rheumatic fever. J Neuropsychiatry Clin Neurosci 18:405–408, 2006

Arnold LM, Auchenbach MB, McElroy SL: Psychogenic excoriation: clinical features, proposed diagnostic criteria, epidemiology and approaches to treatment. CNS Drugs 15:351–359, 2001

Arnold PD, Sicard T, Burroughs E, et al: Glutamate transporter gene SLC1A1 associated with obsessive-compulsive disorder. Arch Gen Psychiatry 63:769–776, 2006

Azrin NH, Nunn RG: Habit reversal: a method of eliminating nervous habits and tics. Behav Res Ther 11:619–628, 1973

Babel TB, Warnke PC, Ostertag CB: Immediate and long term outcome after infrathalamic and thalamic lesioning for intractable Tourette's syndrome. J Neurol Neurosurg Psychiatry 70:666–671, 2001

Baker EFW: Gilles de la Tourette syndrome treated by bimedial leucotomy. Can Med Assoc J 86:746–747, 1962

Baumgardner TL, Singer HS, Denckla MB, et al: Corpus callosum morphology in children with Tourette syndrome and attention deficit hyperactivity disorder. Neurology 47:477–482, 1996

Beckers W: Gilles de la Tourette's disease based on five own observations. Arch Psychiatr Nervenkr 217:169–186, 1973

Berthier ML, Kulisevsky J, Campos VM: Bipolar disorder in adult patients with Tourette's syndrome: a clinical study. Biol Psychiatry 43:364–370, 1998

Bienvenu OJ, Samuels JF, Riddle MA, et al: The relationship of obsessive-compulsive disorder to possible spectrum disorders: results from a family study. Biol Psychiatry 48:287–293, 2000

Bloch MH, Leckman JF, Zhu H, et al: Caudate volumes in childhood predict symptom severity in adults with Tourette syndrome. Neurology 65:1253–1258, 2005

Bloch MH, Landeros-Weisenberger A, Kelmendi B, et al: A systematic review: antipsychotic augmentation with treatment refractory obsessive-compulsive disorder. Mol Psychiatry 11:622–632, 2006a

Bloch MH, Peterson BS, Scahill L, et al: Adulthood outcome of tic and obsessive-compulsive symptom severity in children with Tourette syndrome. Arch Pediatr Adolesc Med 160:65–69, 2006b

Bohlhalter S, Goldfine A, Matteson S, et al: Neural correlates of tic generation in Tourette syndrome: an event-related functional MRI study. Brain 129:2029–2037, 2006

Bohne A, Keuthen NJ, Tuschen-Caffier B, et al: Cognitive inhibition in trichotillomania and obsessive-compulsive disorder. Behav Res Ther 43:923–942, 2005a

Bohne A, Savage CR, Deckersbach T, et al: Visuospatial abilities, memory, and executive functioning in trichotillomania and obsessive-compulsive disorder. J Clin Exp Neuropsychol 27:385–399, 2005b

Carpenter LL, Heninger GR, McDougle CJ, et al: Cerebrospinal fluid interleukin-6 in obsessive-compulsive disorder and trichotillomania. Psychiatry Res 112:257–262, 2002

Castellanos FX, Ritchie GF, Marsh WL, et al: DSM-IV stereotypic movement disorder: persistence of stereotypies of infancy in intellectually normal adolescents and adults. J Clin Psychiatry 57:116–122, 1996

Cavallini MC, Perna G, Caldirola D, et al: A segregation study of panic disorder in families of panic patients responsive to the 35% CO_2 challenge. Biol Psychiatry 46:815–820, 1999

Chae JH, Nahas Z, Wassermann E, et al: A pilot safety study of repetitive transcranial magnetic stimulation (rTMS) in Tourette's syndrome. Cognitive and Behavior Neurology 17:109–117, 2004

Chamberlain SR, Fineberg NA, Blackwell AD, et al: Motor inhibition and cognitive flexibility in obsessive-compulsive disorder and trichotillomania. Am J Psychiatry 163:1282–1284, 2006

Choi JS, Kim SH, Yoo SY, et al: Shape deformity of the corpus striatum in obsessive-compulsive disorder. Psychiatry Res 155:257–264, 2007

Christenson GA, Mackenzie TB, Mitchell JE: Characteristics of 60 adult chronic hair pullers. Am J Psychiatry 148:365–370, 1991

Christenson GA, Mackenzie TB, Reeve EA: Familial trichotillomania. Am J Psychiatry 149:283, 1992

Coetzer R, Stein DJ: Neuropsychological measures in women with obsessive-compulsive disorder and trichotillomania. Psychiatry Clin Neurosci 53:413–415, 1999

Coffey BJ, Miguel EC, Biederman J, et al: Tourette's disorder with and without obsessive-compulsive disorder in adults: are they different? J Nerv Ment Dis 186:201–206, 1998

Comings DE, Comings BG: A controlled study of Tourette syndrome, IV: obsessions, compulsions, and schizoid behaviors. Am J Hum Genet 41:782–803, 1987

Cooper IS: Dystonia reversal by operation in the basal ganglia. Arch Neurol 7:64–74, 1962

Cuker A, State MW, King RA, et al: Candidate locus for Gilles de la Tourette syndrome/obsessive compulsive disorder/chronic tic disorder at 18q22. Am J Med Genet 130:37–39, 2004

DeBakey M, Ochsner W: Bezoars and concretions: a comprehensive review of the literature with an analysis of 303 collected cases and a presentation of 8 additional cases. Surgery 5:934–963, 1939

Dell'Osso B, Altamura AC, Allen A, et al: Brain stimulation techniques in the treatment of obsessive-compulsive disorder: current and future directions. CNS Spectr 10:966–979, 2005

Denys D, van der Wee N, Janssen J, et al: Low level of dopaminergic D2 receptor binding in obsessive-compulsive disorder. Biol Psychiatry 55:1041–1045, 2004

Denys D, Van Nieuwerburgh F, Deforce D, et al: Association between the dopamine D2 receptor TaqI A2 allele and low activity COMT allele with obsessive-compulsive disorder in males. Eur Neuropsychopharmacol 16:446–450, 2006

DeVito TJ, Drost DJ, Pavlosky W, et al: Brain magnetic resonance spectroscopy in Tourette's disorder. J Am Acad Child Adolesc Psychiatry 44:1301–1308, 2005

Diederich NJ, Kalteis K, Stamenkovic M, et al: Efficient internal pallidal stimulation in Gilles de la Tourette syndrome: a case report. Mov Disord 20:1496–1499, 2005

Diefenbach GJ, Tolin DF, Hannan S, et al: Trichotillomania: impact on psychosocial functioning and quality of life. Behav Res Ther 43:869–884, 2005

Diniz JB, Rosario-Campos MC, Shavitt RG, et al: Impact of age at onset and duration of illness on the expression of comorbidities in obsessive-compulsive disorder. J Clin Psychiatry 65:22–27, 2004

Diniz JB, Rosário-Campos MC, Hounie AG, et al: Chronic tics and Tourette syndrome in patients with obsessive compulsive disorder. J Psychiatr Res 40:487–493, 2005

Eapen V, Pauls DL, Robertson MM: Evidence for autosomal dominant transmission in Tourette's syndrome: United Kingdom cohort study. B J Psychiatry 162:593–596, 1993

Eapen V, Robertson MM, Alsobrook JP, et al: Obsessive compulsive symptoms in Gilles de la Tourette syndrome and obsessive compulsive disorder: differences by diagnosis and family history. Am J Hum Genet 74:432–438, 1997

Ferrão YA, Scheidt B: Basal ganglia hemorrhagic ablation causing temporary suppression of trichotillomania symptoms. Rev Bras Psiquiatr 25:262–263, 2003

Ferrão YA, Almeida VP, Bedin NR, et al: Impulsivity and compulsivity in patients with trichotillomania or skin picking compared with patients with obsessive-compulsive disorder. Compr Psychiatry 47:282–288, 2006

Flaherty AW, Williams ZM, Amirnovin R, et al: Deep brain stimulation of the anterior internal capsule for the treatment of Tourette syndrome: technical case report. Neurosurgery 57(suppl):E403, 2005

Garner JP, Weisker SM, Dufour B, et al: Barbering (fur and whisker trimming) by laboratory mice as a model of human trichotillomania and obsessive-compulsive spectrum disorders. Comp Med 54:216–224, 2004

Garvey MA, Perlmutter SJ, Allen AJ, et al: A pilot study of penicillin prophylaxis for neuropsychiatric exacerbations triggered by streptococcal infections. Biol Psychiatry 45:1564–1571, 1999

George MS, Trimble MR, Ring HA, et al: Obsessions in obsessive-compulsive disorder with and without Gilles de la Tourette's syndrome. Am J Psychiatry 150:93–97, 1993

George S, Moselhy H: Cocaine-induced trichotillomania. Addiction (Abingdon, England) 100:255–256, 2005

Gilbert DL: Motor cortex inhibitory function in Tourette syndrome, attention deficit disorder, and obsessive compulsive disorder: studies using transcranial magnetic stimulation. Adv Neurol 99:107–114, 2006

Grados MA, Riddle MA, Samuels JF, et al: The familial phenotype of obsessive-compulsive disorder in relation to tic disorder: the Hopkins OCD family study. Biol Psychiatry 50:559–565, 2001

Greenberg BD, Malone DA, Friehs GM, et al: Three-year outcomes in deep brain stimulation for highly resistant obsessive-compulsive disorder. Neuropsychopharmacology 31:2394, 2006

Greer JM, Capecchi MR: Hoxb8 is required for normal grooming behavior in mice. Neuron 33:23–34, 2002

Hanna GL, Fischer DJ, Chadha KR, et al: Familial and sporadic subtypes of early onset obsessive-compulsive disorder. Biol Psychiatry 57:895–900, 2005

Hasler G, LaSalle-Ricci VH, Ronquillo JG, et al: Obsessive-compulsive disorder symptom dimensions show specific relationships to psychiatric comorbidity. Psychaitry Res 135:121–132, 2005

Hasstedt SJ, Leppert M, Filloux F, et al: Intermediate inheritance of Tourette syndrome, assuming assortive mating. Am J Hum Genet 57:682–689, 1995

Hemmings SM, Kinnear CJ, Lochner C, et al: Early versus late-onset obsessive-compulsive disorder: investigating genetic and clinical correlates. Psychiatry Res 128:175–182, 2004

Himle JA, Fischer DJ, Van Etten ML, et al: Group behavioral therapy for adolescents with tic-related and non-tic-related obsessive-compulsive disorder. Depress Anxiety 17:73–77, 2003

Holzer JC, Goodman WK, McDougle CJ, et al: Obsessive-compulsive disorder with and without a chronic tic disorder: a comparison of symptoms in 70 patients. Br J Psychiatry 164:469–473, 1994

Houeto JL, Karachi C, Mallet L, et al: Tourette's syndrome and deep brain stimulation. J Neurol Neurosurg Psychiatry 76:992–995, 2005

Hounie AG, Pauls DL, do Rosario-Campos MC, et al: Obsessive-compulsive spectrum disorders and rheumatic fever: a family study. Biol Psychiatry 61:266–272, 2007

Hyde TM, Aaronson BA, Randolph C, et al: Relationship of birth weight to the phenotypic expression of Gilles de la Tourette's syndrome in monozygotic twins. Neurology 42:652–658, 1992

Inoff-Germain G, Rodríguez RS, Torres-Alcantara S, et al: An immunological marker (D8/17) associated with rheumatic fever as a predictor of childhood psychiatric disorders in a community sample. J Child Psychol Psychiatry 44:782–790, 2003

Ipser JC, Carey P, Dhansay Y, et al: Pharmacotherapy augmentation strategies in treatment-resistant anxiety disorders. Cochrane Database Syst Rev 18:CD005473, 2006

Jaisoorya TS, Reddy YC, Srinath S: The relationship of obsessive-compulsive disorder to putative spectrum disorders: results from an Indian study. Compr Psychiatry 44:317–323, 2003

Karadenizli Bek D, Dilbaz N, Bayam G: Gilles de la Tourette syndrome: response to electroconvulsive therapy. J ECT 21:246–248, 2005

Karayiorgou M, Sobin C, Blundell ML, et al: Family based association studies support a sexually dimorphic effect of COMT and MAOA on genetic susceptibility to obsessive-compulsive disorder. Biol Psychiatry 45:1178–1189, 1999

Kerbeshian J, Burd L, Klug MG: Comorbid Tourette's disorder and bipolar disorder: an etiologic perspective. Am J Psychiatry 152:1646–1651, 1995

Keuthen NJ, Deckersbach T, Wilhelm S, et al: The Skin Picking Impact Scale (SPIS): scale development and psychometric analyses. Psychosomatics 42:397–403, 2001

Keuthen NJ, Makris N, Schlerf JE, et al: Evidence for reduced cerebellar volumes in trichotillomania. Biol Psychiatry 61:374–381, 2007

Kim SJ, Lee HS, Kim CH: Obsessive-compulsive disorder, factor-analyzed symptom dimensions and serotonin transporter polymorphism. Neuropsychobiology 52:176–182, 2005

Kurlan R, Caine ED, Lichter D, et al: Surgical treatment of severe obsessive-compulsive disorder associated with Tourette syndrome. Neurology 38(suppl):203, 1988

Kurlan R, Kersun J, Ballantine HT Jr, et al: Neurosurgical treatment of severe obsessive-compulsive disorder associated with Tourette's syndrome. Move Disord 5:152–155, 1990

Kurlan R, Eapen V, Stern J, et al: Bilineal transmission in Tourette's syndrome families. Neurology 44:2336–2342, 1994

Leckman JF: Tourette's syndrome. Lancet 360:1577–1586, 2002

Leckman JF, Kim YS: A primary candidate gene for obsessive-compulsive disorder. Arch Gen Psychiatry 63:717–720, 2006

Leckman JF, de Lotbiniere AJ, Marek K, et al: Severe disturbances in speech, swallowing, and gait following stereotactic infrathalamic lesions in Gilles de la Tourette's syndrome. Neurology 43:890–894, 1993

Leckman JF, Walker DE, Goodman WK, et al: "Just-right" perceptions associated with compulsive behavior in Tourette's syndrome. Am J Psychiatry 151:675–680, 1994

Leckman JF, Goodman WK, Anderson GM, et al: Cerebrospinal fluid biogenic amines in obsessive compulsive disorder, Tourette's syndrome, and healthy controls. Neuropsychopharmacology 12:73–86, 1995

Leckman JF, Peterson BS, Pauls DL, et al: Tic disorders. Psychiatr Clin North Am 20:839–862, 1997

Leckman JF, Pauls DL, Zhang H, et al: Obsessive-compulsive symptom dimensions in affected sibling pairs diagnosed with Gilles de la Tourette syndrome. Am J Med Genet 116:60–68, 2003

Lenane MC, Swedo SE, Rapoport JL, et al: Rates of obsessive compulsive disorder in first degree relatives of patients with trichotillomania: a research note. J Child Psychol Psychiatry 33:925–933, 1992

Leonard HL, Lenane MC, Swedo SE, et al: Tics and Tourette's disorder: a 2- to 7-year follow-up of 54 obsessive-compulsive children. Am J Psychiatry 149:1244–1251, 1992

Lochner C, du Toit PL, Zungu-Dirwayi N, et al: Childhood trauma in obsessive-compulsive disorder, trichotillomania, and controls. Depress Anxiety 15:66–68, 2002

Lochner C, Seedat S, Hemmings SMJ, et al: Dissociative experiences in obsessive compulsive disorder and trichotillomania: clinical and genetic findings. Compr Psychiatry 45:384–391, 2004

Lochner C, Seedat S, du Toit PL, et al: Obsessive-compulsive disorder and trichotillomania: a phenomenological comparison. BioMedical Center Psychiatry 5:2, 2005

Lopes AC, de Mathis ME, Canteras MM, et al: Update on neurosurgical treatment for obsessive compulsive disorder. Rev Bras Psiquiatr 26:62–66, 2004

Managoli S, Vilhekar KY: Trichotillomania as an ictal manifestation of partial seizure in a 4-year-old girl. Indian J Pediatr 70:843, 2003

Marsh R, Alexander GM, Packard MG, et al: Habit learning in Tourette syndrome: a translational neuroscience approach to a developmental psychopathology. Arch Gen Psychiatry 61:1259–1268, 2004

McDougle CJ, Goodman WK, Leckman JF, et al: Haloperidol addition in fluvoxamine-refractory obsessive-compulsive disorder. Arch Gen Psychiatry 51:302–308, 1994

McMahon WM, van de Wetering BJM, Filloux F, et al: Bilineal transmission and phenotypic variation of Tourette's disorder in a large pedigree. J Am Acad Child Adolesc Psychiatry 35:672–680, 1996

Mell LK, Davis RL, Owens D: Association between streptococcal infection and obsessive-compulsive disorder, Tourette's syndrome, and tic disorder. Pediatrics 116:56–60, 2005

Mercadante MT, Filho GB, Lombroso PJ, et al: Rheumatic fever and comorbid psychiatric disorders. Am J Psychiatry 157:2036–2038, 2000

Mercadante MT, Diniz JB, Hounie AG, et al: Obsessive-compulsive spectrum disorders in rheumatic fever patients. J Neuropsychiatry Clin Neurosci 17:544–547, 2005

Miguel EC, Coffey BJ, Baer L, et al: Phenomenology of intentional repetitive behaviors in obsessive-compulsive disorder and Tourette's disorder. J Clin Psychiatry 56:246–255, 1995

Miguel EC, Baer L, Coffey BJ, et al: Phenomenological differences appearing with repetitive behaviours in obsessive-compulsive disorder and Gilles de la Tourette's syndrome. Br J Psychiatry 170:140–145, 1997

Miguel EC, Rosário-Campos MC, Prado HS, et al: Sensory phenomena in obsessive-compulsive disorder and Tourette's disorder. J Clin Psychiatry 61:150–156, 2000

Miguel EC, Shavitt RG, Ferrão YA, et al: How to treat OCD in patients with Tourette syndrome. J Psychosom Res 55:49–57, 2003

Miltenberger RG, Fuqua RW, Woods DW: Applying behavior analysis to clinical problems: review and analysis of habit reversal. J Appl Behav Anal 31:447–469, 1998

Moriarty J, Eapen V, Costa DC, et al: HMPAO SPET does not distinguish obsessive-compulsive and tic syndromes in families multiply affected with Gilles de la Tourette's syndrome. Psychol Med 27:737–740, 1997

Mostofsky SH, Wendlandt J, Cutting L, et al: Corpus callosum measurements in girls with Tourette syndrome. Neurology 53:1345–1347, 1999

Munchau A, Bloem BR, Thilo KV, et al: Repetitive transcranial magnetic stimulation for Tourette syndrome. Neurology 59:1789–1791, 2002

Nadvornik P, Sramka M, Lisy L, et al: Experiences with dentatotomy. Confin Neurol 34:320–324, 1972

Nestadt G, Samuels J, Riddle M, et al: A family study of obsessive-compulsive disorder. Arch Gen Psychiatry 57:358–363, 2000

Nestadt G, Addington A, Samuels J, et al: The identification of OCD-related subgroups based on comorbidity. Biol Psychiatry 53:914–920, 2003

Nicolini H, Hanna G, Baxter L, et al: Segregation analysis of obsessive-compulsive and associated disorders: preliminary results. Ursus Medicus 1:25–28, 1991

Niehaus DJ, Knowles JA, van Kradenberg J, et al: D8/17 in obsessive-compulsive disorder and trichotillomania. South Afr Med J 89:755–756, 1999

O'Sullivan RL, Rauch SL, Breiter HC, et al: Reduced basal ganglia volumes in trichotillomania measured via morphometric magnetic resonance imaging. Biol Psychiatry 42:39–45, 1997

Orth M, Kirby R, Richardson MP, et al: Subthreshold rTMS over pre-motor cortex has no effect on tics in patients with Gilles de la Tourette syndrome. Clin Neurophysiol 116:764–768, 2005

Pauls DL, Leckman JF: The inheritance of Gilles de la Tourette's syndrome and associated behaviors: evidence for autosomal dominant transmission. N Engl J Med 315:993–997, 1986

Pauls DL, Towbin KE, Leckman JF, et al: Gilles de la Tourette's syndrome and obsessive-compulsive disorder: evidence supporting a genetic relationship. Arch Gen Psychiatry 43:1180–1182, 1986

Pauls DL, Pakstis AJ, Kurlan R, et al: Segregation and linkage analyses of Gilles de la Tourette's syndrome and related disorders. J Am Acad Child Adolesc Psychiatry 29:195–203, 1990

Pauls DL, Raymond CL, Stevenson JM, et al: A family study of Gilles de la Tourette syndrome. Am J Hum Genet 48:154–163, 1991

Pauls DL, Alsobrook JP, Goodman W, et al: A family study of obsessive-compulsive disorder. Am J Psychiatry 152:76–84, 1995

Perlmutter SJ, Leitman SF, Garvey MA, et al: Therapeutic plasma exchange and intravenous immunoglobulin for obsessive-compulsive disorder and tic disorders in childhood. Lancet 354:1153–1158, 1999

Peterson B, Riddle MA, Cohen DJ, et al: Reduced basal ganglia volumes in Tourette's syndrome using three dimensional reconstruction techniques from magnetic resonance images. Neurology 43:941–949, 1993

Peterson BS, Thomas P, Kane MJ, et al: Basal ganglia volumes in patients with Gilles de la Tourette syndrome. Arch Gen Psychiatry 60:415–424, 2003

Petter T, Richter MA, Sandor P: Clinical features distinguishing patients with Tourette's syndrome and obsessive-compulsive disorder from patients with obsessive-compulsive disorder without tics. J Clin Psychiatry 59:456–459, 1998

Price RA, Kidd KK, Cohen DJ, et al: A twin study of Tourette syndrome. Arch Gen Psychiatry 42:815–820, 1985

Rapoport M, Feder V, Sandor P: Response of major depression and Tourette's syndrome to ECT: a case report. Psychosom Med 60:528–529, 1998

Rauch SL: Neuroimaging research and the neurobiology of obsessive compulsive disorder: where do we go from here? Biol Psychiatry 47:168–170, 2000

Rauch SL, Baer L, Cosgrove GR, et al: Neurosurgical treatment of Tourette's syndrome: a critical review. Compr Psychiatry 36:141–156, 1995

Ravizza L, Maina G, Bogetto F: Episodic and chronic obsessive-compulsive disorder. Depress Anxiety 6:154–158, 1997

Reddy PS, Reddy YC, Srinath S, et al: A family study of juvenile obsessive-compulsive disorder. Can J Psychiatry 46:346–351, 2001

Robertson MM, Trimble MR, Lees AJ: The psychopathology of the Gilles de la Tourette syndrome: a phenomenological analysis. Br J Psychiatry 152:383–390, 1988

Robertson M, Doran M, Trimble M, et al: The treatment of Gilles de la Tourette syndrome by limbic leucotomy. J Neurol Neurosurg Psychiatry 53:691–694, 1990

Rosario-Campos MC, Leckman JF, Mercadante MT, et al: Adults with early onset obsessive-compulsive disorder. Am J Psychiatry 158:1899–1903, 2001

Rosario-Campos MC, Leckman JF, Curi M, et al: A family study of early onset obsessive-compulsive disorder. Am J Med Genet 136:92–97, 2005

Saxena S, Wang D, Bystritsky A, et al: Risperidone augmentation of SRI treatment for refractory obsessive-compulsive disorder. J Clin Psychiatry 57:303–306, 1996

Scahill L, Erenberg G, Berlin CM, et al: Contemporary assessment and pharmacotherapy of Tourette syndrome. NeuroRx 3:192–206, 2006

Seedat S, Stein DJ: Psychosocial and economic implications of trichotillomania: a pilot study in a South African sample. CNS Spectr 3:40–43, 1998

Senturk V, Tanriverdi N: Resistant trichotillomania and risperidone. Psychosomatics 43:429–430, 2002

Seuchter SA, Hebebrand J, Klug B, et al: Complex segregation analysis of families ascertained through Gilles de la Tourette syndrome. Genetics and Epidemiology 18:33–47, 2000

Shavitt RG, Belotto C, Curi M, et al: Clinical features associated with treatment response in obsessive-compulsive disorder. Compr Psychiatry 47:276–281, 2006

Singer HS: Tourette's syndrome: from behavior to biology. Lancet Neurol 4:149–159, 2005

Snider LA, Lougee L, Slattery M, et al: Antibiotic prophylaxis with azithromycin or penicillin for childhood-onset neuropsychiatric disorders. Biol Psychiatry 57:788–792, 2005

Soriano JL, O'Sullivan RL, Baer L, et al: Trichotillomania and self-esteem: a survey of 62 female hair pullers. J Clin Psychiatry 57:77–82, 1996

Stanley MA, Swann AC, Bowers TC, et al: A comparison of clinical features in trichotillomania and obsessive-compulsive disorder. Behav Res Ther 30:39–44, 1992

Stein DJ, Hollander E: Low-dose pimozide augmentation of serotonin reuptake blockers in the treatment of trichotillomania. J Clin Psychiatry 53:123–126, 1992

Stein DJ, Bouwer C, Hawkridge S, et al: Risperidone augmentation of serotonin reuptake inhibitors in obsessive-compulsive and related disorders. J Clin Psychiatry 58:119–122, 1997a

Stein DJ, Coetzer R, Lee M, et al: Magnetic resonance brain imaging in women with obsessive-compulsive disorder and trichotillomania. Psychiatry Res 74:177–182, 1997b

Stein DJ, van Heerden B, Hugo C, et al: Functional brain imaging and pharmacotherapy in trichotillomania: single photon emission computed tomography before and after treatment with the selective serotonin reuptake inhibitor citalopram. Prog Neuropsychopharmacol 26:885–890, 2002

Stern E, Silbersweig DA, Chee KY, et al: A functional neuroanatomy of tics in Tourette syndrome. Arch Gen Psychiatry 57:741–748, 2000

Stevens H: The syndrome of Gilles de la Tourette and its treatment. Med Ann Dist Columbia 36:277–279, 1964

Stewart RS, Nejtek VA: An open-label, flexible-dose study of olanzapine in the treatment of trichotillomania. J Clin Psychiatry 64:49–52, 2003

Strassing M, Riedel M, Muller N: Electroconvulsive therapy in a patient with Tourette's syndrome and co-morbid obsessive compulsive disorder. World J Biol Psychiatry 5:164–166, 2004

Swedo SE: Is trichotillomania an obsessive-compulsive spectrum disorder?, in The Obsessive-Compulsive Related Disorders. Edited by Hollander E. Washington, DC, American Psychiatric Press, 1993

Swedo SE, Leonard HL, Rapoport JL, et al: A double-blind comparison of clomipramine and desipramine in the treatment of trichotillomania (hair pulling). N Engl J Med 321:497–501, 1989

Swedo SE, Rapoport JL, Leonard HL, et al: Regional cerebral glucose metabolism of women with trichotillomania. Arch Gen Psychiatry 48:828–833, 1991

Swedo SE, Leonard H, Mittleman BB, et al: Identification of children with pediatric autoimmune neuropsychiatric disorders associated with streptococcal infections by a marker associated with rheumatic fever. Am J Psychiatry 154:110–112, 1997

Swerdlow NR, Zinner S, Farber RH, et al: Symptoms in obsessive-compulsive disorder and Tourette syndrome: a spectrum? CNS Spectr 4:21–33, 1999

Temel Y, Visser-Vandewalle V: Surgery in Tourette syndrome. Mov Disord 91:3–14, 2004

The Tourette Syndrome Classification Study Group: Definitions and classification of tic disorders. Arch Neurol 50:1013–1016, 1993

Tukel R, Keser V, Karali N, et al: Comparison of clinical characteristics in trichotillomania and obsessive-compulsive disorder. J Anxiety Disord 15:433–441, 2001

Vandewalle V, van der Linden C, Groenewegen HJ, et al: Stereotactic treatment of Gilles de la Tourette syndrome by high frequency stimulation of thalamus. Lancet 353:724, 1999

van Grootheest DS, Cath DC, Beekman AT, et al: Twin studies on obsessive-compulsive disorder: a review. Twin Res Hum Genet 8:450–458, 2005

Wagaman JR, Miltenberger RG, Willians DE: Treatment of a vocal tic by differential reinforcement. J Behav Ther Exp Psychiatry 26:35–39, 1995

Walkup JT, Leckman JF, Price RA, et al: The relationship between Tourette syndrome and obsessive compulsive disorder: a twin study. Psychopharmacol Bull 24:375–379, 1988

Walkup JT, LaBuda MC, Singer HS, et al: Family study and segregation analysis of Tourette syndrome: evidence for a mixed model of inheritance. Am J Hum Genet 59:684–693, 1996

Whiteside SP, Port JD, Abramowitz JS: A meta-analysis of functional neuroimaging in obsessive-compulsive disorder. Psychiatry Res 132:69–79, 2004

Whiteside SP, Port JD, Deacon BJ, et al: A magnetic resonance spectroscopy investigation of obsessive-compulsive disorder and anxiety. Psychiatry Res 146:137–147, 2006

Wilhelm S, Deckersbach T, Coffey BJ, et al: Habit reversal versus supportive psychotherapy for Tourette's disorder: a randomized controlled trial. Am J Psychiatry 1670:1175–1177, 2003

Woods DW, Miltenberger RG, Lumley VA: Sequential application of major habit-reversal components to treat motor tics in children. J Appl Behav Anal 29:483–493, 1996

Woods DW, Piacentini J, Himle MB, et al: Premonitory Urge for Tics Scale (PUTS): initial psychometric results and examination of the premonitory urge phenomenon in youths with tic disorders. J Dev Behav Pediatr 26:397–403, 2005

Woods DW, Flessner CA, Franklin ME, et al: The Trichotillomania Impact Project (TIP): exploring phenomenology, functional impairment, and treatment utilization. J Clin Psychiatry 67:1877–1888, 2006a

Woods DW, Flessner C, Franklin ME, et al: Understanding and treating trichotillomania: what we know and what we don't know. Psychiatr Clin North Am 29:487–501, 2006b

Zhang H, Leckman JF, Pauls DL, et al: Tourette Syndrome Association International Consortium for Genetics: genomewide scan of hoarding in sib pairs in which both sibs have Gilles de la Tourette syndrome. Am J Hum Genet 70:896–904, 2002

Zohar J, Insel TR: Obsessive-compulsive disorder: psychobiological approaches to diagnosis, treatment, and pathophysiology. Biol Psychiatry 22:667–687, 1987

Zuchner S, Cuccaro ML, Tran-Viet KN, et al: SLITRK1 mutations in trichotillomania. Mol Psychiatry 11:887–889, 2006

4

RELATIONSHIP BETWEEN IMPULSE-CONTROL DISORDERS AND OBSESSIVE-COMPULSIVE DISORDER

A Current Understanding and Future Research Directions

Marc N. Potenza, M.D., Ph.D.
Lorrin M. Koran, M.D.
Stefano Pallanti, M.D., Ph.D.

In anticipation of the generation of the next editions of DSM and the *International Classification of Diseases,* the American Psychiatric Association, National Institutes of Health, and World Health Organization have sponsored a series of meet-

This chapter was first published as "The Relationship Between Impulse-Control Disorders and Obsessive-Compulsive Disorder: A Current Understanding and Future Research Directions." *Psychiatry Research* 170:22–31, 2009. Copyright 2009. Used with permission.

Preparation of the original article that constitutes this chapter was supported in part by the National Institute on Drug Abuse (R01-DA019039); the Women's Health Research at Yale University; and the U.S. Department of Veterans Affairs VISN1 MIRECC and REAP.

ings entitled, "The Future of Psychiatric Diagnosis: Refining the Research Agenda." The conference focusing on obsessive-compulsive spectrum disorders (OCSDs) was convened on June 20–22, 2006. Among the topics discussed were which disorders should be considered within the obsessive-compulsive spectrum and whether disorders currently classified elsewhere might be alternatively grouped in a manner supported by empirical data. Among the disorders warranting consideration for grouping within an obsessive-compulsive spectrum were the impulse-control disorders (ICDs), including pathological gambling (PG) and intermittent explosive disorder (IED). Multiple domains representing potential endophenotypes were identified prior to the meeting to foster exploration and discussion of this topic. These domains included phenomenology, comorbidity, course of illness, family history, genetics, brain circuitry, cross-species considerations, pharmacology, treatments and interventions, and cultural influences.

Impulse-Control Disorders: Current Categorization in DSM-IV-TR

ICDs are currently classified within DSM-IV-TR in the category of "Impulse Control Disorders Not Elsewhere Classified" (American Psychiatric Association 2000). As the category name implies, other disorders characterized by impaired impulse control (e.g., substance abuse and dependence, Cluster B personality disorders, and eating disorders) are categorized elsewhere in DSM-IV-TR. Included in the formal ICD category are IED, kleptomania, pyromania, PG, trichotillomania, and ICD not otherwise specified (NOS). Whereas formal criteria for other ICDs have been proposed (e.g., for excessive, problematic or compulsive behavior in the domains of shopping or buying, computer or Internet use, sex, and skin picking [Grant and Potenza 2004; Koran et al. 2006; Lejoyeaux et al. 1996; Liu and Potenza 2007; McElroy et al. 1994; Potenza and Hollander 2002]), clinically significant behaviors in these areas would currently be diagnosed as ICD-NOS. This article focuses on those ICDs with specific diagnostic criteria already defined in DSM because ICDs without clearly defined diagnostic criteria have been less studied.

Common Features of Impulse-Control Disorders: Relationship to Obsessive-Compulsive Disorder

As described in DSM-IV-TR, the essential feature of ICDs is "the failure to resist an impulse, drive, or temptation to perform an act that is harmful to the person or to others." Each ICD is characterized by a recurrent pattern of behavior that has this essential feature within a specific domain. The repetitive engagement in these behaviors ultimately interferes with functioning in other domains. In this respect, ICDs resemble OCD. That is, individuals with OCD often report difficulties resisting the urge to engage in specific behaviors (e.g., cleaning, ordering, or other ritualistic behaviors) that interfere with functioning. However, this resemblance is not unique to OCD. For example, individuals with drug addictions often report difficulty in resisting the urge to use drugs. Perhaps for these reasons, two of the most common conceptualizations of ICDs link them to OCSDs or to addictive disorders (Hollander and Wong 1995; Potenza et al. 2001a, 2001b). Although the categorizations of ICDs as OCSDs or addictive disorders are not mutually exclusive, they have important theoretical and clinical implications given differences in the prevention and treatment strategies for these disorders (Tamminga and Nestler 2006). Heterogeneities in OCD and addictions and changes that occur during the course of these disorders complicate comparisons across disorders, particularly because investigations concurrently examining OCD, substance addictions, and ICDs are scarce.

ICDs and OCD have been conceptualized to lie along an impulsive/compulsive spectrum, with disorders with high harm avoidance, such as OCD, positioned closer to the more compulsive end and those with low harm avoidance, such as many ICDs, positioned closer to the more impulsive end (Hollander and Wong 1995). Although data indicate that individuals with OCD score high on measures of harm avoidance and those with ICDs such as PG score high on measures of impulsivity and related measures such as novelty seeking (Potenza 2007b), recent data suggest a more complex relationship between impulsivity and compulsivity as they relate to OCD and ICDs. For example, individuals with OCD as compared with control subjects demonstrated high levels of cognitive impulsiveness (Ettelt et al. 2007). An association between measures of cognitive impulsiveness and aggressive obsessions and checking suggests that impulsiveness may be particularly relevant to specific subgroups of individuals with OCD (Ettelt et al. 2007). Another study of OCD, PG, and control subjects found that the majority of the gambling and OCD subjects were characterized by high levels of both impulsivity and harm avoidance, suggesting a more complex relationship between impulsivity and compulsivity than originally proposed (Potenza 2007b). More research is needed to examine the extent to which some of these similarities across these disorders might explain similarities in specific clinical phenomena—for example, whether high levels of impulsiveness in PG and OCD account for high levels of suicidality reported across these disorders (Ledgerwood et al. 2005; Torres et al. 2006). Furthermore, the complex relationship between impulsivity and compulsivity may be influenced by different factors in specific populations. For example, gender differences in the relationship between measures of impulsivity and compulsivity have been reported in a sample of high school students (Li and Chen 2007), and the extent to which these findings extend to groups with OCD and/or ICDs has yet to be systematically investigated.

As described in DSM-IV-TR, additional features common to ICDs are feelings of "tension or arousal before committing the act" and "pleasure, gratification or relief at the time of committing the act." There may or may not be feelings of regret, self-reproach, or guilt following the act. In multiple respects, the motivations and sensations preceding and relating to the repetitive acts in ICDs and OCD are different. Among the most striking difference is the ego-dystonic nature typically ascribed to the obsessions and compulsions in OCD as compared with the ego-syntonic feelings typically associated with ICD behaviors such as gambling (Stein and Lochner 2006). The ego-syntonic nature of ICD behaviors is at least superficially more similar to the experience of drug use behaviors in drug dependence. Similarly, the variability in the degree of guilt or remorse following the ICD behavior is reminiscent of the variability observed in individuals with drug addictions. However, the motivational and emotional processes underlying engagement in and experiencing of the repetitive behaviors in ICDs may change over time (Brewer and Potenza 2008; Chambers et al. 2007). For example, individuals with PG often report that although they initially gambled to win money, later they became motivated simply by the experience of gambling itself (to be "in action"). Whereas gambling urges early in the course of the disorder are typically pleasurable, over time they often become less ego-syntonic as people more fully appreciate the negative consequences of their gambling and struggle to refrain. Although these changes appear similar to those reported during the course of the addictive process, they also resemble processes in OCD. That is, as the urge to engage in an ICD behavior and the behavior itself become more ego-dystonic, less driven by seeking of pleasure and more driven by a desire to reduce an anxious or distressing state, the urge and behavior more closely resemble the phenomenological features of obsessions and compulsions, respectively, in OCD. On the other hand, the ego-dystonic quality of OCD symptoms may diminish over time (Rasmussen and Eisen 1992).

Heterogeneity of Impulse-Control Disorders: Unique Features

The behavioral domains covered by the current ICDs include anger management, stealing, fire-setting, gambling, and hair-pulling. Because these domains are in many ways distinct and disparate, a question arises as to whether the disorders should be grouped together. DSM-IV-TR groups some other disorders characterized by excessive or interfering levels of engagement separately according to the specific target behavior (e.g., substance-related and eating disorders). Data examining the extent to which ICDs warrant clustering are sparse. Until recently, ICDs were typically omitted from large epidemiological studies. Although recent studies such as the National Epidemiologic Survey on Alcoholism and Related Conditions (NESARC) and the National Comorbidity Survey Replication Study (NCS-R) included measures of specific ICDs such as PG and IED (Kessler et al. 2006; Petry et al. 2005), the entire group of disorders has not been assessed concurrently in a large, population-based sample. Thus, the extent to which they form a cohesive group has not been directly examined, nor has the extent to which they fit into an empirically supported structure of psychiatric disorders. That is, data indicate that most psychiatric disorders can be categorized into internalizing or externalizing clusters (Kendler et al. 2003; Krueger 1999). Although ICDs often share with externalizing disorders a disinhibited personality style or a lack of constraint (Slutske et al. 2000, 2001, 2005), they also share features with internalizing disorders such as major depression (Potenza 2007a; Potenza et al. 2005). Where OCD and ICDs best fit within this structure warrants direct investigation. Whereas the disabling distress and anxiety associated with OCD contribute to its current classification in DSM-IV-TR as an anxiety disorder, it is categorized separately in the 10th edition of the International Classification of Diseases (World Health Organization 2003).

Existing studies suggest that the ICDs represent a heterogeneous group of disorders. Within a clinical sample of subjects with OCD, pathological skin-picking and nail-biting were frequently endorsed and other ICDs were relatively uncommon (Grant et al. 2006a). OCD subjects with ICDs were more likely than those without OCD to acknowledge hoarding and symmetry obsessions and hoarding and repeating rituals, suggesting a differential association of ICDs with subgroups of individuals with OCD (Grant et al. 2006a). Within a sample of probands with or without OCD, excessive "grooming disorders" including trichotillomania and pathological nail-biting and skin-picking were more common in the individuals with OCD (Bienvenu et al. 2000). In contrast, other ICDs, including PG, pyromania, and kleptomania, were not more commonly identified in individuals with OCD versus those without the disorder. This pattern extended to first-degree relatives, suggesting a heritable component to the overlap between OCD and the grooming-related ICD behaviors. However, a study of individuals with trichotillomania and their family members did not find a close link between OCD and trichotillomania (Lenane et al. 1992). Methodological limitations, including relatively small sample sizes, might be responsible in part for the heterogeneity in findings. Co-occurring ICDs in OCD have been associated with an earlier age at onset of OCD, a more insidious appearance of obsessive-compulsive symptoms, a greater number and severity of those symptoms, and a larger number of therapeutic trials (du Toit et al. 2005; Fontenelle et al. 2005; Grant et al. 2006a; Matsunaga et al. 2005).

An independent study found that OCSDs (including ICDs) in subjects with OCD clustered into the following three groups: 1) a "reward deficiency" group that included trichotillomania, PG, Tourette's disorder, and hypersexual disorder; 2) an "impulsivity" group that included kleptomania, IED, compulsive shopping, and self-injurious behaviors; and 3) a "somatic" group that included body dysmorphic disorder and hypochondriasis (Lochner et al. 2005). The different clusters correlated with different clinical features of the OCD sample. Specifically, cluster 1 was associated with early age at onset of OCD and the presence of tics, cluster 2 with female gender and childhood trauma, and cluster 3 with poor insight. These findings highlight several important points. First, they suggest that ICDs cluster into distinct groups, particularly within subjects with OCD. Second, specific groups of ICDs might be particularly relevant to specific subsets of individuals with OCD. That is, data support the existence of multiple subtypes of OCD with different clinical characteristics and treatment responses (e.g., tic vs. non–tic-related and the relationship to early onset and treatment refractoriness [Denys et al. 2003; Leckman et al. 1994, 2003; McDougle et al. 1994; Rosario-Campos et al. 2005]). Factor-analytic studies have suggested that particular OCD symptom types (aggressive obsessions/checking, religious or sexual obsessions, symmetry/ordering, contamination/cleaning, hoarding) may represent biologically distinct disorders (Leckman et al. 2001), and positron emission tomography studies have found differences in OCD subjects with different symptom clusters (Rauch et al. 1998). Specific ICDs (or clusters thereof) may be particularly relevant to specific subtypes of OCD—for example, IED and aggressive subtypes of OCD. More research is needed to examine the specific categorical and dimensional features of OCD in relation to ICDs in order to clarify these relationships (Lochner and Stein 2006; Stein and Lochner 2006).

Individual Impulse-Control Disorders

Given individual differences between the ICDs, representative ICDs were selected for further consideration according to the potential endophenotype domains identified for the obsessive-compulsive spectrum workgroup meeting: 1) phenomenology and epidemiology; 2) co-occurring disorders; 3) family history and genetics; 4) neurobiology, including animal models and human studies; 5) pharmacological and behavioral treatments and interventions; and 6) cultural considerations. Some aspects relevant to OCD (e.g., important immune system contributions to OCD in a subset of individuals [Snider and Swedo 2004]) are not presently suspected in the etiology of any of the formal ICDs and are not discussed here. Two ICDs, IED and PG, were selected for consideration here because they 1) have been identified as belonging to distinct categories in OCD subjects in a data-driven cluster analysis (Lochner et al. 2005), and 2) have been most thoroughly studied to date. This latter aspect is particularly relevant in that not all ICDs have sufficient empirical data to address adequately all of the domains specified by the workgroup. The third cluster of OCSDs previously identified (the somatic cluster including body dysmorphic disorder [Lochner et al. 2005]) is not addressed here because it does not include formal ICDs and is covered in a separate article derived from the workgroup meeting. The findings from the cluster analysis (Lochner et al. 2005) have limitations; for example, they are obtained from a population with OCD, thereby potentially introducing bias. However, similar studies have not been performed in other populations. Consequently, these data seem the best available to guide decision making regarding which ICDs to cover most extensively here. Although it would be desirable to cover each ICD in similar detail in the following sections, space limitations coupled with the intent to cover adequately the domains identified prevent this.

Intermittent Explosive Disorder

PHENOMENOLOGY AND EPIDEMIOLOGY

Available data suggest that although there are similarities between IED and OCD, substantial differences exist. IED is characterized by recurrent episodes of aggression that are out of proportion to psychosocial stressors and/or provocation and are not better accounted for by another mental disorder, by comorbid medical conditions, or by the physiological effects of a drug or other substance with psychotropic properties (American Psychiatric Association 2000). IED may be repetitive, intrusive, persistent, and recurrent like OCD, but it is often episodic. Unlike compulsions in OCD, aggressive outbursts in IED typically do not occur in response to an obsession. Aggression is typically unplanned and occurs without substantial forethought (Grant and Potenza 2006b). Aggression in IED differs from compulsions in OCD in that it may be gratifying and accompanied by excitement rather than by anxiety reduction; however, like OCD compulsions, aggressive acts can be perceived as distressing (McElroy et al. 1998).

Chart reviews of psychiatric inpatients (Monopolis and Lion 1983) and clinical interviews (Felthous et al. 1991) reported prevalence estimates of IED from 1% to 3% in psychiatric settings (Olvera 2002). A more recent study of adult psychiatric inpatients found that 6.4% and 6.9% had current and lifetime IED, respectively (Grant et al. 2005). A separate study of adolescent psychiatric inpatients found a larger proportion of subjects (12.7%) met criteria for IED (Grant et al. 2007b). In both the adult and adolescent inpatient studies, diagnoses of IED were only identified following active screening and interviewing. These findings suggest that IED, like other ICDs, often goes undiagnosed and thus is often not targeted for treatment. Estimates of IED in community samples suggest that IED is common. For example, one community study found a 11.1% lifetime prevalence and a 3.2% 1-month prevalence (Cocarro et al. 2004). In the NCS-R study, lifetime and 12-month prevalence estimates of DSM-IV-TR IED were 7.3% and 3.9%, respectively (Kessler et al. 2006). Together, these studies suggest that IED is more common than OCD.

In some respects, the clinical characteristics and course of IED resemble those of other disorders characterized by impaired control (e.g., substance use disorders) more than those of OCD. Unlike OCD, in which there is an approximately 1:1

male-to-female ratio (Robins and Regier 1991) or a slight female predominance (Grabe et al. 2006; Mohammadi et al. 2004), IED is characterized by an approximately 2:1 male predominance (Grant and Potenza 2006b; Kessler et al. 2006). Age at onset for DSM-IV-TR IED peaks in the teenage years, is earlier for men than women, and is earlier than for most disorders that frequently co-occur with IED (discussed later), with the possible exception of phobic anxiety disorders (Kessler et al. 2006). Similarly, many individuals (49%) report OCD symptom onset during childhood or adolescence, and a majority (75%) report onset prior to age 25 (Robins and Regier 1991). In IED, aggressive behaviors occur in nearly all decades of life beginning in the first decade, peaking in the third decade, diminishing steadily after the fourth decade, and culminating in little or no reported aggression by the eighth decade (Cocarro et al. 2004). Sociodemographic correlates of lifetime IED include low educational level, being married, and having low family income (Kessler et al. 2006). In contrast, OCD does not show a clear association with educational level, and married individuals are less likely to be afflicted (Robins and Regier 1991).

CO-OCCURRING DISORDERS

Like other ICDs (Potenza 2007), IED frequently co-occurs with other psychiatric disorders including OCD. Initial findings were reported from clinical samples. One study reported OCD in 22% of individuals with IED (McElroy et al. 1998). Estimates of IED in clinical samples of subjects with OCD have ranged from about 2% to about 10% (du Toit et al. 2005; Fontenelle et al. 2005). In the NCS-R, the vast majority (81.8%) of patients with lifetime broadly defined IED met criteria for at least one other lifetime DSM-IV-TR disorder (Kessler et al. 2006). A wide range of psychiatric disorders was found in association with IED including mood, anxiety, impulse-control, and substance use disorders (Kessler et al. 2006). Among individuals with broadly defined IED, 4.4% met criteria for OCD. The odds ratio for broadly defined IED in association with OCD was 2.5 (95% CI, 1.1–5.7). Within the broadly defined group, there was no significant difference in the degree of association between the narrowly defined IED and OCD (OR, 1.1; 95% CI, 0.2–6.9). In contrast, generalized anxiety disorder, all ICDs, and many substance use disorders showed significantly elevated odds ratios for both broadly and narrowly defined IED, suggesting a particularly close relationship between these disorders and both less and more severe forms of IED (Kessler et al. 2006).

FAMILY HISTORY AND GENETICS

Although studies suggest that impulsive and aggressive behaviors demonstrate familial transmission (Halperin et al. 2003; Kreek et al. 2005), few genetic or family history studies have been performed in individuals with IED. Several lines of research have identified familial sociopathy and aggression as salient risk factors for the persistence of childhood aggression into adolescence and adulthood (Cadoret et al. 1995; Frick et al. 1990). A familial pattern of aggressive behaviors has been associated with central serotonin function (see next section, "Neurobiology: Animal Models and Human Studies") (Halperin et al. 2003). The family history of individuals with IED is characterized by high rates of mood, substance use, and other impulse-control disorders (McElroy et al. 1998). A genetic linkage study found an association between an allelic variant of the serotonin $5\text{-}HT_{1B}$ receptor gene *(5HT1B)* and alcoholism in aggressive/impulsive individuals who met criteria either for antisocial personality disorder or IED (Lappalainen et al. 1998). In contrast, *5HT1B* has not been implicated in genetic studies of OCD, although several other serotonin-related genes (e.g., those encoding the $5\text{-}HT_{1D}$ and $5\text{-}HT_{2A}$ receptors and the serotonin transporter) have been implicated in some but not all studies of OCD (Hemmings and Stein 2006).

NEUROBIOLOGY: ANIMAL MODELS AND HUMAN STUDIES

Many neurotransmitter systems and brain regions contribute to impulsive aggression. Animal models have implicated numerous biological systems and neurotransmitters including those involving testosterone, γ-aminobutyric acid, nitric oxide, monoamine oxidase, glutamate, dopamine, and serotonin (Korff and Harvey 2006; Olivier and Young 2002). Within these systems, specific components seem particularly salient. For example, robust data implicate the $5\text{-}HT_{1B}$ receptor in impulsive aggression in mice; knockout mice lacking the receptor show marked physical aggression (Saudou et al. 1994). These findings are consistent with human studies implicating the receptor in impulsive-aggressive alcoholism (Lappalainen et al. 1998). Although some of the same systems (e.g., serotonin, dopamine) are relevant to both IED and OCD, they seem involved in different ways. For example, disruption of the genes encoding the $5\text{-}HT_{2C}$ receptor and the dopamine transporter generates stereotypic behaviors resembling OCD (Korff and Harvey 2006), as compared with the $5\text{-}HT_{1B}$ receptor manipulation more relevant to IED. Genetic variations in commonly occurring serotonin-related gene variants (e.g., of the serotonin transporter) influence serotonin measures associated with impulsive aggression (Mannelli et al. 2006).

Few studies have examined the neurobiology of IED in humans, and those available have not consistently identified between-group differences. For example, a magnetic resonance spectroscopy study that identified differences in adolescent bipolar and control subjects in myoinositol measures found no differences between adolescents with and without IED (Davanzo et al. 2003). Although few studies have been performed in individuals with IED, many have investigated individuals with impulsive aggression. Multiple biological systems, including those involving opiates, vasopressin, testosterone, catecholamines (norepinephrine, dopamine), and serotonin, have been identified as contributing to human aggression (Coccaro and Siever 2002). Among the most widely replicated findings is that of low levels of central measures of serotonin (particularly of the serotonin metabolite 5-hydroxy-indoleacetic acid) in impulsive-aggressive individuals (Coccaro and Siever 2002; Williams and Potenza 2008). Although serotonin systems have been implicated in OCD, the nature of the involvement differs, as judged by the results of pharmacological challenge studies. Administration of the serotonergic drugs meta-chloro-phenylpiperazine (m-CPP, a 5-HT$_1$ and 5-HT$_2$ receptor partial agonist [Potenza and Hollander 2002]) and fenfluramine (a drug inducing serotonin release and having postsynaptic serotonergic action [Curzon and Gibson 1999]) is associated with an exacerbation of obsessive-compulsive symptoms and enhanced prolactin release in subjects with OCD (Gross-Isseroff et al. 2004; Hollander et al. 1991; Monteleone et al. 1997). However, groups of children and adults characterized by impulsive aggression exhibit a blunted prolactin response to m-CPP and fenfluramine (Cocarro et al. 1997; Halperin et al. 2003; New et al. 2004b; Patkar et al. 2006). These findings are consistent with those from primates, in which an inverse relationship between aggression and serotonergic activity has been reported (Tiefenbacher et al. 2003).

Brain imaging studies have yielded insight into the pathophysiology of impulsive aggression in humans. Consistent with a role for the ventromedial prefrontal cortex (vmPFC, a region including the medial orbital frontal cortex [Bechara 2003]) in decision making and social and moral judgments (Anderson et al. 1999; Bechara 2003; Damasio 1994), individuals with impulsive aggression show relatively diminished activation of the vmPFC. For example, among individuals with depression, those with anger attacks showed an inverse correlation between regional cerebral blood flow in the left vmPFC and left amygdala during anger induction, whereas subjects without anger attacks did not (Dougherty et al. 2004). Aspects of vmPFC function as related to impulsive aggression appear linked to serotonin function. Individuals with impulsive aggression as compared with those without show blunted hemodynamic responses to the serotonergic drugs fenfluramine (Siever et al. 1999) and m-CPP (New et al. 2002). Individuals with impulsive aggression also show diminished serotonin availability in the anterior cingulate cortex, including within the ventral portion included in the vmPFC (Frankle et al. 2005). The serotonin reuptake inhibitor fluoxetine increases metabolism within orbitofrontal cortex (New et al. 2004a). Although orbitofrontal cortical function has been implicated in OCD, the nature of its involvement differs from that in impulsive aggression. Specifically, in apparent contrast to the diminished vmPFC activity associated with impulsive aggression, increased activation of cortical-striato-thalamo-cortical circuitry, including orbitofrontal regions involving the vmPFC, has been repeatedly implicated in OCD (Korff and Harvey 2006; Mataix-Cols and van den Heuvel 2006). However, specific subgroups of individuals with OCD show differential activation of this circuitry. For example, during a functional magnctic resonance imaging symptom provocation study, individuals with washing OCD showed strong activation of vmPFC and caudate, those with checking OCD showed strong activation of putamen/globus pallidus, thalamus, and dorsal cortical areas, and those with hoarding OCD showed strong activation of precentral gyrus and orbitofrontal cortex (Mataix-Cols et al. 2004).

PHARMACOLOGICAL AND BEHAVIORAL TREATMENTS AND INTERVENTIONS

Relatively few clinical trials have investigated the efficacy and tolerability of drugs in the treatment of IED. Drugs that block serotonin transport (both relatively selective and nonselective serotonin reuptake inhibitors such as sertraline and venlafaxine, respectively) have been reported in case reports to be helpful in individuals with IED (Feder 1999; McElroy et al. 1998). Although this finding may suggest similarities to the use of serotonin reuptake inhibitors in treating OCD, the dosages employed were often lower than those typically used in OCD (Denys 2006). For example, in one case series involving IED subjects, sertraline was dosed at 50–100 mg/day (Feder 1999) instead of at doses approaching 200 mg/day, as are often used for OCD. A role for serotonin reuptake inhibitors in the treatment of IED is consistent with their efficacy in targeting impulsive aggression (Coccaro and Kavoussi 1997; Reist et al. 2003). Mood-stabilizing drugs such as lithium and valproic acid have been reported helpful in open-label IED treatment studies (McElroy et al. 1998), consistent with findings from some but not all studies of these and other mood stabilizers (carbamazepine, phenytoin) in targeting impulsive aggression (Dell'Osso et al. 2006; Grant and Potenza 2006b; Olvera 2002). However, lithium lacks efficacy as an augmenting agent in the treatment of OCD (McDougle et al. 1991), although some antipsychotic drugs (e.g., olanzapine, risperidone) with mood-stabilizing properties have demonstrated efficacy in augmenting serotonin reuptake inhibitor response in refractory OCD (Denys 2006). Some antipsychotic drugs have also been effective in treating aggression in controlled studies (Buitelaar et al. 2001; Findling et al. 2001). α-Adrenergic agonists and β-adrenergic antagonists have each shown some promise in targeting impulsive aggression (Dell'Osso et al. 2006; Grant and Potenza 2006b; Olvera 2002), whereas no role for these drugs has been demonstrated in the treatment of OCD (Denys 2006). Taken together, although the data for IED are limited, existing information suggests that the similarities in the pharmacological treatments of IED and OCD are outweighed by substantial differences.

Data from psychotherapy trials for individuals with IED are limited, with suggestions that insight-oriented psychotherapy and behavioral therapy might be helpful for some individuals (Grant and Potenza 2006b). Limited studies involving small numbers of subjects have not found significant improvement related to group, couples, or family therapies (McElroy et al. 1998). With respect to aggressive behaviors, controlled studies of behavioral interventions including cognitive-behavioral therapy, group therapy, family therapy, and social skills training report some effectiveness for aggressive patients (Alpert and Spilman 1997). These treatments differ from the exposure and response prevention methods that are effective in the treatment of OCD (Neziroglu et al. 2006). Thus, like the pharmacotherapy data, the behavioral therapy findings suggest significant differences between IED and OCD.

CULTURAL CONSIDERATIONS

Cultural attitudes toward aggressive behaviors warrant consideration in IED, although little systematic research has been performed with respect to the influence of cultural factors. One form of aggression, amok episodes, is characterized by acute, unrestrained violence, typically associated with amnesia and traditionally seen only in southeastern Asian countries (American Psychiatric Association 2000). The extent to which IED resembles amok episodes or perceptions thereof warrants examination. Although OCD occurs across racial/ethnic groups and geographic locations (Karno et al. 1988; Mohammadi et al. 2004), cultural differences are important to consider because cultural norms relating to a range of ritualistic behaviors may differ (American Psychiatric Association 2000). Although cultural considerations exist for both IED and OCD, the nature of the associations between specific cultural factors and the two disorders appears to differ.

Pathological Gambling

PHENOMENOLOGY AND EPIDEMIOLOGY

Pathological gambling has been hypothesized to represent both an OCSD and an addiction without a drug, and data exist to support each categorization (Hollander and Wong 1995; Potenza et al. 2001a, 2001b). Although these categorizations are not mutually exclusive, they have important theoretical and clinical implications (Tamminga and Nestler 2006). Repetitive, intrusive thoughts about gambling in this disorder share features with obsessions in OCD. Like OCD, PG is characterized by repetitive behaviors; gambling and gambling-related behaviors (e.g., handicapping, getting money to gamble) are performed repeatedly (Potenza et al. 2001a, 2001b). As with OCD, the behaviors typically interfere significantly with major areas of functioning (American Psychiatric Association 2000). In contrast to the ego-dystonic behaviors related to OCD, gambling in PG is often initially ego-syntonic or hedonic in nature, although over time the pleasure derived from gambling may diminish. In this respect, the gambling in this disorder may be similar to drug use in drug dependence, and this and other phenomenological similarities have suggested that PG may represent a "behavioral addiction" (Holden 2001; Petry 2006; Potenza 2006). A telescoping phenomenon has been reported for this disorder and in drug and alcohol dependence in which women on average initially engage in disorder-related behavior at a later age but progress more quickly ("telescope") to problematic levels than do men (Potenza et al. 2001a, 2001b; Tavares et al. 2001). The ratio of men to women with PG (about 2:1) also resembles that for drug and alcohol dependence more than that for OCD (about 1:1) (Petry 2006; Potenza 2006; Potenza et al. 2001a, 2001b). The existing data on the clinical courses of PG and substance dependence also suggest similarities, with negligible rates in childhood, high rates in adolescence and young adulthood, and lower rates in older adults (Chambers and Potenza 2003; Potenza 2006). These patterns differ from those observed in OCD. For example, in OCD, onset during childhood is relatively common (American Psychiatric Association 2000). Many inclusionary diagnostic criteria for PG are more reflective of those for substance dependence, including aspects of tolerance, withdrawal, repeated unsuccessful attempts to cut back or quit, and interference in major areas of life functioning. Personality measures suggest that individuals with PG, like those with substance dependence, are impulsive and sensation seeking (Blaszczynski et al. 1997; Potenza et al. 2003b), whereas those with OCD are more harm avoidant (Hollander and Wong 1995; Anholt et al. 2004). Thus, although there are phenomenological similarities between PG and OCD, those between PG and substance dependence appear more robust.

CO-OCCURRING DISORDERS

Studies of clinical samples indicate high rates of co-occurrence between PG and a broad range of internalizing and externalizing disorders, including both Axis I and Axis II conditions (Crockford and el-Guebaly 1998; Potenza 2007a). Data from community samples also indicate high rates of co-occurring disorders. For example, data from the St. Louis Epidemiologic Catchment Area study found elevated odds ratios between problem/pathological gambling and major depression, anxiety disorders (phobias, somatization), drug use disorders (nicotine dependence and alcohol abuse/dependence), psychotic disorders, and antisocial personality disorder (Cunningham-Williams et al. 1998). A non-elevated odds ratio of 0.6 was observed between problem/pathological gambling and OCD (Cunningham-Williams et al. 1998). Other large community samples (e.g., the sample of male twins in the Vietnam Era Twin Registry) have also shown elevated associations between PG and mood, anxiety, substance use, and antisocial personality disorders (Potenza et al. 2005). More recently, data from the NESARC indicated elevated odds ratios for PG in association with numerous Axis I and Axis II disorders including alcohol, nicotine, and other drug dependence; mood disorders (including manic and depressive episodes); anxiety disorders (including panic, phobic, and generalized anxiety); and personality disorders (including avoidant, dependent, obsessive-compulsive, paranoid, schizoid, histrionic, and antisocial) (Petry et al. 2005). In neither the NESARC nor the Vietnam Era Twin Registry samples were diagnostic assessments of OCD obtained. Thus, existing community-based data suggest a stronger connection between PG and a broad range of other psychiatric disorders than is found between PG and OCD.

FAMILY HISTORY AND GENETICS

Twin studies indicate that PG has a high rate of heritability. A study of 3,359 male twin pairs concluded that heredity explained from 35% to 54% of the liability for PG (Eisen et al. 1998; Shah et al. 2005). These findings are consistent with a smaller family history study in which estimates of PG in relatives of probands with PG were 9%, substantially higher than the 1% rate typically observed in the general population (Black et al. 2003). Consistent with the existing data on co-occurring disorders, family history studies do not indicate high rates of PG among family members of probands with OCD (Bienvenu et al. 2000; Hollander et al. 1997). Also consistent with patterns of co-occurring disorders seen in population-based samples (Cunningham-Williams et al. 1998; Petry et al. 2005), data from the Vietnam Era Twin Registry indicate significant genetic and environmental contributions to PG and to its co-occurrence with alcohol dependence (Slutske et al. 2000) and antisocial behaviors (Slutske et al. 2001). In comparison, the overlap between PG and major depression is predominantly attributable to shared genetic factors (Potenza et al. 2005). Similar studies probing the relationship between PG and OCD have not been reported.

Candidate gene studies have suggested that multiple commonly occurring allelic variants contribute to PG (Ibanez et al. 2003; Shah et al. 2004). The Taq-A1 polymorphism of the gene encoding the D_2 dopamine receptor has been associated with PG, attention-deficit/hyperactivity disorder, Tourette's syndrome, alcohol and drug abuse/dependence, antisocial behaviors, and poor inhibitory control (Blum et al. 1996; Comings 1998; Ponce et al. 2003; Rodriguez-Jimenez et al. 2006). Other allelic variants including those in genes coding for the D_1 dopamine receptor, monoamine oxidase A enzyme, and the serotonin transporter, among others, have been implicated in PG (Comings 1998; Comings et al. 2001; Ibanez et al. 2003; Perez de Castro et al. 1997, 1999; Shah et al. 2004; Williams and Potenza 2008). Although some of the same allelic variants (e.g., variants of the serotonin transporter gene) have been implicated in OCD and PG, the nature of the association has differed, with the long allele found in association with OCD and the short allele found in association with PG (Hemmings and Stein 2006; Ibanez et al. 2003). Moreover, the findings in OCD have been inconsistent, with several studies implicating the allele and others not (Hemmings and Stein 2006). Numerous limitations exist in the candidate gene studies performed to date in PG. For example, some studies have not included diagnostic assessments or considered differences in racial/ethnic compositions between groups. As a result, these studies should be regarded as preliminary, with more work needed to identify the specific genetic contributions to PG and how they compare and contrast with those underlying OCD.

NEUROBIOLOGY: ANIMAL MODELS AND HUMAN STUDIES

Although animal models of PG per se have not been established, frontostriatal circuitry has been implicated across species in tasks involving impulsive choice (Everitt and Robbins 2005; Jentsch and Taylor 1999; Schultz et al. 2000). This circuitry has also been implicated in human studies of PG (Potenza 2001, 2006; Williams and Potenza 2008). Brain imaging studies of individuals with PG have implicated vmPFC during gambling urges (Potenza et al. 2003b), cognitive control (Potenza et al. 2003a), and simulated gambling (Reuter et al. 2005). In non-PG subjects, this brain region is involved in cognitive processes relevant to gambling, including reward processing (Knutson et al. 2001; McClure et al. 2004) and risk-reward decision making (Bechara 2003; Bechara et al. 1998, 1999). Studies of performance on neuro-cognitive tasks targeting these processes have revealed differences between PG and control comparison subjects (Cavedini et al. 2002a; Petry 2001; Petry and Casarella 1999). Differences between PG and control subjects in decision-making task performance have been found (Cavedini et al. 2002a), and these differences are similar to those between OCD and control subjects (Cavedini et al. 2002b) and those between drug-dependent and control subjects (Bechara 2003). However, the brain activations underlying these between-subject-group differences on decision-making tasks have not been directly examined. Given that increased activation of frontostriatal circuitry has been repeatedly observed in OCD (Mataix-Cols and van den Heuvel 2006) and diminished activation seen in PG (Potenza 2006; Reuter et al. 2005), concurrent investigation of PG, OCD, drug-dependent, and control subjects on the neural correlates of cognitive processes relevant to these subject groups is needed.

Pharmacological challenge studies have implicated multiple neurotransmitter systems in PG, including serotonin, dopamine, norepinephrine, opioid, and other systems (Chambers and Potenza 2003; Potenza 2001; Potenza and Hollander 2002). Many of these systems are implicated in other psychiatric disorders, including OCD, in which data indicating involvement of serotonin and dopamine systems are well substantiated (Pauls et al. 2002). However, data suggest differences in the nature of the involvement of these systems in PG and OCD. Studies in OCD subjects of pro-serotonergic agents such as *m*-CPP indicate that a substantial proportion (about 50%) report a transient worsening of symptoms following drug challenge (Pauls et al. 2002). In contrast, individuals with PG are more likely to report a euphoric or "high" response to pro-serotonergic agents (Potenza and Hollander 2002). These findings not only complement brain imaging findings in which similar paradigms suggest between-group differences of opposite valences in OCD and PG (Potenza et al. 2003b) but also suggest that specific components of impulsivity (e.g., those related to euphoria in relationship to disinhibition) may be linked to specific components of the serotonin system.

PHARMACOLOGICAL AND BEHAVIORAL TREATMENTS AND INTERVENTIONS

Over the past decade our understanding of safe and effective treatments for PG has advanced considerably (Brewer et al. 2008; Grant and Potenza 2004, 2007). Both similarities and differences are evident with respect to pharmacological treatments for PG and OCD. First-line pharmacotherapy for OCD involves the use of serotonin reuptake inhibitors, drugs that have been shown in multiple placebo-controlled, randomized clinical trials to be effective (Denys 2006). The role for serotonin reuptake inhibitors in the treatment of PG is less clear. Although several randomized, controlled trials have found serotonin reuptake inhibitors such as fluvoxamine and paroxetine to be superior to placebo in the treatment of PG (Hollander et al. 2000; Kim et al. 2002), others have not found a statistically significant effect (Blanco et al. 2002; Grant et al. 2003). These findings suggest that there exist significant individual factors related to treatment outcome in groups of individuals with PG. Considering co-occurring disorders might be one method for guiding pharmacotherapies (Hollander et al. 2004; Potenza 2007a). For example, a recent study of escitalopram in the treatment of PG and co-occurring anxiety found concurrent reduction in anxiety and gambling symptoms during open-label treatment (Grant and Potenza 2006a). In subjects receiving active drug during the double-blind discontinuation phase, clinical response was maintained; in contrast, placebo treatment was associated with symptom worsening (Grant and Potenza 2006a). Emerging data suggest roles for glutamatergic therapies in the treatment of both OCD and PG (Denys 2006; Grant 2006). However, the results from these and most other pharmacotherapy trials of PG should be considered cautiously given such limitations as small sample sizes and short-term treatment durations. Particular caution is warranted with respect to open-label findings, given high placebo response rates observed in PG studies (Grant and Potenza 2004).

Results of other pharmacotherapy trials suggest differences between PG and OCD. For example, opioid antagonists such as naltrexone and nalmefene have been found to be superior to placebo in the treatment of PG (Grant et al. 2006b; Kim et al. 2000). In contrast, the opioid antagonist naloxone has been associated with symptom exacerbation with OCD (Insel and Pickar 1983; Keuler et al. 1996). Whereas mood stabilizers such as lithium may be helpful in groups of subjects with PG (Hollander et al. 2005), their efficacy in OCD seems questionable (McDougle et al. 1991). Whereas antipsychotic drugs that antagonize D_2 dopamine receptors (e.g., haloperidol, risperidone and olanzapine) have shown efficacy as augmenting agents in OCD (Denys 2006), existing data do not support a role for these drugs in the treatment of PG (Grant and Potenza 2004).

Data suggest that behavioral therapies have important roles in the treatment of PG and OCD. However, the specific behavioral interventions differ. In PG, the 12-Step program Gamblers Anonymous is arguably the most widely used intervention, and existing data suggest that those who attend fare better than those who do not (Brewer et al. 2008; Petry 2005). The extent to which this represents a true treatment effect or reflects selection bias (i.e., those motivated to stay in Gamblers Anonymous are also motivated not to gamble) warrants more investigation. Gamblers Anonymous, an intervention with limited economic burden, is modeled after Alcoholics Anonymous. No similarly organized 12-Step program is established for or believed to be helpful for individuals with OCD. Behavioral therapies helpful for individuals with PG include motivational enhancement or interviewing and cognitive-behavioral therapy (Brewer et al. 2008; Grant and Potenza 2007; Hodgins et al. 2001; Petry et al. 2006; Sylvain et al. 1997). These approaches tend to be modeled after the ones with demonstrated efficacy in the treatment of drug addiction (Carroll et al. 1998; Miller 1995) rather than the exposure and response prevention strategies that are effective for treating OCD (Hohagen et al. 1998; Neziroglu et al. 2006).

CULTURAL CONSIDERATIONS

Both PG and OCD are present across cultures. Cultural differences relating to social acceptability and availability of legalized gambling might influence rates of PG (Shaffer et al. 1999). As with OCD, largely similar estimates of PG prevalence have been observed in studies around the world (Abbott et al. 2004; Cunningham-Williams and Cottler 2001). Nonetheless, certain populations (e.g., southeast Asian immigrants [Petry 2003]) have particularly high rates of gambling problems. The precise reasons for these findings require additional investigation. Environmental contributions that might differ across cultures and contribute to PG are likely to differ from those contributing to OCD, but more research is needed to investigate this notion directly.

Conclusions, Existing Limitations, and Future Directions

Although ICDs resemble OCD in some domains, existing data suggest substantial differences between ICDs and OCD. Although progress has been made over the past decade in understanding ICDs and OCD, existing data are often limited and include methodological concerns that are sometimes severe and complicate interpretation and comparisons across subject groups. Methodological limitations include ascertainment bias affecting the samples evaluated, small study samples, error-prone methods of data gathering (e.g., gathering family history from probands without confirmatory interviews of family members), differing methods of establishing diagnoses (e.g., structured versus unstructured interviews) and differing methods of examining biological characteristics (e.g., different methods of brain imaging). For many data domains (e.g., genetics, neurobiology, and immune function) there exist little or no data for many of the ICDs and only limited data for OCD. The group of ICDs as a whole remains understudied, and specific ICDs (e.g., pyromania and kleptomania) receive particularly little attention from the research and clinical communities. Other proposed ICDs (including compulsive buying or shopping, compulsive computer use or problematic Internet use, compulsive sexual behavior, compulsive skin-picking/nail-biting) need further examination. For these ICDs, it is recommended that diagnostic criteria be derived for DSM-V from examinations of large samples of clinical cases or of subjects ascertained through random-sample community surveys (Aboujaoude et al. 2006; Koran et al. 2006). ICDs, when present, often go unrecognized within clinical settings (Grant et al. 2005; Grant et al. 2007b), and this underrecognition is associated with suboptimal treatment outcomes in multiple domains (Potenza 2007a). Thus, increased efforts to identify ICDs are needed to enhance clinical care (Chamberlain et al. 2007).

Numerous gaps exist in our understanding of ICDs and their relationships with OCD and other psychiatric disorders. Additional research is needed to obtain evidence for clustering individual ICDs together or to support alternate categorizations (Lochner et al. 2005). From a broader perspective, it is important to examine the relationships between non-ICD psychiatric disorders and individual ICDs or empirically derived groups thereof. These investigations will have not only theoretical implications for grouping the disorders but also direct clinical relevance given the high rates of co-occurring disorders observed in individuals with ICDs (Potenza 2007a). Because ICDs often have elements consistent with relationships with several psychiatric disorders (e.g., addictions and OCD [Grant et al. 2007a]), investigations of dimensional as well as categorical measures of psychiatric symptomatology are needed (Muthen 2006; Saxena et al. 2005). Within each ICD, identification of individual characteristics that differentiate subgroups of individuals with unique treatment needs is important. Identification of relevant endophenotypes that can facilitate prevention and treatment advances is needed and should include an understanding of specific environmental, genetic, and interactive influences (Gottesman and Gould 2003; Kreek et al. 2005). The potential clinical utilities of these specific individual differences or endophenotypes in targeting behavioral and pharmacological interventions and for identifying high- versus low-risk individuals require direct examination. Among the most salient needs is an improved understanding of the pathophysiology of ICDs. Additional large-scale molecular genetic and brain imaging studies are needed to better understand the biological underpinnings of the disorders and to translate this information into clinical advances in prevention and treatment.

References

Abbott MW, Volberg RA, Ronnberg S: Comparing the New Zealand and Swedish national surveys of gambling and problem gambling. J Gambl Stud 20:237–258, 2004

Aboujaoude E, Koran LM, Gamel N, et al: Potential markers for problematic internet use: a telephone survey of 2513 adults. CNS Spectr 11:750–755, 2006

Alpert JE, Spilman MK: Psychotherapeutic approaches to aggressive and violent patients. Psychiatr Clin North Am 20:453–471, 1997

American Psychiatric Association: Diagnostic and Statistical Manual of Mental Disorders, 4th Edition, Text Revision. Washington, DC, American Psychiatric Association, 2000

Anderson S, Bechara A, Damasio H, et al: Impairment of social and moral behavior related to early damage in human prefrontal cortex. Nat Neurosci 2:1032–1037, 1999

Anholt GE, Emmelkamp PMG, Cath DC, et al: Do patients with OCD and pathological gambling have similar dysfunctional cognitions? Behav Res Ther 42:529–537, 2004

Bechara A: Risky business: emotion, decision-making, and addiction. J Gambl Stud 19:23–51, 2003

Bechara A, Damasio H, Tranel D, et al: Dissociation of working memory from decision making within the human prefrontal cortex. J Neurosci 18:428–437, 1998

Bechara A, Damasio H, Damasio AR, et al: Different contributions of the human amygdala and ventromedial prefrontal cortex to decision-making. J Neurosci 19:5473–5481, 1999

Bienvenu O, Samuels JF, Riddle MA, et al: The relationship of obsessive–compulsive disorder to possible spectrum disorders: results from a family study. Biol Psychiatry 48:287–293, 2000

Black DW, Moyer T, Schlosser S: Quality of life and family history in pathological gambling. J Nerv Ment Dis 191:124–126, 2003

Blanco C, Petkova E, Ibanez A, et al: A pilot placebo-controlled study of fluvoxamine for pathological gambling. Ann Clin Psychiatry 14:9–15, 2002

Blaszczynski A, Steel Z, McConaghy N: Impulsivity in pathological gambling: the antisocial impulsivist. Addiction 92:75–87, 1997

Blum K, Cull JG, Braverman ER, et al: Reward deficiency syndrome. Am Sci 84:132–145, 1996

Brewer JA, Potenza MN: The neurobiology and genetics of impulse control disorders: relationships to drug addictions. Biochem Pharmacol 75:63–75, 2008

Brewer JA, Grant JE, Potenza MN: The treatment of pathological gambling. Addict Disord Their Treat 7:1–13, 2008

Buitelaar JK, Van der Gaag RJ, Cohen-Kettenis P, et al: A randomized controlled trial of risperidone in the treatment of aggression in hospitalized adolescents with subaverage cognitive abilities. J Clin Psychiatry 62:239–248, 2001

Cadoret RJ, Yates WR, Troughton E, et al: Genetic-environmental interaction in the genesis of aggressivity and conduct disorders. Arch Gen Psychiatry 52:916–924, 1995

Carroll K, Connors GJ, Cooney NL, et al: A Cognitive Behavioral Approach: Treating Cocaine Addiction. Rockville, MD, National Institute on Drug Abuse, 1998

Cavedini P, Riboldi G, Keller R, et al: Frontal lobe dysfunction in pathological gambling. Biol Psychiatry 51:334–341, 2002a

Cavedini P, Riboldi G, D'Annucci A, et al: Decision making heterogeneity in obsessive-compulsive disorder: ventromedial prefrontal cortex function predicts different treatment outcomes. Neuropsychologia 40:205–211, 2002b

Chamberlain SR, Menzies L, Sahakian BJ, et al: Lifting the veil on trichotillomania. Am J Psychiatry 164:568–574, 2007

Chambers RA, Potenza MN: Neurodevelopment, impulsivity and adolescent gambling. J Gambl Stud 19:53–84, 2003

Chambers RA, Bickel WK, Potenza MN: A scale-free systems theory of motivation and addiction. Neurosci Biobehav Rev 31:1017–1045, 2007

Coccaro EF, Kavoussi RJ: Fluoxetine and impulsive aggressive behavior in personality-disordered subjects. Arch Gen Psychiatry 54:1081–1088, 1997

Coccaro EF, Siever LJ: Pathophysiology and treatment of aggression, in Neuropsychopharmacology: The 5th Generation of Progress. Edited by Charney D, Davis KL, Coyle JT, et al. Philadelphia, PA, Lippincott Williams and Wilkins, 2002, pp 1709–1723

Cocarro EF, Kavoussi RJ, Trestman RL, et al: Serotonin function in human subjects: intercorrelations among central 5-HT indices and aggressiveness. Psychiatry Res 73:1–14, 1997

Cocarro EF, Schmidt CA, Samuels JF, et al: Lifetime and 1-month prevalence of intermittent explosive disorder in a community sample. J Clin Psychiatry 65:820–824, 2004

Comings DE: The molecular genetics of pathological gambling. CNS Spectr 3:20–37, 1998

Comings DE, Gade-Andavolu R, Gonzalez N, et al: The additive effect of neurotransmitter genes in pathological gambling. Clin Genet 60:107–116, 2001

Crockford DN, el-Guebaly N: Psychiatric comorbidity in pathological gambling: a critical review. Can J Psychiatry 43:43–50, 1998

Cunningham-Williams RM, Cottler LB: The epidemiology of pathological gambling. Semin Clin Neuropsychiatry 6:155–166, 2001

Cunningham-Williams RM, Cottler LB, Compton WM 3rd, et al: Taking chances: problem gamblers and mental health disorders. Results from the St. Louis Epidemiologic Catchment Area Study. Am J Public Health 88:1093–1096, 1998

Curzon G, Gibson EL: The serotonergic appetite suppressant fenfluramine. Advances in Experimental Medical Biology 467:95–100, 1999

Damasio AR: Descartes' Error: Emotion, Reason and the Human Brain. New York, Crosset/Putnam, 1994

Davanzo P, Yue K, Thomas MA, et al: Proton magnetic resonance spectroscopy of bipolar disorder versus intermittent explosive disorder in children and adolescents. Am J Psychiatry 160:1442–1452, 2003

Dell'Osso B, Altamura AC, Allen A, et al: Epidemiologic and clinical updates on impulse control disorder: a critical review. Eur Arch Psychiatry Clin Neurosci 256:464–475, 2006

Denys D: Pharmacotherapy of obsessive-compulsive disorder and obsessive-compulsive spectrum disorders. Psychiatr Clin North Am 29:553–584, 2006

Denys D, Burger H, van Megen H, et al: A score for predicting response to pharmacotherapy in obsessive-compulsive disorder. Int Clin Psychopharmacol 18:315–322, 2003

Dougherty RS, Deckersbach T, Marci C, et al: Ventromedial prefrontal cortex and amygdala dysfunction during an anger induction positron emission tomography study in patients with major depressive disorder with anger attacks. Arch Gen Psychiatry 61:795–804, 2004

du Toit PL, van Kradenburg J, Niehaus D, et al: Comparison of obsessive-compulsive disorder in patients with and without putative obsessive compulsive disorder using a structured clinical interview. Compr Psychiatry 45:291–300, 2005

Eisen SA, Lin N, Lyons MJ, et al: Familial influences on gambling behavior: an analysis of 3359 twin pairs. Addiction 93:1375–1384, 1998

Ettelt S, Ruhrmann S, Barnow S, et al: Impulsiveness in obsessive-compulsive disorder: results from a family study. Acta Psychiatr Scand 115:41–47, 2007

Everitt B, Robbins TW: Neural systems of reinforcement for drug addiction: from actions to habits to compulsion. Nat Neurosci 8:1481–1489, 2005

Feder R: Treatment of intermittent explosive disorder with sertraline in 3 patients. J Clin Psychiatry 60:195–196, 1999

Felthous AR, Bryant G, Wingerter CB, et al: The diagnosis of intermittent explosive disorder in violent men. Bull Am Acad Psychiatry Law 19:71–79, 1991

Findling RL, McNamara NK, Branicky LA, et al: A double-blind pilot study of risperidone in the treatment of conduct disorder. J Am Acad Child Adolesc Psychiatry 39:509–516, 2001

Fontenelle LF, Mendlowicz MV, Versiani M: Impulse control disorders in patients with obsessive-compulsive disorder. Psychiatr Clin Neurosci 59:30–37, 2005

Frankle WG, Lombardo I, New AS, et al: Brain serotonin transporter distribution in subjects with impulsive aggressivity: a positron emission study with [11C]McN 5652. Am J Psychiatry 162:915–923, 2005

Frick PJ, Lahey BB, Loeber R, et al: Familial risk factors to oppositional defiant disorder and conduct disorder: parental psychopathology and maternal parenting. J Consult Clin Psychol 60:49–55, 1990

Gottesman I, Gould TD: The endophenotype concept in psychiatry: etymology and strategic intentions. Am J Psychiatry 160:636–645, 2003

Grabe HJ, Ruhrmann S, Ettelt S, et al: Familiality of obsessive–compulsive disorder in nonclinical and clinical subjects. Am J Psychiatry 163:1986–1992, 2006

Grant JE: N-acetyl cysteine treatment of pathological gambling. Presented at the International Society for Research on Impulsivity, Paris, France, September 2006

Grant JE, Potenza MN: Impulse control disorders: clinical characteristics and pharmacological management. Ann Clin Psychiatry 16:27–34, 2004

Grant JE, Potenza MN: Escitalopram treatment of pathological gambling with co-occurring anxiety: an open-label pilot study with double-blind discontinuation. Int Clin Psychopharmacol 21:203–209, 2006a

Grant JE, Potenza MN (eds): Impulse Control Disorders: A Clinical Text of Men's Mental Health. Washington, DC, American Psychiatric Publishing, 2006b

Grant JE, Potenza MN: Treatments for pathological gambling and other impulse control disorders, in A Guide to Treatments That Work. Edited by Gorman J, Nathan P. Oxford, United Kingdom, Oxford University Press, 2007, pp 561–577

Grant JE, Kim SW, Potenza MN, et al: Paroxetine treatment of pathological gambling: a multi-center randomized controlled trial. Int Clin Psychopharmacol 18:243–249, 2003

Grant JE, Levine L, Kim D, et al: Impulse control disorders in adult psychiatric inpatients. Am J Psychiatry 162:2184–2188, 2005

Grant JE, Mancebo M, Pinto A, et al: Impulse control disorders in adults with obsessive compulsive disorder. J Psychiatry Res 40:494–501, 2006a

Grant JE, Potenza MN, Hollander E, et al: Multicenter investigation of the opioid antagonist nalmefene in the treatment of pathological gambling. Am J Psychiatry 163:303–312, 2006b

Grant JE, Odlaug BL, Potenza MN: Addicted to hairpulling? How an alternate model of trichotillomania may improve treatment outcome. Harv Rev Psychiatry 15:80–85, 2007a

Grant JE, Williams KA, Potenza MN: Impulse control disorders in adolescent inpatients: co-occurring disorders and sex differences. J Clin Psychiatry 68:1584–1592, 2007b

Gross-Isseroff R, Cohen R, Sasson Y, et al: Serotonergic dissection of obsessive compulsive symptoms: a challenge study with m-chlorophenylpiperazine and sumatriptan. Neuropsychobiology 50:200–205, 2004

Halperin JM, Schulz KP, McKay KE, et al: Familial correlates of central serotonin function in children with disruptive behavior disorders. Psychiatry Res 119:205–216, 2003

Hemmings SMJ, Stein DJ: The current status of association studies in obsessive-compulsive disorder. Psychiatr Clin North Am 29:411–444, 2006

Hodgins DC, Currie SR, el-Guebaly N: Motivational enhancement and self-help treatments for problem gambling. J Clin Consult Psychol 69:50–57, 2001

Hohagen F, Winkelmann G, Rasche-Ruchle H, et al: Combination of behaviour therapy with fluvoxamine in comparison with behaviour therapy and placebo. results of a multi-centre study. Br J Psychiatry Suppl 35:71–78, 1998

Holden C: 'Behavioral' addictions: do they exist? Science 294:980–982, 2001

Hollander E, Wong CM: Obsessive-compulsive spectrum disorders. J Clin Psychiatry 56(suppl):3–6, 1995

Hollander E, DeCaria C, Gully R, et al: Effects of chronic fluoxetine treatment on behavioral and neuroendocrine responses to meta-chlorophenylpiperazine in obsessive-compulsive disorder. Psychiatry Res 36:1–17, 1991

Hollander E, Stein DJ, Kwon JH, et al: Psychosocial function and economic costs of obsessive-compulsive disorder. CNS Spectr 2:16–25, 1997

Hollander E, DeCaria CM, Finkell JN, et al: A randomized double-blind fluvoxamine/placebo crossover trial in pathological gambling. Biol Psychiatry 47:813–817, 2000

Hollander E, Kaplan A, Pallanti S: Pharmacological treatments, in Pathological Gambling: A Clinical Guide to Treatment. Edited by Grant JE, Potenza MN. Washington, DC, American Psychiatric Publishing, 2004, pp 189–206

Hollander E, Pallanti S, Allen A, et al: Does sustained release lithium reduce impulsive gambling and affective instability versus placebo in pathological gamblers with bipolar spectrum disorders? Am J Psychiatry 162:137–145, 2005

Ibanez A, Blanco C, de Castro IP, et al: Genetics of pathological gambling. J Gambl Stud 19:11–22, 2003

Insel TR, Pickar D: Naloxone administration in obsessive–compulsive disorder: report of two cases. Am J Psychiatry 140:1219–1220, 1983

Jentsch J, Taylor JR: Impulsivity resulting from frontostriatal dysfunction in drug abuse: implications for the control of behavior by reward-related stimuli. Psychopharmacology 146:373–390, 1999

Karno M, Golding JM, Sorenson SB, et al: The epidemiology of obsessive-compulsive disorder in five US communities. Arch Gen Psychiatry 45:1094–1099, 1988

Kendler KS, Prescott C, Myers J, et al: The structure of genetic and environmental risk factors for common psychiatric and substance use disorders in men and women. Arch Gen Psychiatry 60:929–937, 2003

Kessler RC, Coccaro EF, Fava M, et al: The prevalence and correlates of DSM-IV intermittent explosive disorder in the national comorbidity survey replication. Arch Gen Psychiatry 63:669–678, 2006

Keuler DJ, Altemus M, Michelson D, et al: Behavioral effects of naloxone infusion in obsessive-compulsive disorder. Biol Psychiatry 40:154–156, 1996

Kim SW, Grant JE, Adson DE, et al: Double-blind naltrexone and placebo comparison study in the treatment of pathological gambling. Biol Psychiatry 49:914–921, 2000

Kim SW, Grant JE, Adson DE, et al: A double-blind, placebo-controlled study of the efficacy and safety of paroxetine in the treatment of pathological gambling disorder. J Clin Psychiatry 63:501–507, 2002

Knutson B, Fong GW, Adams CM, et al: Dissociation of reward anticipation and outcome with event-related fMRI. NeuroReport 12:3683–3687, 2001

Koran LM, Faber RJ, Aboujaoude E, et al: Estimated prevalence of compulsive buying in the United States. Am J Psychiatry 163:1806–1812, 2006

Korff S, Harvey BH: Animal models of obsessive–compulsive disorder: rational to understanding psychobiology and pharmacology. Psychiatr Clin North Am 29:371–390, 2006

Kreek MJ, Nielsen DA, Butelman ER, et al: Genetic influences on impulsivity, risk-taking, stress responsivity and vulnerability to drug abuse and addiction. Nat Neurosci 8:1450–1457, 2005

Krueger RF: The structure of common mental disorders. Arch Gen Psychiatry 56:921–926, 1999

Lappalainen J, Long JC, Eggert M, et al: Linkage of antisocial alcoholism to the serotonin 5-HT1B receptor gene in 2 populations. Arch Gen Psychiatry 55:989–994, 1998

Leckman JF, Grice DE, Barr LC, et al: Tic-related versus non-tic-related obsessive compulsive disorder. Anxiety 1:208–215, 1994

Leckman JF, Zhang H, Alsobrook JP, et al: Symptom dimension in obsessive-compulsive disorder: toward quantitative phenotypes. Am J Med Genet 105:28–30, 2001

Leckman JF, Pauls DL, Zhang H, et al: Obsessive–compulsive symptom dimensions in affected sibling pairs with Gilles de Tourette syndrome. Am J Med Genet 116B:60–68, 2003

Ledgerwood DM, Steinberg MA, Wu R, et al: Self-reported gambling-related suicidality among gambling helpline callers. Psychol Addict Behav 19:175–183, 2005

Lejoyeaux M, Ades J, Tassain V, et al: Phenomenology and psychopathology of uncontrolled buying. Am J Psychiatry 153:1524–1529, 1996

Lenane MC, Swedo SE, Rapoport JL, et al: Rates of obsessive compulsive disorder in first degree relatives of patients with trichotillomania: a research note. J Child Psychol Psychiatry 33:925–933, 1992

Li C-SR, Chen S-H: Obsessive-compulsiveness and impulsivity in a non-clinical population of adolescent males and females. Psychiatry Res 149:129–138, 2007

Liu T, Potenza MN: Problematic internet use: clinical implications. CNS Spectr 12:453–466, 2007

Lochner C, Stein DJ: Does work on obsessive-compulsive spectrum disorders contribute to the understanding of the heterogeneity of obsessive-compulsive disorder? Prog Neuropsychopharmacol Biol Psychiatry 30:353–361, 2006

Lochner C, Hemmings SMJ, Kinnear CJ, et al: Cluster analysis of obsessive-compulsive spectrum disorder in patients with obsessive-compulsive disorder: clinical and genetic correlates. Compr Psychiatry 46:14–19, 2005

Mannelli P, Patkar AA, Peindl K, et al: Polymorphism in the serotonin transporter gene and moderators of prolactin response to meta-chlorophenylpiperazine in African-American cocaine abusers and controls. Psychiatry Res 144:99–108, 2006

Mataix-Cols D, van den Heuvel OA: Common and distinct neural correlates of obsessive-compulsive disorder and related disorders. Psychiatr Clin North Am 29:391–410, 2006

Mataix-Cols D, Wooderson S, Lawrence N, et al: Distinct neural correlates of washing, checking, and hoarding symptom dimensions in obsessive-compulsive disorder. Arch Gen Psychiatry 61:564–576, 2004

Matsunaga H, Kiriike N, Matsui T, et al: Impulsive disorders in Japanese adult patients with obsessive-compulsive disorder. Compr Psychiatry 46:105–110, 2005

McClure S, Laibson DI, Loewenstein G, et al: Separate neural systems value immediate and delayed monetary rewards. Science 306:503–507, 2004

McDougle CJ, Price LH, Goodman WK, et al: A controlled trial of lithium augmentation in fluvoxamine-refractory obsessive compulsive disorder: lack of efficacy. J Clin Psychopharmacol 11:175–184, 1991

McDougle CJ, Goodman WK, Leckman JF, et al: Haloperidol addition in fluvoxamine-refractory obsessive compulsive disorder: a double-blind, placebo-controlled study in patients with and without tics. Arch Gen Psychiatry 51:302–308, 1994

McElroy SL, Keck PE, Pope HG Jr, et al: Compulsive buying: a report of 20 cases. J Clin Psychiatry 55:242–248, 1994

McElroy SL, Soutullo CA, Beckman DA, et al: DSM-IV intermittent explosive disorder: a report of 27 cases. J Clin Psychiatry 69:203–210, 1998

Miller WR: Motivational enhancement therapy with drug abusers, 1995. Available at: http://motivationalinterview.org/clinical/METDrugAbuse.PDF. Accessed January 15, 2005

Mohammadi MR, Ghanizadeh A, Rahgozar M, et al: Prevalence of obsessive-compulsive disorder in Iran. BMC Psychiatry 4:2, 2004

Monopolis S, Lion JR: Problems in the diagnosis of intermittent explosive disorder. Am J Psychiatry 140:1200–1202, 1983

Montelcone P, Catapano F, Bortolotti F, et al: Plasma prolactin response to D-fenfluramine in obsessive-compulsive patients before and after fluvoxamine treatment. Biol Psychiatry 42:175–180, 1997

Muthen B: Should substance use disorders be considered as categorical or dimensional? Addiction 101:S6–S16, 2006

New AS, Hazlett EA, Buchsbaum MS, et al: Blunted prefrontal cortical 18-fluorodeoxyglucose positron emission tomography response to meta-chlorophenylpiperazine in impulsive aggression. Arch Gen Psychiatry 59:621–629, 2002

New AS, Buchsbaum M, Hazlett EA, et al: Fluoxetine increases relative metabolic rate in prefrontal cortex in impulsive aggression. Psychopharmacology 176:451–458, 2004a

New AS, Trestman RF, Mitropoulou V, et al: Low prolactin response to fenfluramine in impulsive aggression. J Psychiatr Res 38:223–230, 2004b

Neziroglu F, Henricksen J, Yaryura-Tobias JA: Psychotherapy of obsessive-compulsive disorder and spectrum: established facts and advances, 1995–2005. Psychiatr Clin North Am 29:585–604, 2006

Olivier B, Young LJ: Animal models of aggression, Neuropsychopharamcology: The 5th Generation of Progress. Edited by in Charney D, Davis KL, Coyle JT, et al. Philadelphia, PA, Lippincott Williams and Wilkins, 2002, pp 1699–1708

Olvera RL: Intermittent explosive disorder: epidemiology, diagnosis and management. CNS Drugs 16:517–526, 2002

Patkar AA, Mannelli P, Hill KP, et al: Relationship of prolactin response to meta-chlorophenylpiperazine with severity of drug use in cocaine dependence. Human Psychopharmacol 21:367–375, 2006

Pauls DL, Mundo E, Kennedy JL: The pathophysiology and genetics of obsessive-compulsive disorder, in Neuropsychopharmacology: the 5th Generation of Progress. Philadelphia, PA, Lippincott Williams and Wilkins, 2002, pp 1609–1619

Perez de Castro I, Ibanez A, Torres P, et al: Genetic association study between pathological gambling and a functional DNA polymorphism at the D4 receptor gene. Pharmacogenetics 7:345–348, 1997

Perez de Castro I, Ibanez A, Saiz-Ruiz J, et al: Genetic contribution to pathological gambling: possible association between a DNA polymorphism at the serotonin transporter gene (5HTT) and affected men. Pharmacogenetics 9:397–400, 1999

Petry NM: Pathological gamblers, with and without substance use disorders, discount delayed rewards at high rates. J Abnorm Psychol 110:482–487, 2001

Petry NM: Gambling participation and problems among Southeast Asian refugees. Psychiatr Serv 54:1142–1148, 2003

Petry NM: Gamblers anonymous and cognitive–behavioral therapies for pathological gamblers. J Gambl Stud 21:27–33, 2005

Petry NM: Should the scope of addictive behaviors be broadened to include pathological gambling? Addiction 101:152–160, 2006

Petry NM, Casarella T: Excessive discounting of delayed rewards in substance abusers with gambling problems. Drug Alcohol Depend 56:25–32, 1999

Petry NM, Stinson FS, Grant BF: Co-morbidity of DSM-IV pathological gambling and other psychiatric disorders: results from the National Epidemiologic Survey on Alcohol and Related Conditions. J Clin Psychiatry 66:564–574, 2005

Petry NM, Alessi SM, Carroll KM, et al: Cognitive-behavioral therapy for pathological gamblers. J Consult Clin Psychol 74:555–567, 2006

Ponce G, Jiminez-Ariero MA, Rubio G, et al: The A1 allele of the DRD 2 gene (Taq1 A polymorphism) is associated with antisocial personality in a sample of alcohol-dependent patients. Eur Psychiatry 18:356–360, 2003

Potenza MN: The neurobiology of pathological gambling. Semin Clin Neuropsychiatry 6:217–226, 2001

Potenza MN: Should addictive disorders include non-substance-related conditions? Addiction 101:142–151, 2006

Potenza MN: Impulse control disorders and co-occurring disorders: dual diagnosis considerations. J Dual Diagn 3:47–57, 2007a

Potenza MN: Impulsivity and compulsivity in pathological gambling and obsessive-compulsive disorder. Revista Brasileira de Psiquiatria 29:105–106, 2007b

Potenza MN, Hollander E: Pathological gambling and impulse control disorders, in Neuropsychopharmacology: the 5th Generation of Progress. Edited by Charney D, Davis KL, Coyle JT, et al. Philadelphia, PA, Lippincott Williams and Wilkins, 2002

Potenza MN, Kosten TR, Rounsaville BJ: Pathological gambling. JAMA 286:141–144, 2001a

Potenza MN, Steinberg MA, McLaughlin SD, et al: Gender-related differences in the characteristics of problem gamblers using a gambling helpline. Am J Psychiatry 158:1500–1505, 2001b

Potenza MN, Leung H-C, Blumberg HP, et al: An fMRI Stroop study of ventromedial prefrontal cortical function in pathological gamblers. Am J Psychiatry 160:1990–1994, 2003a

Potenza MN, Steinberg MA, Skudlarski P, et al: Gambling urges in pathological gamblers: an fMRI study. Arch Gen Psychiatry 60:828–836, 2003b

Potenza MN, Xian H, Shah K, et al: Shared genetic contributions to pathological gambling and major depression in men. Arch Gen Psychiatry 62:1015–1021, 2005

Rasmussen SA, Eisen JL: The epidemiology and clinical features of obsessive compulsive disorder. Psychiatr Clin North Am 15:743–758, 1992

Rauch SL, Dougherty DD, Shin LM, et al: Neural correlates of factor-analyzed OCD symptom dimensions: a PET Study. CNS Spectr 3:37–43, 1998

Reist C, Nakamura K, Sagart E, et al: Impulsive aggressive behavior: open-label treatment with escitalopram. J Clin Psychiatry 64:81–85, 2003

Reuter J, Raedler T, Rose M, et al: Pathological gambling is linked to reduced activation of the mesolimbic reward system. Nat Neurosci 8:147–148, 2005

Robins L, Regier DA: Psychiatric Disorders in America. New York, Free Press, 1991

Rodriguez-Jimenez R, Avila C, Ponce G, et al: The Taq1A polymorphism linked to the DRD2 gene is related to lower attention and less inhibitory control in alcoholic patients. Eur Psychiatry 21:66–69, 2006

Rosario-Campos MC, Leckman JF, Curi M, et al: A family study of early onset obsessive-compulsive disorder. Am J Med Genet 136B:92–97, 2005

Saudou F, Amara DA, Dierich A, et al: Enhanced aggressive behavior in mice lacking 5-HT$_{1B}$ receptor. Science 265:1875–1878, 1994

Saxena S, Brody AL, Maidment KM, et al: Cerebral glucose metabolism in obsessive-compulsive hoarding. Am J Psychiatry 162:1038–1048, 2005

Schultz W, Tremblay L, Hollerman JR: Reward processing in primate orbitofrontal cortex and basal ganglia. Cereb Cortex 10:272–284, 2000

Shaffer HJ, Hall MN, Vander Bilt J: Estimating the prevalence of disordered gambling in the United States and Canada: a research synthesis. Am J Public Health 89:1369–1376, 1999

Shah KR, Potenza MN, Eisen SA: Biological basis for pathological gambling, in Pathological Gambling: A Clinical Guide to Treatment. Edited by Grant JE, Potenza MN. Washington, DC, American Psychiatric Publishing, 2004, pp 127–144

Shah KR, Eisen SA, Xian H, et al: Genetic studies of pathological gambling: a review of methodology and analyses of data from the Vietnam Era Twin (VET) Registry. J Gambl Stud 21:177–201, 2005

Siever LJ, Buchsbaum MS, New AS, et al: D,L-fenfluramine response in impulsive personality disorder assessed with [18F]-fluorodeoxyglucose positron emission tomography. Neuropsychopharmacology 20:413–423, 1999

Slutske WS, Eisen S, True WR, et al: Common genetic vulnerability for pathological gambling and alcohol dependence in men. Arch Gen Psychiatry 57:666–674, 2000

Slutske WS, Eisen S, Xian H, et al: A twin study of the association between pathological gambling and antisocial personality disorder. J Abnorm Psychol 110:297–308, 2001

Slutske WS, Caspi A, Moffitt TE, et al: Personality and problem gambling: a prospective study of a birth cohort of young adults. Arch Gen Psychiatry 62:769–775, 2005

Snider LA, Swedo SE: PANDAS: current status and directions for research. Mol Psychiatry 9:900–907, 2004

Stein DJ, Lochner C: Obsessive-compulsive spectrum disorders: a multidimensional approach. Psychiatr Clin North Am 29:343–351, 2006

Sylvain C, Ladouceur R, Boisvert JM: Cognitive and behavioral treatment of pathological gambling: a controlled study. J Consult Clin Psychol 65:727–732, 1997

Tamminga CA, Nestler EJ: Pathological gambling: focusing on the addiction, not the activity. Am J Psychiatry 163:180–181, 2006

Tavares H, Zilberman ML, Beites FJ, et al: Gender differences in gambling progression. J Gambl Stud 17:151–160, 2001

Tiefenbacher S, Davenport MD, Novak MA, et al: Fenfluramine challenge, self-injurious behavior, and aggression in rhesus monkeys. Physiol Behav 80:327–331, 2003

Torres AR, Prince MJ, Bebbington PE, et al: Obsessive-compulsive disorder: prevalence, comorbidity, impact, and help-seeking in the British National Psychiatric Morbidity Survey of 2000. Am J Psychiatry 163:1978–1985, 2006

Williams WA, Potenza MN: The neurobiology of impulse control disorders. Revista Brasiliera Psiquiatria 30(suppl):S24–S30, 2008

World Health Organization: International Statistical Classification of Diseases and Related Health Problems, 10th Revision. Geneva, Switzerland, World Health Organization, 2003

5

SYMPTOM DIMENSIONS IN OBSESSIVE-COMPULSIVE DISORDER

Implications for DSM-V

James F. Leckman, M.D.
Scott L. Rauch, M.D.
David Mataix-Cols, Ph.D.

Obsessive-compulsive disorder (OCD) is a chronic and potentially disabling condition affecting from 1% to 3% of the general population. Patients with OCD describe the sudden intrusion into consciousness of unwanted thoughts or unpleasant images. Frequently, these obsessions are accompanied by a profound sense of dread and the urge to complete specific compulsions. Compulsions are repetitive acts, typically performed a certain number of times or according to certain private rules, that the individual is driven to complete, even though these acts are perceived as excessive.

DSM-IV-TR (American Psychiatric Association 2000) and other standard diagnostic classifications, such as ICD-10 (World Health Organization 1992) catego-

This chapter was first published as "Symptom Dimensions in Obsessive-Compulsive Disorder: Implications for the DSM-V." *CNS Spectrums* 12:376–387, 2007. Copyright 2009. Used with permission.

rize OCD as a unitary nosological entity. Although this parsimony has a certain formal appeal, it is misleading. The symptoms used to define OCD are heterogeneous and include various intrusive thoughts and preoccupations, rituals, and compulsions. Two individuals with OCD may have totally different and non-overlapping symptom patterns.

From as far back as the earliest descriptions of OCD, investigators have attempted to dissect the phenotype into homogeneous subtypes. For example, Falret made the distinction between *folie du doute* (madness of doubt) and *délire du toucher* (delusion of touch) in 1869 (Hantouche and Lancrenon 1996). Most commonly investigators have distinguished "washers" from "checkers" (Horesh et al. 1997; Khanna and Mukherjee 1992; Matsunaga et al. 2001; Rachman and Hodgson 1980). With a few notable exceptions, these attempts had limited success in relating the identified subtypes to biological markers, genetic factors, or treatment response, in part because pure subtypes of patients are rare, and the recruitment of sufficient sample sizes of each subtype is difficult and highly impractical.

The following review considers an alternative approach to obsessive-compulsive symptoms that aims to identify valid quantitative dimensions for use in genetic, neurobiological, and treatment-outcome studies. The review proceeds to examine the potential value of a dimensional approach from a developmental perspective.

Quantitative Obsessive-Compulsive Disorder Phenotypes: Initial Studies Using Factor Analysis

The first study to factor-analyze the Yale-Brown Obsessive Compulsive Scale Symptom Checklist (Y-BOCS-SC; Goodman et al. 1989) was that of Baer (1994). He factor-analyzed the 13 major categories of the Y-BOCS-SC in a sample of 107 patients and identified three factors, accounting for 48% of the variance; these were named "symmetry/hoarding," "contamination/cleaning," and "pure obsessions." Following Baer's seminal work, Leckman et al. (1997) evaluated the 13 *a priori* categories used to group types of obsessions and compulsions in the Y-BOCS-SC in two large groups of OCD patients totaling more than 300 cases (Leckman et al. 1994; Pauls et al. 1995). A principal components factor analysis was performed with a Varimax rotation separately using the symptom information from each group of OCD patients. In an effort to identify valid "traits," they included any OCD symptoms that patients "ever" experienced over the course of their lifetimes, as opposed to limiting these analyses to current symptoms. Remarkably, both data sets yielded nearly identical results. Four factors were identified that in total accounted for more than 60% of the variance in each data set (Leckman et al. 1997). The first factor included obsessions about aggressive behavior toward self or others, sexual obsessions, obsessions related to moral rightness or religion, and related check-ing compulsions (Factor I). This factor accounted for 30.1% of the variance. A sec-ond factor accounted for 13.8% of the variance and included obsessions con-cerning a need for symmetry or exactness, repeating rituals, counting compulsions, and ordering/arranging compulsions (Factor II). A third factor that accounted for 10.2% of the variance was composed of contamination obsessions and cleaning and washing compulsions (Factor III). The fourth factor included hoarding and collecting obsessions and compulsions, accounting for 8.5% of the variance (Fac-tor IV).

Summerfeldt et al. (1999) evaluated existing models of OCD symptom struc-ture in 203 individuals. Using confirmatory factor analyses, they examined four mod-els: a single-factor (i.e., OCD as a single dimension), a two-factor (i.e., obsessions and compulsions), the three-factor model of Baer (1994), and Leckman et al.'s (1997) four-factor model. Adequate fit was found solely for our four-factor model speci-fying aggressive, sexual, and religious obsessions and checking compulsions; sym-metry/ordering; contamination/cleaning; and hoarding. However, parameter esti-mates showed within-factor heterogeneity as well as overlap between factors, most notably between Factors I and III.

One review published in 2005 identified 12 factor-analytic studies involving more than 2,000 patients (Mataix-Cols et al. 2005). Since then, at least five more large studies have been conducted in adults (Denys et al. 2004a, 2004b; Hasler et al. 2005, 2006; Kim et al. 2005; Summerfeldt et al. 2004) and two in children (Delorme et al. 2006; McKay et al. 2006). Although the factorial studies available to date have been fairly consistent, the number of factors has ranged from three to six. Some of the symptom dimensions have been consistently replicated across studies (e.g., contamination/washing, symmetry/ordering, hoarding), but the ag-gressive/checking and sexual/religious dimensions need further study, because it is unclear whether they form a unique factor (Cavallini et al. 2002; Leckman et al. 1997, 2003; McKay et al. 2004; Summerfeldt et al. 1999, 2004) or can be broken down into multiple separate dimensions (Baer 1994; Foa et al. 2002; Hantouche and Lancrenon 1996; Mataix-Cols et al. 1999, 2002a; Tek and Ulug 2001). Sim-ilarly, it is unclear how to regard somatic obsessions and miscellaneous obsessions, because they loaded on the contamination/washing factor in two studies (Baer 1994; Hantouche and Lancrenon 1996), on the obsessions/checking factor in three other studies (Leckman et al. 1997, 2003), and just with sexual obsessions in two other studies (Feinstein et al. 2003; Mataix-Cols et al. 2002a).

There is some controversy as to whether the same dimensional structure is pres-ent in children as is found in adults. One study (McKay et al. 2006) using data from a group of 137 5- to 17-year-olds found four factors that were different in content from those commonly observed in a large number of adult studies. In contrast, two other studies (Delorme et al. 2006) using data from a total of 327 children and ad-olescents found evidence of a four-factor solution: 1) symmetry, ordering, repeating, and checking; 2) contamination and cleaning as well as aggressive and somatic symptoms; 3) hoarding; and 4) sexual and religious obsessions. These data are largely congruent with the factor structure that has been consistently observed in adult studies of OCD. With the newly developed Dimensional Y-BOCS (DY-BOCS; Rosario-Campos et al. 2006), children and adolescents were found to have slightly lower scores for severity of their sexual and religious obsessions and related compulsions than did adults; otherwise the data comparing adults and children were remarkably similar.

Temporal Stability of Obsessive-Compulsive Disorder Symptom Dimensions

Preliminary data are available that support the temporal stability of the obsessive-compulsive symptom dimensions in adult patients. Rettew et al. (1992) assessed the longitudinal course of obsessive-compulsive symptoms in 76 children and adolescents with OCD followed over a period of 2–7 years, using the categories of the Y-BOCS-SC. They found that none of the patients maintained the same constellation of symptoms from baseline to follow-up. Nevertheless, the authors acknowledged that these changes could have occurred within rather than between symptom dimensions, although they did not test this hypothesis.

Two other studies with larger samples have found that patients maintain their symptoms across time intervals as long as 6 years and that the most robust predictor of having a particular symptom was having had that symptom in the past (Mataix-Cols et al. 2002b; Rufer et al. 2005). For those symptoms that changed across time, changes typically occurred within rather than between previously identified symptom dimensions, suggesting that the symptoms of adult OCD patients are more stable than is often assumed. Longitudinal studies following patients from childhood to adulthood are needed to gain a more complete understanding of the natural history of obsessive-compulsive symptoms.

Obsessive-Compulsive Symptom Dimensions and the Vulnerability to Develop Specific Comorbid Disorders?

OCD shares a relatively high comorbidity with a number of other psychiatric conditions, including other anxiety disorders, panic disorder, specific phobias, affective disorders, body dysmorphic disorder, eating disorders, and tic disorders. How useful are obsessive-compulsive symptom dimensions in sorting out comorbid disorders and obsessive-compulsive spectrum disorders? Baer (1994) reported that patients with high scores on his symmetry/hoarding factor were more likely to have a comorbid diagnosis of chronic tics and obsessive-compulsive personality disorder. Similarly, Leckman et al. (1997) found that patients with high scores on the obsessions/checking and symmetry/ordering factors were more likely to present with tics. Mataix-Cols et al. (1999) found that male but not female OCD patients with chronic tics scored higher than patients without tics on the symmetry/ordering dimension. More recently, Hasler et al. (2005) found that aggressive, sexual, religious, and somatic obsessions and checking compulsions were broadly associated with comorbid anxiety disorders and depression, whereas symmetry and repeating obsessions and counting and ordering/arranging compulsions were associated with bipolar disorders and panic disorder/agoraphobia. In the initial characterization of the DY-BOCS, depression and anxiety symptoms were also found to correlate with the severity of the aggressive obsessions and related compulsions (Rosario-Campos et al. 2006).

There also seems to be a clear overlap with eating disorders. For example, Halmi et al. (2003) reported that ~70% of patients with anorexia nervosa had lifetime obsessive-compulsive symptoms, especially symmetry and somatic obsessions and ordering and hoarding compulsions. In a more recent study, Halmi et al. (2005) emphasized the importance of "perfectionism" as well as OCD and obsessive-compulsive personality disorder. In contrast, Hasler et al. (2005) reported an association between eating disorders and contamination obsessions and cleaning compulsions.

Mataix-Cols et al. (2000) examined the presence of all DSM-III-R (American Psychiatric Association 1987) Axis II diagnoses and their relation to obsessive-compulsive symptom dimensions in a sample of 75 OCD patients. They found that hoarding symptoms were strongly related to the presence and number of all personality disorders, especially from the anxious-fearful cluster. Similarly, Frost et al. (2000) found that hoarding was associated with higher levels of comorbidity (i.e., anxiety, depression, personality disorders) as well as work and social disability compared with non-hoarding OCD and other anxiety disorders. In another study (Samuels et al. 2002), the presence of hoarding was associated with male gender, earlier age of onset, comorbid social phobia, personality disorders, and pathological grooming conditions (skin-picking, nail-biting, and trichotillomania). Although Samuels et al. (2002) found that hoarding was associated with greater overall illness severity, another study did not replicate this finding (Saxena et al. 2002).

Taken together, these studies suggest that a symptom-based dimensional approach may be useful in efforts to integrate previous attempts at classification based on age of onset, gender, or presence of comorbid and obsessive-compulsive spectrum conditions. A dimensional approach has the advantage of allowing each patient to have scores in one or more symptom dimension. It also permits studies that cut across traditional diagnostic boundaries. This approach may be particularly valuable for genetic studies where it increasingly seems that some vulnerability genes may be shared by more than a single disorder and subthreshold cases are likely to be found in family members. An initial confirmation of this approach comes from the recent study of Hasler et al. (2007), which collected data from 418 sibling pairs with OCD. Among potentially relevant comorbid conditions for genetic studies, they found that bipolar I/II and major depressive disorder were strongly associated with Factor I ($P<0.001$), whereas attention-deficit/hyperactivity disorder, alcohol dependence, and bulimia were associated with Factor II ($P<0.01$).

Initial Validation From Family Genetic Studies

Like many other psychiatric disorders, twin and family studies suggest that genetic factors play a role in the expression of OCD (Alsobrook and Pauls 1998). Recent advances in molecular genetics have greatly increased the capacity to localize disease genes on the human genome. These methods are now being applied to complex disorders, including OCD. Although earlier studies have indicated that the vertical transmission of OCD in families is consistent with the effects of a single major autosomal gene (Cavallini et al. 1999; Nicolini et al. 1991), it is likely that there are a number of vulnerability genes involved. One of the major difficulties in the application of these approaches is the likely etiological heterogeneity of OCD and related phenotypes. Heterogeneity reduces the power of gene-localization methods, such as linkage analysis (Alcais and Abel 1999; Gu et al. 1998; Zhang and Risch 1996). Etiological heterogeneity may be reflected in phenotypic variability, making it highly desirable to dissect the syndrome, at the level of the phenotype, into valid quantitative heritable components.

Alsobrook et al. (1999) were the first to use obsessive-compulsive symptom dimensions in a genetic study. They found that the relatives of OCD probands who had high scores on the obsessions/checking and symmetry/ordering factors were at greater risk for OCD than were relatives of probands who had low scores on those factors. This finding has been replicated in a second independent family study (Hanna et al. 2005).

Using data collected by the Tourette Syndrome Association International Consortium for Genetics Affected Sibling Pair Study, Leckman et al. (2003) selected all available affected Tourette's syndrome pairs and their parents for which these obsessive-compulsive symptom dimensions (factor scores) could be generated using the four factor algorithm first presented by Leckman et al. (1997). Remarkably, 50% of the siblings with Tourette's syndrome were found to have comorbid OCD and more than 30% of mothers and 10% of fathers also had a diagnosis of OCD. The scores for both Factor I (aggressive, sexual, and religious obsessions and checking compulsions) and Factor II (symmetry and ordering) were significantly correlated in sibling pairs concordant for Tourette's syndrome. In addition, the mother–child correlations, but not father–child correlations, were significant for these two factors. Based on the results of the complex segregation analyses, significant evidence for genetic transmission was obtained for all factors.

A genome scan of the hoarding dimension was completed using the same data set (Zhang et al. 2002). The analyses were conducted for hoarding as both a dichotomous trait and a quantitative trait. Not all sibling pairs in the sample were concordant for hoarding. Standard linkage analyses were performed using GENE-HUNTER and Haseman-Elston methods. In addition, novel analyses with a recursive-partitioning technique were employed. Significant allele sharing was observed for both the dichotomous and the quantitative hoarding phenotypes for markers at 4q34, 5q35.2 and 17q25. The 4q site is in proximity to D4S1625, which was identified as a region linked to the Tourette's syndrome phenotype. A recursive-partitioning analytic technique also examined multiple markers simultaneously. Results suggest joint effects of specific loci on 5q and 4q.

A recent study of 418 sibling pairs with OCD (Hasler et al. 2007) found robust sibling-sibling intraclass correlations (after controlling for sex, age, and age of onset) for Factor IV (hoarding obsessions and compulsions; $P=0.001$) and Factor I (aggressive, sexual, and religious obsessions and checking compulsions; $P=0.002$). A smaller, but still significant, sib-sib intraclass correlation was found for Factor III (contamination/cleaning; $P=0.02$) and Factor II (symmetry/ordering/arranging; $P=0.04$). Limiting the sample to female subjects more than doubled the sib-sib intraclass correlations for Factor II ($P=0.003$).

Two studies (Cavallini et al. 2002; Hasler et al. 2006) have genotyped OCD patients for the functional polymorphism in the promoter region of the serotonin transporter gene *(5-HTTLPR)* and both found that the frequencies of the S allele and the SS genotype were associated with obsessions regarding symmetry and compulsions involving repeating, counting, and ordering/arranging (Factor II). This is promising given that Hu et al. (2006) suggested that *5-HTTLPR* remains a major candidate gene for OCD. This observation may also be consistent with the findings of Sutcliffe et al. (2005). They reported that males with autism who had prominent compulsive disorders, including ordering, symmetry, and arranging, were also more likely to have coding substitutions at highly conserved positions and 15 other variants in 5′ noncoding and other intronic regions within the *5-HTTLPR* locus.

In summary, the use of quantitative traits that are familial may provide a powerful approach to detect the genetic susceptibility loci that contribute to OCD presentations. Thus far, this approach has provided promising leads with regard to the hoarding obsessive-compulsive phenotype. Next steps include, first, the use of these symptom dimensions in large multigenerational families in order to refine the initial genetic linkage results for the hoarding phenotype. Obviously, if specific loci are identified this will provide compelling evidence for the validity of this multidimensional approach to OCD. Second, genome scans must be conducted using the remaining obsessive-compulsive symptom dimensions. Families segregating for Tourette's syndrome or early onset OCD may be especially valuable in this enterprise. Given the high mother–child correlations in the study by Leckman et al. (2003), it may also be valuable to examine the linkage results for alleles that are identical by descent from the mother. Third, twin and cross-fostering studies are needed to further evaluate the heritability of these symptom dimensions within the general population. Finally, future genetic studies will also need to examine the relationship between these dimensions and other closely related phenotypes, including various eating disorders (Halmi et al. 2003) and body dysmorphic disorder.

Despite our enthusiasm for the identification of dimension specific OCD vulnerability genes, it should also be noted that environmental factors doubtless play an important role in the transmission of these traits across generations. Indeed, the bulk of the evidence concerning familial risk has come from affected sibling-pair studies and genetic family studies. In contrast to twin and adoption studies, the design of these studies simply tests for familial transmission; they do not exclude the likely role of nongenetic familial transmission, in which family members can serve as models for dysfunctional behaviors. More work is needed to identify the environmental factors that foster the onset and course of these symptoms.

Neuropsychological Findings

Relatively few studies have examined the utility of the obsessive-compulsive symptom dimensions as they relate to neuropsychological functions. Recently, Lawrence et al. (2006) studied 39 OCD patients and 40 control subjects using tests of decision making and set shifting. OCD patients and control subjects showed comparable decision making, but patients with prominent hoarding symptoms (Factor IV) showed impaired decision making. OCD patients as a group had poorer set shifting abilities than control subjects, and symmetry/ordering symptoms (Factor II) were negatively associated with set shifting. These results support recent neuroimaging data that suggest dissociable neural mechanisms involved in mediating the different OCD symptom dimensions.

Hints at Validation From In Vivo Neuroimaging Studies

Functional neuroimaging studies have the potential to increase our understanding of the neural mechanisms underlying OCD. Taken as a whole, these studies strongly link obsessive-compulsive symptoms with activation of the orbitofrontal cortex, with less consistent involvement of anterior cingulate gyrus, lateral frontal and temporal cortices, caudate nucleus, thalamus, amygdala, and insula (Saxena and Rauch 2000). We would predict that if a dimensional approach is useful, then a significant portion of the individual variation seen in these studies may be accounted for by the unique mix of symptom dimensions seen in any given patient. Initial studies generally support this conclusion.

In the first such study, using positron emission tomography, Rauch et al. (1998) found that checking symptoms correlated with increased, and symmetry/ordering with reduced, regional cerebral blood flow in the striatum, whereas washing symptoms correlated with increased regional cerebral blood flow in the bilateral anterior cingulate and left orbitofrontal cortex. Phillips et al. (2000) compared OCD patients with mainly washing ($n=7$) or checking ($n=7$) symptoms while viewing pictures of either normally disgusting scenes or washer-relevant pictures using functional magnetic resonance imaging. When viewing washing-related pictures, only washers demonstrated activations in regions implicated in emotion and disgust perception (i.e., visual regions and insular cortex), whereas checkers demonstrated activations in frontostriatal regions and the thalamus. In a similar study (Shapira et al. 2003), eight OCD patients with predominantly washing symptoms demonstrated greater activation than control subjects in the right insula, ventrolateral prefrontal cortex, and parahippocampal gyrus when viewing disgust-inducing pictures. Another study (Van den Heuvel et al. 2004) found increased amygdala activation in a group of 11 washers during the presentation of contamination-related pictures.

Saxena et al. (2004) found that 12 patients with predominantly hoarding symptoms showed reduced glucose metabolism in the posterior cingulate gyrus (vs. control subjects) and the dorsal anterior cingulate cortex (vs. non-hoarding OCD) and that severity of hoarding in the whole patient group ($n=45$) correlated negatively with metabolism in the latter region. One recent functional magnetic resonance imaging study (Mataix-Cols et al. 2004b) used a symptom provocation paradigm to examine, within the same patients, the neural correlates of washing, checking, and hoarding symptom dimensions of OCD. Each of these dimensions was mediated by distinct but partially overlapping neural systems. Although patients and control subjects activated similar brain regions in response to symptom provocation, patients showed greater activations in the bilateral ventromedial prefrontal regions (washing experiment); putamen/globus pallidus, thalamus, and dorsal cortical areas (checking experiment); and left precentral gyrus, and right orbitofrontal cortex (hoarding experiment). These results were further supported by correlation analyses within the patient group, which revealed highly specific positive associations between subjective anxiety, questionnaire scores, and neural response in each experiment.

Another recent study (Lawrence et al. 2007) demonstrated that eight patients with predominant washing symptoms showed increased neural responses to disgusting (but not fearful) faces, compared with non-washing OCD patients ($n=8$) and healthy control subjects ($n=19$). Specifically, washers showed greater activation in the left ventrolateral prefrontal cortex (Brodmann area 47) compared with the other two groups. Finally, a study by Rauch et al. (2007) tested for associations between OCD symptom factors and regional brain activation during an implicit learning task. They found that activation within right caudate was inversely correlated with symmetry/arranging and contamination/washing factors; left orbitofrontal activation was directly correlated with the sexual/religious/aggressive/counting factor symptom severity.

Structural neuroimaging OCD studies have been remarkably inconsistent. Only one recent study examined the correlations between symptom scores and gray matter volumes. Pujol et al. (2004) found that patients with high scores on the aggressive/checking dimension had reduced gray matter volume in the right amygdala. The significance of this finding is unclear, especially because the convergent validity of the aggressive/checking factor of the Y-BOCS-SC is poor (Mataix-Cols et al. 2004a).

Taken together, these studies raise the question of whether the inconsistencies in previous imaging studies of OCD could be accounted for by phenotypic variations among their subjects. If these preliminary findings are confirmed, and a consistent pattern of results can be documented by symptom factor, this would suggest that discrete neural systems are activated in association with the evocation of specific obsessive-compulsive symptoms.

Prediction of Treatment Response: Pharmacotherapy

Although controlled trials with selective serotonin reuptake inhibitors (SSRIs) have demonstrated a selective efficacy in OCD, 40%–60% of patients do not have a satisfactory outcome (Hollander et al. 2002). Nonresponse to treatment in OCD is associated with serious social disability. These differences in treatment outcome emphasize the heterogeneity of OCD and the need for identifying predictors of treatment response. Although definitive studies have not been undertaken, recent studies have suggested that a symptom-based dimensional approach may prove to be valuable for identifying significant predictors of treatment outcome. For example, at least five studies (Black et al. 1998; Erzegovesi et al. 2001; Mataix-Cols et al. 1999; Saxena et al. 2002; Winsberg et al. 1999) have shown that patients with high scores on the hoarding dimension respond more poorly to SSRIs. In contrast, Saxena et al. (2007) recently reported that compulsive hoarders and non-hoarding OCD patients improved significantly with paroxetine treatment.

In another study, high scores on the sexual/religious obsessions factor identified by Mataix-Cols et al. (1999) were associated with poorer long-term outcome with SSRIs and behavior therapy in 66 adult outpatients who were followed for 1–5 years (Alonso et al. 2001). Two other groups have recently reported that the presence of sexual obsessions ($P=0.002$) was a predictor of nonresponse to SSRIs (Ferrão et al.

2006; Shetti et al. 2005). Shetti et al. (2005) also found washing and contamination obsessions were associated with nonresponse to SSRIs. Another study (Erzegovesi et al. 2001) reported that patients with somatic obsessions had poorer insight and responded less well to SSRIs.

Other somatic treatments may also help patients with specific symptoms. For example, one study (Jenike et al. 1997) found that patients with symmetry and unusual somatic obsessions may respond well to monoamine oxidase inhibitors. In another study (Baer et al. 1995), the presence of symmetry obsessions, ordering compulsions, and hoarding rituals predicted better response in refractory cases treated with cingulotomy.

Compliance and Response to Behavioral Interventions

In many respects cognitive-behavioral therapy (CBT) for OCD is based on a dimensional perspective (McKay et al. 2004). The efficacy of CBT for OCD has been demonstrated in numerous controlled and meta-analytic studies. However, a significant number of patients still remain unimproved or simply refuse or drop out from this treatment. Some studies have suggested that checking rituals may respond less well to CBT (Basoglu et al. 1988; Rachman and Hodgson 1980), but others found no differences in outcome between washers and checkers (Basoglu et al. 1988). Foa and Goldstein (1978), however, reported that washers and checkers responded at different rates to behavioral treatments, with checkers being slower to respond. It is often assumed that patients with "pure" obsessions and mental rituals respond less well to classic behavioral interventions, although data supporting these assumptions are sparse. In a meta-analysis, patients with primary obsessive thoughts without rituals tended to improve less with CBT than those who had overt motor rituals (Christensen et al. 1987). In a study by Alonso et al. (2001), the presence of sexual and/or religious obsessions predicted poorer long-term outcome, but because most patients had received both SSRIs and CBT, it was not clear from this study whether these symptoms predicted poorer outcome with SSRIs, CBT, or both.

Patients with hoarding symptoms have been described as having poor compliance with and response to CBT (Abramowitz et al. 2003; Ball et al. 1996; Mataix-Cols et al. 2002a; Rufer et al. 2006). For example, using a dimensional approach, Mataix-Cols et al. (2002a) examined 153 OCD outpatients who participated in a randomized, controlled trial of CBT. Results showed that high scorers on the hoarding dimension were more likely to drop out prematurely from the trial and also tended to improve less than non-hoarding OCD patients. In addition, high scorers on the sexual/religious dimension responded less well to CBT. Interestingly, patients with mental rituals did as well as other OCD patients in this study. Therefore, it seems that CBT is mostly indicated for patients with contamination/washing, aggressive/checking, and symmetry/ordering symptoms. Besides, previous anecdotal accounts of unsuccessful CBT in patients with hoarding symptoms may be due in part to their propensity to drop out earlier from treatment.

A Developmental Perspective

Children engage in a significant amount of ritualistic, repetitive, and compulsive-like activity that is part of their normal behavioral repertoire. Clinically, this phenomenon reaches a peak at about 24 months of age (Gesell and Ilg 1943). Using a parent-report questionnaire, the Childhood Routines Inventory, to assess compulsive-like behavior in young children, we collected data from 1,492 parents with children between 8 and 72 months of age (Evans et al. 1997). The Childhood Routines Inventory was found to have a strong internal consistency and a two-factor structure. The first factor accounted for 33% of the variance and included items such as "lines up objects in straight lines or symmetrical patterns," "arranges objects or performs certain behaviors until they seem 'just right,'" and "prefers to have things done in a particular order."

Evans et al. (1997) found an early emergence of specific behaviors that resemble the symptom dimensions observed in OCD patients. For example, parents reported that their children arranged objects or performed certain behaviors until they seemed "just right," on average, beginning at 22–25 months of age (Factor II). Similarly, behaviors resembling those associated with the contamination/washing dimension identified with such questions as "Seemed very concerned with dirt or cleanliness" were found to have their mean age of onset from 22 to 24 months of age (Factor III). Finally, parents reported that their children on average began to "collect or store objects" (resembling the hoarding dimension) from 25 to 27 months of age (Factor IV). Although direct evidence linking the emergence of these behaviors to the later development of OCD is lacking, investigators have found that aspects of these ritualistic and compulsive-like behaviors are correlated with children's fears and phobias (Evans et al. 1999; Zohar and Felz 2001). Further exploration of the factors that underlie the emergence and resolution of these behaviors in normally developing children may provide valuable insights into their neurobiological substrates and evolutionary origins.

Evolutionary Perspectives

The ultimate causes of many neuropsychiatric disorders, including OCD, are likely built into the genetic and neurobiological mechanisms that underlie highly conserved behavioral and cognitive repertoires (Bracha 2006; Feygin et al. 2006;

Leckman and Mayes 1998; Leckman et al. 1999). In the case of OCD and its composite dimensions, such an evolutionary perspective seems particularly apt. Indeed, we hypothesize that each of these obsessive-compulsive dimensions corresponds to unconscious neural evaluation of specific threats (Table 5–1). During the evolution of our species, it is likely that, had our forbearers not been acutely attuned to potential external threats posed by other humans, by predators, by the external manifestations of microbial disease, or by periods of privation due to drought, natural disasters, or internecine conflict, our species would not have survived.

Specifically, it is probable that during our evolutionary history there were times of great privation such that hoarding was adaptive and likely increased the chances of survival and reproductive success. A similar argument can be made for each of the other dimensions (e.g., that compulsive checking to see that items in the home environment were "just right" and not out of place, or ensuring that food and key aspects of the home environment were free of contamination) would have served families well at some points in what Darwin called "the struggle for life" (Darwin 1859).

The possible evolutionary origins of obsessions and compulsions related to fears about harm befalling a close family member are of particular interest, because they may reveal something of the normal states of heightened preoccupation that are associated with formation of intimate interpersonal relationships. For example, for expectant parents, the immediate perinatal period involves an altered mental state characterized by excitement and heightened sensitivity to environmental and emotive cues. The infant becomes an increasingly exclusive focus of thought and action toward the end of pregnancy and the early postpartum period. Cues from the infant before and after birth as well as the infant's proximity, physical appearance, and temperament provide a major stimulus for these preoccupations and associated behaviors. Guided by this perspective, Leckman et al. (1999) recently completed a prospective longitudinal study of 80 expectant parents. Consistent with their *a priori* hypothesis, the content of the parents' preoccupations involved anxious-intrusive thoughts and harm-avoidant behaviors that closely resemble some obsessions seen in OCD patients with aggressive symptoms; namely, worries about aggressive behavior, unintentional or intentional, that would lead to the baby being harmed were commonplace. Consistently, such intrusive thoughts were relieved by the performance of compulsive-checking behaviors that the parents may regard as excessive or unnecessary.

Viewed from an evolutionary perspective, it seems self-evident that the behavioral repertoires associated with early parenting skills would be subject to intense selective pressure. For one's genes to self-replicate, sexual intimacy must occur and the progeny of such unions must survive. Pregnancy and the early years of an infant's life are fraught with mortal dangers. Indeed, it has only been during the past century that infant mortality rates have fallen from more than 100 per 1,000 live

TABLE 5–1. Threat domains, conserved behaviors, and developmental epochs associated with heightened sensitivity and obsessive-compulsive—like behaviors

Threat domain	Focus of concern	Mental state	Behavioral response	Developmental epochs
Harm from aggressive behavior from conspecifics	Well-being of self and close family members	Intrusive images or thoughts that contain feared outcomes of separation or loss; among older children and adults, a heightened sense of responsibility	Physical proximity; checking to ensure the safety of close family members; avoidance of danger	Early childhood—formation of attachment to caregivers; Early family life—pregnancy, delivery, and care of young children; Threats to family members due to injury or other external threats
Physical security	Immediate home environment	Heightened attention to the placement of specific objects in the environment	Checking to ensure that things look "just right" and are in their expected places; arranging/ordering objects	Early childhood—initial period of exploration of the home environment by infants and toddlers; Early family life—pregnancy, delivery, and early childhood; Threats to family members due to injury or other external threats

TABLE 5–1. Threat domains, conserved behaviors, and developmental epochs associated with heightened sensitivity and obsessive-compulsive–like behaviors *(continued)*

Threat domain	Focus of concern	Mental state	Behavioral response	Developmental epochs
Environmental cleanliness	Personal hygiene Hygiene of family members Cleanliness of the home	Preoccupation with intrusive images or thoughts that contain feared outcomes of being dirty or causing others to be ill; among older children and adults, a heightened sense of responsibility	Washing; checking to ensure cleanliness; avoidance of shared or disgusting items	Early childhood—initial period of selection of items of food and drink by toddlers Early family life—pregnancy, delivery and care of young children Threats to family members due to injury or other external threats
Privation	Essential resources	Preoccupation with intrusive images or thoughts that contain feared outcomes of privation; a heightened sense of responsibility	Collecting items; checking to ensure the sufficient supplies are available	Latency—initial period of collecting Early family life—pregnancy, delivery and care of young children

births in 1900 to about 10 per 1,000 at present. Little wonder, then, that a specific state of heightened sensitivity on the part of new parents would be evolutionarily conserved.

Consistent with the emerging data from brain imaging studies, this evolutionary perspective suggests that each of the obsessive-compulsive symptom dimensions is based on overlapping brain-based alarm systems that have the potential to become dysregulated due to genetic vulnerability, adverse environmental change during the course of development (maladaptive learning leading to brain changes), or brain injury. Viewed in this light, the diverse behaviors and mental states encountered in OCD are not in themselves pathological. It is only in the distress they cause, their persistence, and their tendency to occupy time to the exclusion of more normal activities that they become pathological.

Although some may view this evolutionary perspective as reductionistic and naïve, in our view, invoking the Darwinian principle of natural selection and discussing the role of neural systems is in no way inconsistent with an awareness that environmental factors are doubtless important in the development of OCD in all of its variety. Nor is it inconsistent with prevailing cognitive-behavioral models of OCD that emphasize the role of the internal subjective experience of patients, the power of will, and the crucial role of learning and memory both in the generation and the treatment of these symptoms (McKay et al. 2004).

Limitations

Although much of the available data concerning a dimensional approach to OCD symptoms are promising, many questions remain unresolved. Principal among these is how best to measure these putative dimensional traits in patients and populations. The patient-based methods have relied on *a priori* symptom categories derived from the Y-BOCS-SC, whereas the population-based studies have been based on parent report. Furthermore, is it best to conceptualize these dimensions as measuring individual differences in the degree of obsessive worry and alarm (and related compulsive behaviors), or is there some converse set of "anti-obsessional" or "carelessness" traits that belong on these dimensions as well?

Other issues include the accuracy of the four-factor solution, in which some investigators suggest that the factor that includes aggressive, sexual, and religious obsessions and related checking compulsions is divisible within two separate domains: aggressive obsessions and related checking compulsions versus obsessions with either sexual or religious content. Other problems relate to the method of analysis itself. Principal components analysis is limited in that there is no probability model, it is sensitive to variable scaling, and it depends on the decision rules to retain the factors. As Summerfeldt et al. (1999) noted, most factorial studies of the Y-BOCS-SC used *a priori*-defined symptom groupings rather than its individual symptoms. Indeed, when individual items have been examined, the results have not always been consistent with the prevailing factor structures. For example, Feinstein et al. (2003) reported that some of the symptoms typically found in the contamination and washing dimension loaded on the aggressive/checking dimension, whereas others formed their own unique category. Another challenge concerns miscellaneous obsessions and compulsions. In many instances, these symptoms were not included in the analyses.

A further limitation relates to the convergent and divergent validity of the Y-BOCS-SC. In one study (Mataix-Cols et al. 2004a), the Y-BOCS-SC factor scores correlated poorly with scores on the Padua Inventory, a self-administered measure of obsessive-compulsive symptoms.

Conclusion

Despite these limitations, a strong case can be made to support the continued use of a dimensional approach to obsessive-compulsive symptoms. It is consistent with an emerging theory of OCD, which posits that obsessive-compulsive symptoms arise when evolutionarily conserved neural threat-detection systems are damaged or become dysregulated. The conceptual framework of this evolutionarily based model provides a powerful foundation for understanding disease pathogenesis and should permit the integration of new knowledge from a broad range of scientific disciplines, from genetics and neurobiology to the development of safe and effective treatments, perhaps ones specifically tailored to specific dimensions. The quantitative nature of these dimensions should also prove to be another important asset because it will add statistical power and readily allow the inclusion of subthreshold cases across a broad range of studies, including population-based studies (Maser and Patterson 2002).

Aspects of this approach may permit a deeper empathic understanding of our patients. For example, if some forms of OCD bear some relationship to the conserved mental states with highly conserved behavioral repertoires typically encountered in expectant parents, it should be easier for clinicians to have a deeper emotional empathy for the anguish the patient is experiencing as they relate the patient's symptoms to emotional experiences in their own lives.

Future Directions

In addition to continuing to explore the heuristic value and utility of a dimensional approach, there are at least two other directions for future research efforts. First, we need to acknowledge that a dimensional approach is not mutually exclusive of other methods to parse the larger spectrum of obsessive-compulsive-like disorders.

The most promising subtypes have been identified based on clinical characteristics, such as age of onset or comorbid diagnoses, particularly tic disorders and obsessive-compulsive personality disorder (Coles et al. 2008; de Mathis et al. 2006; Grados et al. 2001; Leckman et al. 1994–1995; Mataix-Cols et al. 1999; McDougle et al. 1993, 1994; Pauls et al. 1995; Rosario-Campos et al. 2001; Wewetzer et al. 2001). Future studies will need to explore the value of combining these methods. Second, it is clear that new clinical rating instruments such as the DY-BOCS (Rosario-Campos et al. 2006) must be used to further explore the dimensional structure of obsessive-compulsive symptoms and measure the severity of symptoms within each dimension. Practically, by dividing symptoms by their respective dimensions, it is possible to inquire about symptom types that at present are inherently ambiguous. For example, checking compulsions can be inquired about in several domains: checking related to sexual and religious obsessions versus checking to confirm that surfaces or objects are not contaminated. The same is true of the understudied area of mental rituals in OCD and how they relate to specific dimension dimensions (McKay et al. 2004). Indeed, in the DY-BOCS inquiries about checking symptoms, mental rituals, and avoidance are included within each symptom domain. The DY-BOCS and other new instruments should permit the development of better quantitative traits for genetic analyses (based on lifetime symptoms) as well as more discriminating data for use in clinical trials. For example, a patient with contamination worries and hoarding compulsions might show a consistent and marked benefit for the treatment of his or her contamination symptoms but little or no benefit in the treatment of his or her hoarding.

Provisional Recommendations for DSM-V

- DSM-V will be enriched by adding a dimensional perspective.
- A categorical approach should be maintained in DSM-V and ICD-11, giving full weight to the potential value of a dimensional approach.
- Although a multidimensional "map" of vulnerability may be too complex for a useable nosology, it will be important to document their presence through the use of specifiers (e.g., "OCD with prominent contamination obsessions and cleaning compulsions").
- If specifiers are to be used in DSM-V, limit the number to those for which this information has important clinical relevance: hoarding (Factor IV); symmetry, ordering, doing, and redoing (Factor II); obsessions concerning harm and related compulsions (Factor IA); and contamination and washing (Factor III).
- There are suggestive data that specifying other dimensions (religious, sexual, and somatic) may be clinically valuable, but additional research is needed.

References

Abramowitz JS, Franklin ME, Schwartz SA, et al: Symptom presentation and outcome of cognitive-behavioral therapy for obsessive-compulsive disorder. J Consult Clin Psychol 71:1049–1057, 2003

Alcais A, Abel L: Maximum-Likelihood-Binomial method for genetic model-free link-age analysis of quantitative traits in sibships. Genet Epidemiol 17:102–117, 1999

Alonso MP, Menchón JM, Pifarré J, et al: Long-term follow-up and predictors of clinical outcome in obsessive-compulsive patients treated with serotonin reuptake inhibitors and behavioral therapy. J Clin Psychiatry 62:535–540, 2001

Alsobrook II JP, Pauls DL: Molecular approaches to child psychopathology. Hum Biol 70:413–432, 1998

Alsobrook II JP, Leckman JF, Goodman WK, et al: Segregation analysis of obsessive-compulsive disorder using symptom-based factor scores. Am J Med Genet 88:669–675, 1999

American Psychiatric Association: Diagnostic and Statistical Manual of Mental Disorders, 3rd Edition Revised. Washington, DC, American Psychiatric Association, 1987

American Psychiatric Association: Diagnostic and Statistical Manual of Mental Disorders, 4th Edition, Text Revision. Washington, DC, American Psychiatric Association, 2000

Baer L: Factor analysis of symptom subtypes of obsessive-compulsive disorder and their relation to personality and tic disorders. J Clin Psychiatry 55(suppl):18–23, 1994

Baer L, Rauch SL, Ballantine HT, et al: Cingulotomy for intractable obsessive compulsive disorder: prospective long-term follow-up of 18 patients. Arch Gen Psychiatry 52:384–392, 1995

Ball SG, Baer L, Otto MW: Symptom subtypes of obsessive-compulsive disorder in behavioral treatment studies: a quantitative review. Behav Res Ther 34:47–51, 1996

Basoglu M, Lax T, Kasvikis Y, et al: Predictors of improvement in obsessive-compulsive disorder. J Anxiety Disord 2:299–317, 1988

Black DW, Monahan P, Gable J, et al: Hoarding and treatment response in 38 nondepressed subjects with obsessive-compulsive disorder. J Clin Psychiatry 59:420–425, 1998

Bracha HS: Human brain evolution and the "Neuroevolutionary Time-depth Principle": implications for the reclassification of fear-circuitry-related traits in DSM-V and for studying resilience to war zone-related posttraumatic stress disorder. Prog Neuropsychopharmacol Biol Psychiatry 30:827–853, 2006

Cavallini MC, Pasquale L, Bellodi L, et al: Complex segregation analysis for obsessive-compulsive disorder and related disorders. Am J Med Genet 88:38–43, 1999

Cavallini MC, Di Bella D, Siliprandi F, et al: Exploratory factor analysis of obsessive-compulsive patients and association with 5-HTTLPR polymorphism. Am J Med Genet 114:347–353, 2002

Christensen H, Hadzai-Pavlovic D, Andrews G, et al: Behavior therapy and tricyclic medication in the treatment of obsessive-compulsive disorder: a quantitative review. J Consult Clin Psychol 55:701–711, 1987

Coles ME, Pinto A, Mancebo MC, et al: OCD with comorbid OCPD: a subtype of OCD? J Psychiatr Res 42:289–296, 2008

Darwin CR: On the Origin of the Species By Means of Natural Selection, or the Preservation of Favored Races in the Struggle for Life. London, England, John Murray, 1859 de Mathis MA, Diniz JB, do Rosario MC, et al: What is the optimal way to subdivide obsessive-compulsive disorder? CNS Spectr 11:762–779, 2006

Delorme R, Bille A, Betancur C, et al: Exploratory analysis of obsessive compulsive symptom dimensions in children and adolescents: a prospective follow-up study. BMC Psychiatry 6:1, 2006

Denys D, de Geus F, van Megen HJ, et al: Symptom dimensions in obsessive-compulsive disorder: factor analysis on a clinician-rated scale and a self-report measure. Psychopathology 37:181–189, 2004a

Denys D, de Geus F, van Megen HJ, et al: Use of factor analysis to detect potential phenotypes in obsessive-compulsive disorder. Psychiatry Res 128:273–280, 2004b

Erzegovesi S, Cavallini MC, Cavedini P, et al: Clinical predictors of drug response in obsessive-compulsive disorder. J Clin Psychopharmacol 21:488–492, 2001

Evans DW, Leckman JF, Carter A, et al: Ritual, habit, and perfectionism: the prevalence and development of compulsive like behavior in normal young children. Child Dev 68:58–68, 1997

Evans DW, Gray FL, Leckman JF: The rituals, fears and phobias of young children: insights from development, psychopathology and neurobiology. Child Psychiatry Hum Dev 29:261–276, 1999

Feinstein SB, Fallon BA, Petkova E, et al: Item-by-item factor analysis of the Yale-Brown Obsessive Compulsive Scale Symptom Checklist. J Neuropsychiatry Clin Neurosci 15:187–193, 2003

Ferrão YA, Shavitt RG, Bedin NR, et al: Clinical features associated to treatment response in obsessive-compulsive disorder. J Affect Disord 94:199–209, 2006

Feygin DL, Swain JE, Leckman JF: The normalcy of neurosis: evolutionary origins of obsessive-compulsive disorder and related behaviors. Prog Neuropsychopharmacol Biol Psychiatry 30:854–864, 2006

Foa EB, Goldstein A: continuous exposure and complete response prevention in the treatment of obsessive-compulsive neurosis. Behav Ther 9:821–829, 1978

Foa EB, Huppert JD, Leiberg S, et al: The Obsessive-Compulsive Inventory: development and validation of a short version. Psychol Assess 14:485–496, 2002

Frost RO, Steketee G, Williams LF, et al: Mood, personality disorder symptoms and disability in obsessive-compulsive hoarders: a comparison with clinical and nonclinical controls. Behav Res Ther 38:1071–1081, 2000

Gesell A, Ilg F: Infant and Child in the Culture of Today: The Guidance of Development in Home and Nursery School. New York, Harper and Brothers Publishers, 1943

Goodman WK, Price LH, Rasmussen SA, et al: The Yale-Brown Obsessive Compulsive Scale, I: development, use, and reliability. Arch Gen Psychiatry 46:1006–1011, 1989

Grados MA, Riddle MA, Samuels JF, et al: The familial phenotype of obsessive-compulsive disorder in relation to tic disorders: the Hopkins OCD family study. Biol Psychiatry 50:559–565, 2001

Gu C, Province M, Todorov A, et al: Meta-analysis methodology for combining non-parametric sibpair linkage results: genetic homogeneity and identical markers. Genet Epidemiol 15:609–626, 1998

Halmi KA, Sunday SR, Klump K, et al: Obsessions and compulsions in anorexia nervosa subtypes. Int J Eat Disord 33:308–319, 2003

Halmi KA, Tozzi F, Thornton LM, et al: The relation among perfectionism, obsessive-compulsive personality disorder and obsessive-compulsive disorder in individuals with eating disorders. Int J Eat Disord 38:371–374, 2005

Hanna GL, Fischer DJ, Chadha KR, et al: Familial and sporadic sub-types of early onset obsessive-compulsive disorder. Biol Psychiatry 57:895–900, 2005

Hantouche EG, Lancrenon S: Modern typology of symptoms and obsessive-compulsive syndromes: results of a large French study of 615 patients [French]. Encephale 22:9–21, 1996

Hasler G, LaSalle-Ricci VH, Ronquillo JG, et al: Obsessive-compulsive disorder symptom dimensions show specific relationships to psychiatric comorbidity. Psychiatry Res 135:121–132, 2005

Hasler G, Kazuba D, Murphy DL: Factor analysis of obsessive-compulsive disorder Y-BOCS-SC symptoms and association with 5-HTTLPR SERT polymorphism. Am J Med Genet B Neuropsychiatr Genet 141:403–408, 2006

Hasler G, Pinto A, Greenberg BD, et al: Familiality of factor analysis-derived Y-BOCS dimensions in OCD-affected sibling pairs from the OCD Collaborative Genetics Study. Biol Psychiatry 61:617–625, 2007

Hollander E, Bienstock CA, Koran LM, et al: Refractory obsessive-compulsive disorder: state-of-the-art treatment. J Clin Psychiatry 63:20–29, 2002

Horesh N, Dolberg OT, Kirschenbaum-Aviner N, et al: Personality differences between obsessive-compulsive disorder subtypes: washers versus checkers. Psychiatry Res 71:197–200, 1997

Hu XZ, Lipsky RH, Zhu G, et al: Serotonin transporter promoter gain-of-function genotypes are linked to obsessive-compulsive disorder. Am J Hum Genet 78:815–826, 2006

Jenike MA, Baer L, Minichiello WE, et al: Placebo-controlled trial of fluoxetine and phenelzine for obsessive-compulsive disorder. Am J Psychiatry 154:1261–1264, 1997

Khanna S, Mukherjee D: Checkers and washers: valid subtypes of obsessive compulsive disorder. Psychopathology 25:283–288, 1992

Kim BN, Lee CB, Hwang JW, et al: Effectiveness and safety of risperidone for children and adolescents with chronic tic or Tourette disorders in Korea. J Child Adolesc Psychopharmacol 15:318–324, 2005

Lawrence NS, Wooderson S, Mataix-Cols D, et al: Decision making and set shifting impairments are associated with distinct symptom dimensions in obsessive-compulsive disorder. Neuropsychology 20:409–419, 2006

Lawrence NS, An SK, Mataix-Cols D, et al: Neural responses to facial expressions of disgust but not fear are modulated by washing symptoms in OCD. Biol Psychiatry 61:1072–1080, 2007

Leckman JF, Mayes LC: Understanding developmental psychopathology: how useful are evolutionary perspectives? J Am Acad Child Adolesc Psychiatry 37:1011–1021, 1998

Leckman JF, Walker WK, Goodman WK, et al: "Just right" perceptions associated with compulsive behaviors in Tourette's syndrome. Am J Psychiatry 151:675–680, 1994

Leckman JF, Grice DE, Barr LC, et al: Tic-related vs. non-tic-related obsessive compulsive disorder. Anxiety 1:208–215, 1994–1995

Leckman JF, Grice DE, Boardman J, et al: Symptoms of obsessive-compulsive disorder. Am J Psychiatry 154:911–917, 1997

Leckman JF, Mayes LC, Feldman R, et al: Early parental preoccupations and behaviors and their possible relationship to the symptoms of obsessive-compulsive disorder. Acta Psychiatr Scand Suppl 396:1–26, 1999

Leckman JF, Pauls DL, Zhang H, et al: Obsessive-compulsive symptom dimensions in affected sibling pairs diagnosed with Gilles de la Tourette syndrome. Am J Med Genet B Neuropsychiatr Genet 116:60–68, 2003

Maser JD, Patterson T: Spectrum and nosology: implications for DSM-V. Psychiatr Clin North Am 25:855–885, 2002

Mataix-Cols D, Rauch SL, Manzo PA, et al: Use of factor-analyzed symptom dimensions to predict outcome with serotonin reuptake inhibitors and placebo in the treatment of obsessive-compulsive disorder. Am J Psychiatry 156:1409–1416, 1999

Mataix-Cols D, Baer L, Rauch SL, et al: Relation of factor-analyzed symptom dimensions of obsessive-compulsive disorder to personality disorders. Acta Psychiatr Scand 102:199–202, 2000

Mataix-Cols D, Marks IM, Greist JH, et al: Obsessive-compulsive symptom dimensions as predictors of compliance with and response to behaviour therapy: results from a controlled trial. Psychother Psychosom 71:255–262, 2002a

Mataix-Cols D, Rauch SL, Baer L, et al: Symptom stability in adult obsessive compulsive disorder: data from a naturalistic two-year follow-up study. Am J Psychiatry 159:263–268, 2002b

Mataix-Cols D, Fullana MA, Alonso P, et al: Convergent and discriminant validity of the Yale-Brown Obsessive-Compulsive Scale Symptom Checklist. Psychother Psychosom 73:190–196, 2004a

Mataix-Cols D, Wooderson S, Lawrence N, et al: Distinct neural correlates of washing, checking, and hoarding symptom dimensions in obsessive-compulsive disorder. Arch Gen Psychiatry 61:564–576, 2004b

Mataix-Cols D, Rosario-Campos MC, Leckman JF: A multidimensional model of obsessive-compulsive disorder. Am J Psychiatry 162:228–238, 2005

Matsunaga H, Kiriike N, Matsui T, et al: A comparative study of clinical features between pure checkers and pure washers categorized using a lifetime symptom rating method. Psychiatry Res 105:221–229, 2001

McDougle CJ, Goodman WK, Leckman JF, et al: The efficacy of fluvoxamine in obsessive-compulsive disorder: effects of comorbid chronic tic disorder. J Clin Psychopharmacol 13:354–358, 1993

McDougle CJ, Goodman WK, Leckman JF, et al: Haloperidol addition in fluvoxamine-refractory obsessive-compulsive disorder: a double-blind, placebo-controlled study in patients with and without tics. Arch Gen Psychiatry 51:302–308, 1994

McKay D, Abramowitz JS, Calamari JE, et al: A critical evaluation of obsessive-compulsive disorder subtypes: symptoms versus mechanisms. Clin Psychol Rev 24:283–313, 2004

McKay D, Piacentini J, Greisberg S, et al: The structure of childhood obsessions and compulsions: dimensions in an outpatient sample. Behav Res Ther 44:137–146, 2006

Nicolini H, Kuthy I, Hernandez E, et al: A family study of obsessive-compulsive disorder in Mexican population. Am J Hum Genet Suppl 49:477–447, 1991

Pauls DL, Alsobrook J, Goodman W, et al: A family study of obsessive compulsive disorder. Am J Psychiatry 152:76–84, 1995

Phillips ML, Marks IM, Senior C, et al: A differential neural response in obsessive-compulsive patients with washing compared with checking symptoms to disgust. Psychiatr Med 30:1037–1050, 2000

Pujol J, Soriano-Mas C, Alonso P, et al: Mapping structural brain alterations in obsessive-compulsive disorder. Arch Gen Psychiatry 61:720–730, 2004

Rachman SJ, Hodgson RJ: Obsessions and Compulsions. Englewood Cliffs, NJ, Prentice-Hall, 1980

Rauch SL, Dougherty DD, Shin LM, et al: Neural correlates of factor-analyzed OCD symptom dimension: a PET study. CNS Spectr 3:37–43, 1998

Rauch SL, Wedig MM, Wright CI, et al: Functional magnetic resonance imaging study of regional brain activation during implicit sequence learning in obsessive-compulsive disorder. Biol Psychiatry 61:330–336, 2007

Rettew DC, Swedo SE, Leonard HL, et al: Obsessions and compulsions across time in 79 children and adolescents with obsessive-compulsive disorder. J Am Acad Child Adolesc Psychiatry 31:1050–1056, 1992

Rosario-Campos MC, Leckman JF, Mercadante MT, et al: Adults with early onset obsessive-compulsive disorder. Am J Psychiatry 158:1899–1903, 2001

Rosario-Campos MC, Miguel EC, Quatrano S, et al: The Dimensional Yale-Brown Obsessive-Compulsive Scale (DY-BOCS): an instrument for assessing obsessive-compulsive symptom dimensions. Mol Psychiatry 11:495–504, 2006

Rufer M, Grothusen A, Mass R, et al: Temporal stability of symptom dimensions in adult patients with obsessive-compulsive disorder. J Affect Disord 88:99–102, 2005

Rufer M, Fricke S, Moritz S, et al: Symptom dimensions in obsessive-compulsive disorder: prediction of cognitive-behavior therapy outcome. Acta Psychiatr Scand 113:440–446, 2006

Samuels J, Bienvenu OJ 3rd, Riddle MA, et al: Hoarding in obsessive compulsive disorder: results from a case-control study. Behav Res Ther 40:517–528, 2002

Saxena S, Rauch SL: Functional neuroimaging and the neuroanatomy of obsessive-compulsive disorder. Psychiatr Clin North Am 23:563–586, 2000

Saxena S, Maidment KM, Vapnik T, et al: Obsessive-compulsive hoarding: symptom severity and response to multimodal treatment. J Clin Psychiatry 63:21–27, 2002

Saxena S, Brody AL, Maidment KM, et al: Cerebral glucose metabolism in obsessive-compulsive hoarding. Am J Psychiatry 161:1038–1048, 2004

Saxena S, Brody AL, Maidment KM, et al: Paroxetine treatment of compulsive hoarding. J Psychiatr Res 41:481–487, 2007

Shapira NA, Liu Y, He AG, et al: Brain activation by disgust-inducing pictures in obsessive-compulsive disorder. Biol Psychiatry 54:751–756, 2003

Shetti CN, Reddy YC, Kandavel T, et al: Clinical predictors of drug nonresponse in obsessive-compulsive disorder. J Clin Psychiatry 66:1517–1523, 2005

Summerfeldt LJ, Richter MA, Antony MM, et al: Symptom structure in obsessive-compulsive disorder: a confirmatory factor-analytic study. Behav Res Ther 37:297–311, 1999

Summerfeldt LJ, Kloosterman PH, Antony MM, et al: The relationship between miscellaneous symptoms and major symptom factors in obsessive-compulsive disorder. Behav Res Ther 42:1453–1467, 2004

Sutcliffe JS, Delahanty RJ, Prasad HC, et al: Allelic heterogeneity at the serotonin transporter locus (SLC6A4) confers susceptibility to autism and rigid-compulsive behaviors. Am J Hum Genet 77:265–279, 2005

Tek C, Ulug B: Religiosity and religious obsessions in obsessive-compulsive disorder. Psychiatry Res 104:99–108, 2001

Van den Heuvel OA, Veltman DJ, Groenewegen HJ, et al: Amygdala activity in obsessive-compulsive disorder with contamination fear: a study with oxygen-15 water positron emission tomography. Psychiatry Res 132:225–237, 2004

Wewetzer C, Jans T, Muller B, et al: Long-term outcome and prognosis of obsessive-compulsive disorder with onset in childhood or adolescence. Eur Child Adolesc Psychiatry 10:37–46, 2001

Winsberg ME, Cassic KS, Koran LM: Hoarding in obsessive-compulsive disorder: a report of 20 cases. J Clin Psychiatry 60:591–597, 1999

World Health Organization: International Classification of Diseases, 10th Edition. Geneva, Switzerland, World Health Organization, 1992

Zhang H, Risch N: Mapping quantitative-trait loci in humans by use of extreme concordant sib pairs: selected sampling by parental phenotypes. Am J Hum Genet 59:951–957, 1996

Zhang H, Leckman JF, Tsai CP, et al: Genomewide scan of hoarding in sib pairs in which both sibs have Gilles de la Tourette syndrome. Am J Hum Genet 70:896–904, 2002

Zohar AH, Felz L: Ritualistic behavior in young children. J Abnorm Child Psychol 29:121–128, 2001

6

OVERVIEW OF GENETICS AND OBSESSIVE-COMPULSIVE DISORDER

Humberto Nicolini, M.D., Ph.D.
Paul Arnold, M.D., Ph.D., FRCP
Gerald Nestadt, M.D., M.P.H.
Nuria Lanzagorta, BSPSY
James L. Kennedy, M.D.

Ultimately, nosology ought to be guided by etiology. The development of classification systems in psychiatry is a complex task, but it is critical for both research and clinical practice. Therefore, there is interest in the prospects that genetic studies may be a useful approach for understanding the place of obsessive-compulsive disorder (OCD) in future psychiatric nomenclatures such as DSM-V. For a revised and refined classification to be most effective, ambiguities in the diagnostic criteria, the possibility of distinct clinical subtypes, and the high rate of comorbidity need to be resolved, and then we will have better phenotypes for genetic research.

OCD is heterogeneous; symptoms are experienced within multiple potentially overlapping dimensions, and it will be important to document their presence as

This chapter was first published as "Overview of Genetics and Obsessive-Compulsive Disorder." *Psychiatry Research* 170:7–14, 2009. Copyright 2009. Used with permission.

specifiers in DSM-V (Mataix et al. 2007). This remarkably diverse clinical presentation hampers the interpretation of findings and complicates the search for vulnerability genes. Variability in clinical subtypes in genetic research translates into variability of phenotypic expression. A combined symptom dimensional approach within distinctive clinical subgroups is proposed as probably the most effective way of helping to identify the heritable components of OCD (Miguel et al. 2005). Therefore, we need indicators of processes mediating between phenotype and genotype, the so-called endophenotypes or intermediate phenotypes, which in turn may be less influenced by environmental factors (Gottesman and Gould 2003).

The following sections discuss what has been learned from the different molecular genetic/family studies of OCD to date. Several of these approaches provide information relevant for diagnostic refinements. The additional sections provide an overview of additional genetic studies in OCD. Finally, there is a review of some data derived from attempts to evaluate the environmental contribution to OCD, by means of epidemiological, family, and twin studies.

Evidence From Family Studies in Obsessive-Compulsive Disorder

There have been many family studies in OCD over the past 75 years. The majority of them, in particular those prior to 1991, used the "family history" method, an approach that indirectly gathers information in all relatives. The "family study" method may also rely on direct structured interviews that obtain information directly from the subjects assessed (Nicolini et al. 1999; Pauls et al. 1999). The general conclusion of these family studies is that rates of OCD are significantly greater in relatives. In addition, the type of obsessions and compulsions displayed by probands (e.g., ordering, checking, and symmetry) adds homogeneity to the phenotype, increasing as a consequence the rates of OCD in relatives (Alsobrook et al. 1999; Hanna et al. 2005b; Miguel et al. 2005).

The concept of a spectrum is not new in psychiatry. The schizophrenia spectrum disorders have been well documented and mainly supported in family studies (Barch 2008). There may be an "OCD spectrum" of related disorders that share some of the same vulnerability genes, but the extent of this "spectrum" remains unknown. Similarities in symptomatology, course of illness, patient population, and neurocircuitry of OCD and obsessive-compulsive spectrum disorders (OCSD) are supported by comorbidity, family, and neurological studies, which also offer a critical reevaluation of the relationship between OCD and anxiety disorders (Hollander et al. 2007). However, there is compelling evidence supporting the family genetic OCSD association among OCD, tic disorders, body dysmorphic disorder, somatoform disorders, and grooming behaviors (Bienvenu et al. 2000; Grados et al. 2001; Pauls et al. 1995; Phillips et al. 2005).

The prevalence of OCD in relatives of probands is clearly elevated: 12% in first-degree relatives compared with 2% in relatives of normal control subjects (Alsobrook et al. 1999; Pauls et al. 1995). For the anxiety disorders, there is no elevation in rates for specific or social phobia, but there are higher rates of generalized anxiety disorder (GAD), separation anxiety disorder, panic disorder, and agoraphobia in first-degree relatives of probands with OCD (Grabe et al. 2006; Grados et al. 2003; Nestadt et al. 2000b). When one controls for the presence of these disorders in the probands, GAD and agoraphobia still remain significantly higher in first-degree relatives, suggesting that GAD and agoraphobia are strongly related to the OCD phenotype (Nestadt et al. 2000b). Although major depressive disorder (MDD) is elevated (in contrast to bipolar and dysthymic disorders), the elevation is no longer significant when adjusted for MDD in the probands, suggesting that MDD in relatives may be secondary to OCD (Arnold et al. 2004; Grabe et al. 2006; Nestadt et al. 2000b). This could be taken as a further hint that a specific gene does not cause OCD but that a disposition to develop any anxiety disorder may be genetically based.

The rates of affected relatives with OCD tend to vary depending on several factors related to proband definition, such as comorbidity with tics or earlier age at onset, that significantly increase such rates (Hanna et al. 2005c; Nestadt et al. 2000b; Rosario-Campos et al. 2006). There were higher rates of tics in relatives of probands with OCD, and rates of OCD were higher in relatives of probands with tics (Nestadt et al. 2000b; Pauls et al. 1995). The familiality of OCD is even stronger when there is comorbidity with tics and an earlier onset (Miguel et al. 2005). Family members are also more likely to have the types of obsessions and compulsions displayed by the probands, such as ordering, checking, and symmetry (Alsobrook et al. 1999; Mataix-Cols et al. 2004). In addition, age at onset was associated with a higher probability of having comorbidity with tic, anxiety, somatoform, eating, and impulse-control disorders (de Mathis et al. 2008).

It has been hypothesized that genetic and environmental factors relate to psychiatric disorders through the effect of intermediate vulnerability traits called endophenotypes. One example of this kind of research is the work of Delorme et al. (2005), who investigated blood serotonin abnormalities in the unaffected parents of OCD patients. They found lower whole blood 5-HT concentration, fewer platelet 5-HTT binding sites, and higher platelet IP3 content in OCD probands and their unaffected parents compared with control subjects. The only parameter that appeared to discriminate affected and unaffected subjects was 5-HT$_{2A}$ receptor binding characteristics, with increased receptor number and affinity in parents and no change in OCD probands.

In summary, published family studies support the contention that OCD, alone or comorbid with other disorders, is a condition influenced by genetic factors.

Evidence From Twin Studies in Obsessive-Compulsive Disorder

There have been only a few twin studies of OCD, and these all support the presence of significant genetic influence. Most of the largest studies have been based on samples of nonclinical twins in which obsessive-compulsive symptoms have been assessed through self-report measures and not through a psychiatric diagnosis. Hettema et al. (2001) conducted a meta-analysis of data from family and twin studies of panic disorder, GAD, phobias, and OCD to explore the roles of genetic and environmental factors in their etiology. For family studies, odds ratios predicting association of illness in first-degree relatives with affection status of the proband (disorder present or absent) were homogeneous across studies for all disorders. Panic disorder, GAD, phobias, and OCD all have significant familial aggregation. The role of nonshared environmental experience was relevant, underscoring the importance of identifying putative environmental risk factors that predispose individuals to anxiety. In the most recent study of adults, Jonnal et al. (2000) studied 527 pairs from the Virginia Twin Registry. Principal component analyses suggested two meaningful factors corresponding roughly to obsessions and compulsions, with heritabilities of 33% and 26%, respectively. Van Grootheest et al. (2005) conducted an extensive review of more than 70 years of twin research on OCD. The authors concluded that only the studies using structural equation modeling have convincingly shown that, in children, obsessive-compulsive symptoms are heritable, with genetic influences in the range of 45%–65%. In contrast, adult studies have suggested a somewhat lower genetic influence on symptoms, ranging from 27% to 47%.

Evidence From Segregation Analyses in Obsessive-Compulsive Disorder

The purpose of segregation analyses is to statistically assess the mode of inheritance for a particular disorder. In this case, segregation analysis has been used to assess the mode of inheritance of OCD in families ascertained through OCD and OCD-subtype probands. Segregation analysis has suggested that there is evidence of a single gene (autosomal dominant) for the following OCD subtypes: symptom-based groupings such as symmetry and ordering (Alsobrook et al. 1999), OCD with eating disorders (Cavallini et al. 2000), gender-specific OCD (Nestadt et al. 2000a), and early age at onset (Hanna et al. 2005a; Nicolini et al. 1991). Somewhat surprisingly, the main results provided by this methodology supported the hypothesis that OCD may be caused by the effect of a single major gene, with residual family effects (possibly caused by polygenic influences). This is true when ascertaining via pediatric or adult probands (Cavallini et al. 1999; Hanna et al. 2005a; Nestadt et al. 2000a; Nicolini et al. 1991). Nonetheless, Mendelian factors only partially explain the familial aggregation of the phenotype. It is important to note that the results cannot determine whether the same genetic locus is segregating across all families, or the number of genetic loci segregating in OCD, or the extent to which genetic heterogeneity is present in the disorder. However, stratification of the sample by the sex of probands provides further evidence of genetic heterogeneity (Nestadt et al. 2000a). In the specific case of tics or Tourette's syndrome comorbid with OCD, when probands are primary Tourette's syndrome with comorbid OCD, the most parsimonious model is an autosomal dominant gene (Pauls et al. 1990); however, when probands are diagnosed with primary OCD, this finding does not hold true (Cavallini et al. 1999). In conclusion, segregation analyses suggest both evidence for genes of major effect and/or a polygenic inheritance.

Genome Scans

There are only two published genome scans of OCD per se conducted to date (Hanna et al. 2002; Shugart et al. 2006). Hanna et al. (2002) found suggestive linkage on chromosome 9p24. This finding was replicated in a linkage study of the 9p24 region by Willour et al. (2004). However, this 9p24 finding was not replicated in the genome-wide screen conducted with the sample that included the subset of families in the Willour et al. sample. This is a demonstration of an important lesson in genetic studies; namely, that this could therefore be considered either evidence of nonreplication or may demonstrate evidence for heterogeneity and that a subset of the larger sample had a different genetic etiology from that of the entire larger sample.

The strongest linkage signal in the second genome scan (300 families) was in 3q27–28 (Shugart et al. 2006), a region that contains the gene encoding the serotonin 5-HT_{3C} receptor, suggesting a candidate gene not previously investigated in OCD. There were several additional linkage signals that deserve further follow-up. Also, a genome-wide linkage scan was performed for the phenotype of compulsive hoarding (Samuels et al. 2007), and significant linkage was found on chromosome 14. It is important to point out that the hoarding study used a subset of the sample that had been reported for the OCD genome scan.

Candidate Gene Studies

There have been many reports over the past 10 years regarding genetic polymorphisms associated with OCD. However, a great majority of these studies had small sample sizes that may have led to false positives. Methodologies to assess association have varied from case control to family based transmission tests. Also, in many of these studies, positive results are obtained only if the cases are subtyped into smaller and supposedly more homogenous subsamples. The following genes are among the main ones that have been studied thus far.

CATECHOL-O-METHYLTRANSFERASE

Catechol-O-methyltransferase (COMT) is an enzyme which metabolizes mono-amine neurotransmitters; it is encoded by a gene in the 22q11 region. Interestingly, microdeletions of 22q11 have been associated with obsessive-compulsive symptoms in adults (Gothelf et al. 2004) and children (Arnold et al. 2001). The first finding of an association between *COMT* and OCD was reported by Karayiorgou et al. (1997), who described a functional allele of the gene, Val158Met, wherein the met variant resulted in a three- to fourfold reduction in enzyme activity. The met allele was significantly associated in a recessive manner with susceptibility to OCD, particularly in males. Since that publication there have been several others with mixed results (Alsobrook et al. 2002; Meira-Lima et al. 2004; Niehaus et al. 2001). Azzam and Mathews (2003) conducted a systematic review and meta-analysis of both the published literature and unpublished data. Available data were stratified according to the original study design as either case-control or family based, and two separate meta-analyses were conducted. These analyses showed insufficient evidence to support an association between the COMT gene polymorphism and OCD. Subgroup stratification based on gender generated no statistically significant associations. Finally, Poyurovsky et al. (2005) could not support the hypothesis that the *COMT* Val158Met gene polymorphism is associated with liability to schizo-obsessive syndrome. Additional work is required to definitively rule in or out the role of *COMT,* particularly using newer markers and haplotypes that provide more extensive information regarding the participation of this gene in the etiology of OCD.

MONOAMINE OXIDASE A

Monoamine oxidase A (MAO-A) is a major catabolic enzyme for monoamines, and thus influences levels of serotonin, dopamine, and norepinephrine in the brain. Regarding OCD, the literature suggests a significant association of the MAO-A low enzymatic activity allele in OCD, particularly in females with comorbid depression (Camarena et al. 1998, 2001a; Hemmings et al. 2003; Karayiorgou et al. 1999). However, these studies are not large enough to provide compelling evidence to support this association.

DOPAMINE SYSTEM

The dopamine system has been implicated in OCD from pharmacologic studies using dopamine receptor blocking agents that ameliorate some symptoms of the disorder. Several genes in this system have been studied in OCD such as the dopamine transporter *(DAT)* and dopamine receptors *(DRD1, DRD2, DRD3* and *DRD4)* with some positive associations, particularly with *DRD4*. However, findings have been mixed, with no conclusively identified markers (Billett et al. 1998; Cruz-Fuentes et al. 1997; Hemmings et al. 2003; Millet et al. 2003; Nicolini et al. 1996).

SEROTONIN SYSTEM

The serotonin transporter gene *(SERT)* is probably the most widely studied gene in psychiatry (Graff-Guerrero et al. 2005). In particular, the most widely studied *SERT* variant consists of an insertion (long allele, "L") or deletion (short allele, "S") of a 44 base pair sequence in the promoter region. Although the results in OCD suggest an effect of the "L" allele, the literature still remains controversial (Bengel et al. 1999; Camarena et al. 2001b; Hu et al. 2006; Meira-Lima et al. 2004). In the case of Hu et al. (2006) a single nucleotide polymorphism that converts the long allele to a functionally short one was important in determining the significance of *SERT* in OCD. The long allele containing the A variant of the single nucleotide polymorphism was associated with OCD, while the long-G and short alleles were not. Thus other groups should investigate this in their analyses. Other genes, such as the 5-HT$_{2A}$ receptor promoter polymorphism *(5HT2A)* and *5HT1B* have been extensively studied, although for only a small number of single nucleotide polymorphisms, with positive associations for both of them (Camarena et al. 2004; Hemmings et al. 2003; Hu et al. 2006; Levitan et al. 2006; Meira-Lima et al. 2004; Mundo et al. 2000, 2002; Walitza et al. 2002), but also negative findings (Di Bella et al. 2002a, 2002b; Frisch et al. 2000; Walitza et al. 2004).

GLUTAMATE SYSTEM

The glutamate *N*-methyl-D-aspartic acid (NMDA) subunit receptor gene was associated with OCD in a family based association study (Arnold et al. 2004). The glutamate transporter gene *SLC1A1* is a promising positional and functional candidate gene given its location within a linkage peak on 9p24 and its potential functional significance due to its role in glutamate neurotransmission. Three groups have now identified associations with this gene (Arnold et al. 2006; Dickel et al. 2006; Stewart et al. 2007a), with no negative findings reported to date. Delorme et al. (2004) recently examined the kainate receptor genes *GRIK2* and *GRIK3*, resulting in a weak association with *GRIK2* that requires replication.

OTHER GENES

Other genes that have been less studied but may be promising are those for brain-derived neurotrophic factor *(BDNF)*, with both positive (Hall et al. 2003) and negative (Mossner et al. 2000; Zai et al. 2005b) findings; γ-aminobutyric acid *(GABA)* type B receptor 1 (Zai et al. 2005a); myelin oligodendrocyte glycoprotein *(MOG;* Zai et al. 2004); the μ opioid receptor (Urraca et al. 2004); and the myelin regulatory gene *Olig2* (Stewart et al. 2007b). On the other hand interesting genes that have been studied with negative results are those for tumor necrosis factor α *(TNFα;* ; Zai et al. 2006) and apolipoprotein E *(ApoE;* Nicolini et al. 2001). Also, it is noteworthy that no genetic studies with prospective measures of medication response in OCD have been done. This is a very interesting endophenotype, possibly more homogeneous and more closely connected to the biological function of the candidate genes.

More than 60 candidate gene studies have been conducted. Most studies have focused on genes in the serotonergic and dopaminergic pathways. Unfortunately, none have achieved genome-wide significance and, with the exception of the glutamate transporter gene, none have been reliably replicated (Pauls 2008). Future research will require much larger samples and the collaboration of researchers to be able to identify susceptibility loci for OCD.

Although OCD appears to have a genetic component, additional innovative research, such as whole-genome association studies, are needed to unravel the genetic influences in the disorder. Two whole-genome association scans that cover the entire genome with more than 1,200,000 single nucleotide polymorphism markers in one experiment are in progress. This methodology is purported to be more useful in detecting common genetic variants with only moderate effect size.

Alternate and Intermediate Phenotypes

Results from family studies have suggested that OCD is a genetically heterogeneous disorder and have emphasized the importance of identifying valid subgroups of patients, such as early onset, sex effects, symptom clustering, neuropsychological performance, neuroimaging, and response to treatment. Such clinical subgroups, also called *alternate phenotypes,* do not necessarily represent true biological entities. However, a major challenge in OCD genetic research is to demonstrate processes mediating between DSM-IV-TR (American Psychiatric Association 2000) OCD phenotype and genotype, becoming true intermediate phenotypes or endophenotypes (Miguel et al. 2005). Endophenotypes represent simpler clues to genetic underpinnings than the disease syndrome itself. The interaction between genes and environment (epigenetics) may also be of critical importance for modifying the development of the OCD phenotype. Endophenotypes would ideally have genetic routes. A clinical subtype or a biological marker may not necessarily reflect genetic underpinnings but may rather reflect associated findings. Therefore, the endophenotype is heritable, is state independent, co-segregates with the illness, and is found in unaffected family members at a higher rate than in the general population (Gottesman and Gould 2003).

EARLY ONSET

Early onset OCD appears to be a particular subtype that exhibits distinct clinical features and is associated with greater familial loading (Chabane et al. 2005; do Rosario-Campos et al. 2005; Hemmings et al. 2004). In addition, in an early onset form of the disorder triggered by infection (OCD with pediatric autoimmune neuropsychiatric disorders associated with Streptococcus [PANDAS]), which is more of an environmental form of the disorder, it has been shown that rates of tic disorders and OCD in first-degree relatives of pediatric probands with PANDAS are higher than those reported in the general population and are similar to those reported for tic disorders and OCD (Lougee et al. 2000).

NEUROPSYCHOLOGY AND NEUROIMAGING

Chamberlain et al. (2007) demonstrated deficits in cognitive flexibility and motor inhibition that were present in both OCD-affected individuals and their unaffected relatives, suggesting another potential endophenotype. Other neuropsychological tasks associated with OCD might serve as endophenotypes, although there are no published reports based on unaffected relatives. Examples include executive functioning (Kuelz et al. 2004), procedural or implicit learning (Joel et al. 2005), or visual memory encoding (Penades et al. 2005).

There are some studies that have assessed brain imaging as an endophenotype in OCD. Using magnetic resonance imaging (MRI) and behavioral performance on a response inhibition task (Stop-Signal), Menzies et al. (2007) found that OCD patients and their relatives both had delayed response inhibition on the Stop-Signal task compared with healthy control subjects. This finding was significantly associated with reduced gray matter in orbitofrontal and right inferior frontal regions and increased gray matter in cingulate, parietal, and striatal regions. A novel permutation test indicated significant familial effects on variation of the MRI markers of inhibitory processing, supporting the candidacy of these brain structural systems as endophenotypes of OCD. These authors concluded that structural variation in large-scale brain systems related to motor inhibitory control may mediate genetic risk for OCD, providing evidence for a neurocognitive endophenotype of OCD.

Obsessive-compulsive hoarding may be a well-defined subgroup or variant of OCD in addition to its symptoms, but compelling data supported by neuroimaging studies suggest that the "compulsive hoarding syndrome" may be a neurobiologically distinct entity (An et al. 2009; Mataix et al. 2007; Saxena et al. 2004).

GENDER

It has been suggested that gender may contribute to the clinical and biological heterogeneity of OCD. Besides different clinical presentations, gender has been associated with distinct candidate gene associations for at least four genes: *MAOA, COMT, 5HT1Dβ*, and *SLC1A1,* as well as one linkage study that detected a significant linkage signal in the region of 11p15 at D11S4146 in the families of male probands (Arnold et al. 2006; Camarena et al. 2001a, 2004; Dickel et al. 2006; Karayiorgou et al. 1999; Lochner et al. 2004; Wang et al. 2009).

SYMPTOM

There have been several factor-analytic studies of OCD that consistently found three to five factors that explained nearly 70% of the variance (Cullen et al. 2008; do Rosario-Campos et al. 2005; Pinto et al. 2008). These symptom factors are consistent between adult and child samples (Stewart et al. 2007c). Those dimensions are cleaning and contamination, hoarding, symmetry and ordering, and sexual and religious obsessions. There is a high familial risk if probands present high scores on obsessions/checking and symmetry/ordering factors for OCD and Tourette's syndrome, as well as an increased allele sharing at three loci in chromosomes 4, 5, and 17 in hoarder patients (Alsobrook et al. 1999; Leckman et al. 2003; Lochner et al. 2005). As noted earlier, hoarding has also been associated with distinct findings on a genome scan on OCD (Samuels et al. 2007). In addition, there is an association with the serotonin transporter in patients with OCD and tics that also presents the repeating/counting factor (Cavallini et al. 2002).

PERSONALITY

Little is known about personality disorders and normal personality dimensions in relatives of patients with OCD or if personality may serve as an endophenotype. However, there are some interesting data. Neuroticism and obsessive-compulsive personality disorder may share a common familial etiology with OCD (Samuels et al. 2000). Perfectionism appears to be more closely associated with obsessive-compulsive personality symptoms rather than OCD (Halmi et al. 2005), and there is a relation of temperament and character dimensions with the severity of obsessive-compulsive symptoms. On the Temperament and Character Inventory, OCD subjects displayed increased harm avoidance and lower self-directedness and cooperativeness (Cruz-Fuentes et al. 2004). There is an extensive amount of research that shows associations with personality and several candidate genes, some of which have also been associated with OCD (Ebstein 2006), although the usefulness of personality as an endophenotype remains to be further studied.

DRUG RESPONSE

There are not many studies exploring the pharmacogenetics of OCD. However, this may be a useful endophenotype for future research (Billett et al. 1997). OCD symptoms respond differently to drug treatments (Shetti et al. 2005); moreover, there are polymorphisms associated with the mechanism of action of anti-obsessional drugs that may in fact be vulnerability genes to the disorder. Also, genes associated with susceptibility to OCD may represent future targets for drug development.

The most studied polymorphism is again the promoter region of the serotonin transporter. However, no differences among the genotypes and response to serotonin reuptake inhibitors have been demonstrated (Di Bella et al. 2002a, 2002b). On the other hand, there is some evidence that response in venlafaxine-treated OCD patients is associated with the S/L genotype of the *5-HTTLPR* polymorphism and in paroxetine-treated OCD patients with the G/G genotype of the *5HT2A* polymorphism (Denys et al. 2007). Nonetheless, there is still a lack of studies in this area; additional research is needed to better understand if treatment response may constitute an endophenotype.

Environment and Obsessive-Compulsive Disorder

There are some reports that have attempted to evaluate environment contribution to OCD. One important strategy has been through twin studies, which can assess genetic as well as environmental contributions to the OCD phenotype. For instance, Santangelo et al. (1996), in a study of Tourette's syndrome patients, found that labor complications, excessive consumption of caffeine or alcohol by the mother, and maternal smoking all correlated with the development of OCD. Hudziak et al. (2004) assessed cultural differences in a large twin dataset by determining whether the genetic/environmental contributions differ by country (United States or Netherlands). They found a unique environmental contribution of the nonshared type using nonclinical measures of DSM-IV-TR OCD and concluded that some environmental possibilities that may lead to the expression of OCD are PANDAS, differences in parenting, and school activities. However, they did not directly test for them. Other researchers evaluated prenatal, perinatal, and postnatal risk factors in OCD. They concluded that edema during pregnancy and prolonged labor were the most significant risk factors (Salema et al. 2007). Also there is some evidence that shows an increase in postpartum OCD. However, most studies are retrospective in nature, thus not answering questions about the overall prevalence of such symptoms. In addition, the neurobiological basis of this phenomenon remains unknown (Abramowitz et al. 2003).

Discussion

As we can see from the numerous studies listed earlier, multiple genetic and environmental factors may be involved in OCD etiology. This is complicated by the probability of genetic heterogeneity for this phenotype, which needs further exploration of gene–gene and gene–environment interactions. In addition, the exploration of alternate phenotypes based on symptom expression, age at onset, or comorbid conditions may be crucial in finding good candidate genes. However, there is some compelling evidence. First OCD is a spectrum disorder phenotype, with many alternate forms that deserve further research; based on family genetic studies, OCD, tics, body dysmorphic disorder and grooming behaviors seem to be part of it. In addition there is good evidence that a polygenic etiology is supported by segregation analysis. This evidence is further supported by the signals of genome scans. Many candidate genes have been found in association with OCD; however, the glutamate and serotonin system genes have been the most replicated. Among all alternative phenotypes described, the most compelling evidence to be considered points to neuroimaging studies and the hoarding subtype and performance on a response inhibition task as well as deficits in cognitive flexibility and motor inhibition. Finally, environment needs further study because it contributes to several interesting forms of the disorder (e.g., PANDAS).

OCD is remarkably diverse and can vary both within and across patients over time. This variability in the phenotypic expression means that OCD is a heterogeneous disorder and this heterogeneity complicates the search for vulnerability genes. In order to find valid endophenotypes for OCD we need several approaches. Phenotype needs to be narrowed by identifying biologically valid subgroups of patients, such as the ones reviewed before. By identifying heritable components of OCD, it should be possible to find genes for these separate components.

A goal of genetic research is to provide improved and earlier diagnosis of OCD. It may be that multiple genes combined together in an algorithm will be used for prediction, or risk models that include both genetic and environmental factors. Once risk genes for OCD are confirmed, "high-risk" individuals (e.g., children who are exhibiting early symptoms or have a strong family history) could be genotyped for risk alleles and followed prospectively. Such an approach would be the most valid design for identifying environmental factors that interact with genotype to confer susceptibility to OCD. Furthermore, prevention programs could be designed and targeted to children with high genetic risk, a more cost-effective strategy than offering it to all children or even all children with a positive family history of OCD. Identification of susceptibility genes, and a better understanding of how environment interacts with them, should refine our classification of OCD and OCSDs, because our current syndrome-based diagnosis likely represents a heterogeneous group of disorders that may have different associated features and respond to different treatment approaches. This is analogous to infectious diseases, in which a variety of conditions that could only previously be identified by nonspecific symptoms (e.g., fever) were found to be the result of different infectious agents and to respond to different medications. Conversely, the identification of susceptibility genes will likely be enhanced by more refined definition of the clinical phenotype. For example, as noted earlier, factor analyses have identified symptom dimensions that may have distinct genetic correlates.

In summary, genetic findings have already informed our understanding of the diagnosis of OCD and OCSDs, and future research promises to enhance our diagnostic system even more. Genetic technology is rapidly advancing, making it feasible to genotype most of human genetic variation. This capability will allow us not only to understand genes better but also how environment interacts with the genome.

References

Abramowitz JS, Schwartz SA, Moore KM, et al: Obsessive-compulsive symptoms in pregnancy and the puerperium: a review of the literature. J Anxiety Disord 17:461–478, 2003

Alsobrook J, Leckman J, Goodman W, et al: Segregation analysis of obsessive-compulsive disorder using symptom-based factor scores. Am J Med Genet B Neuropsychiatr Genet 88:669–675, 1999

Alsobrook JP II, Zohar AH, Leboyer M, et al: Association between the COMT locus and obsessive-compulsive disorder in females but not males. Am J Med Genet 114:116–120, 2002

American Psychiatric Association: Diagnostic and Statistical Manual of Mental Disorders, 4th Edition, Text Revision. Washington, DC, American Psychiatric Association 2000

An SK, Mataix-Cols D, Lawrence NS, et al: To discard or not to discard: the neural basis of hoarding symptoms in obsessive-compulsive disorder. Mol Psychiatry 14:318–331, 2009

Arnold PD, Siegel-Bartelt J, Cytrynbaum C, et al: Velocardiofacial syndrome: implications of microdeletion 22q11 for schizophrenia and mood disorders. Am J Med Genet 105:354–362, 2001

Arnold PD, Summerfeldt LJ, Sicard T, et al: A family based association study of novel serotonin polymorphisms in OCD and OCD symptom subgroups. Am J Med Genet B Neuropsychiatr Genet 130B:69, 2004

Arnold PD, Sicard T, Burroughs E, et al: Glutamate transporter gene SLC1A1 associated with obsessive-compulsive disorder. Arch Gen Psychiatry 63:769–776, 2006

Azzam A, Mathews CA: Meta-analysis of the association between the catecholamine-O-methyltransferase gene and obsessive-compulsive disorder. Am J Med Genet 123B:64–69, 2003

Barch DM: Emotion, motivation, and reward processing in schizophrenia spectrum disorders: what we know and where we need to go. Schizophr Bull 34:816–818, 2008

Bengel D, Greenberg BD, Cora-Locatelli G, et al: Association of the serotonin transporter promoter regulatory region polymorphism and obsessive-compulsive disorder. Mol Psychiatry 4:463–466, 1999

Bienvenu OJ, Samuels JF, Riddle MA, et al: The relationship of obsessive-compulsive disorder to possible spectrum disorders: results from a family study. Biol Psychiatry 48:287–293, 2000

Billett EA, Richter MA, King N, et al: Obsessive compulsive disorder, response to serotonin reuptake inhibitors and the serotonin transporter gene. Mol Psychiatry 2:403–406, 1997

Billett EA, Richter MA, Sam F, et al: Investigation of dopamine system genes in obsessive-compulsive disorder. Psychiatr Genet 8:163–169, 1998

Camarena B, Cruz-Fuentes C, De la Fuente JR, et al: A higher frequency of a low activity-related allele of the MAO-A gene in females with obsessive-compulsive disorder. Psychiatr Genet 8:255–257, 1998

Camarena B, Rinetti G, Cruz-Fuentes C, et al: Additional evidence that genetic variation of MAO-A gene supports a gender subtype in obsessive-compulsive disorder. Am J Med Genet B Neuropsychiatr Genet 105:279–282, 2001a

Camarena B, Rinetti G, Cruz-Fuentes C, et al: Association study of the serotonin transporter gene polymorphism in obsessive-compulsive disorder. Int J Neuropsychopharmacol 4:269–272, 2001b

Camarena B, Aguilar A, Loyzaga C, et al: A family based association study of the 5-HT-1D receptor gene in obsessive-compulsive disorder. Int J Neuropsychopharmacol 7:49–53, 2004

Cavallini MC, Pasquale L, Bellodi L, et al: Complex segregation analysis for obsessive compulsive disorder and related disorders. Am J Med Genet 88:38–43, 1999

Cavallini MC, Bertelli S, Chiapparino D, et al: Complex segregation analysis of obsessive-compulsive disorder in 141 families of eating disorder probands, with and without obsessive-compulsive disorder. Am J Med Genet 96:384–391, 2000

Cavallini MC, Di Bella D, Siliprandi F, et al: Exploratory factor analysis of obsessive-compulsive patients and association with 5-HTTLPR polymorphism. Am J Med Genet 114:347–353, 2002

Chabane N, Delorme R, Millet B, et al: Early onset obsessive-compulsive disorder: a subgroup with a specific clinical and familial pattern? J Child Psychol Psychiatry 46:881–887, 2005

Chamberlain SR, Fineberg NA, Menzies LA, et al: Impaired cognitive flexibility and motor inhibition in unaffected first-degree relatives of patients with obsessive-compulsive disorder. Am J Psychiatry 164:335–338, 2007

Cruz-Fuentes C, Camarena B, King N, et al: Increased prevalence of the seven-repeat variant of the dopamine D4 receptor gene in patients with obsessive-compulsive disorder with tics. Neurosci Lett 231:1–4, 1997

Cruz-Fuentes C, Blas C, Gonzalez L, et al: Severity of obsessive-compulsive symptoms is related to self-directedness character trait in obsessive-compulsive disorder. CNS Spectr 9:607–612, 2004

Cullen B, Samuels J, Grados M, et al: Social and communication difficulties and obsessive-compulsive disorder. Psychopathology 41:194–200, 2008 de Mathis MA, do Rosario MC, Diniz JB, et al: Obsessive-compulsive disorder: influence of age at onset on comorbidity patterns. Eur Psychiatry 23:187–194, 2008

Delorme R, Krebs MO, Chabane N, et al: Frequency and transmission of glutamate receptors GRIK2 and GRIK3 polymorphisms in patients with obsessive compulsive disorder. Neuroreport 15:699–702, 2004

Delorme R, Betancur C, Callebert J, et al: Platelet serotonergic markers as endophenotypes for obsessive-compulsive disorder. Neuropsychopharmacology 30:1539–1547, 2005

Denys D, Van Nieuwerburgh F, Deforce D, et al: Prediction of response to paroxetine and venlafaxine by serotonin-related genes in obsessive-compulsive disorder in a randomized, double-blind trial. J Clin Psychiatry 68:747–753, 2007

Di Bella D, Cavallini MC, Bellodi L: No association between obsessive-compulsive disorder and the 5-HT1D-beta receptor gene. Am J Psychiatry 159:1783–1785, 2002a

Di Bella D, Erzegovesi S, Cavallini MC, et al: Obsessive-compulsive disorder, 5-HTTLPR polymorphism and treatment response. Pharmacogenomics J 2:176–181, 2002b

Dickel DE, Veenstra-VanderWeele J, Cox NJ, et al: Association testing of the positional and functional candidate gene SLC1A1/EAAC1 in early onset obsessive-compulsive disorder. Arch Gen Psychiatry 63:778–785, 2006

do Rosario-Campos MC, Leckman JF, Curi M, et al: A family study of early onset obsessive-compulsive disorder. Am J Med Genet B Neuropsychiatr Genet 136B:92–97, 2005

Ebstein RP: The molecular genetic architecture of human personality: beyond self-report questionnaires. Mol Psychiatry 11:427–445, 2006

Frisch A, Michaelovsky E, Rockah R, et al: Association between obsessive-compulsive disorder and polymorphisms of genes encoding components of the serotonergic and dopaminergic pathways. Eur Neuropsychopharmacol 10:205–209, 2000

Gothelf D, Presburger G, Zohar AH, et al: Obsessive-compulsive disorder in patients with velocardiofacial (22q11 deletion) syndrome. Am J Med Genet B Neuropsychiatr Genet 126:99–105, 2004

Gottesman II, Gould T: The endophenotype concept in psychiatry; etymology and strategic intentions. Am J Psychiatry 160:636–645, 2003

Grabe HJ, Ruhrmann S, Ettelt S, et al: Familiality of obsessive-compulsive disorder in nonclinical and clinical subjects. Am J Psychiatry 163:1986–1992, 2006

Grados MA, Riddle MA, Samuels JF, et al: The familial phenotype of obsessive-compulsive disorder in relation to tic disorders: the Hopkins OCD family study. Biol Psychiatry 50:559–565, 2001

Grados MA, Walkup J, Walford S: Genetics of obsessive-compulsive disorders: new findings and challenges. Brain Dev 25(suppl):S55–S61, 2003

Graff-Guerrero A, de la Fuente-Sandoval C, Camarena B, et al: Frontal and limbic metabolic differences in subjects selected according to genetic variation of the SLC6A4 gene polymorphism. Neuroimage 25:1197–1204, 2005

Hall D, Dhilla A, Charalambous A, et al: Sequence variants of the brain-derived neurotrophic factor (BDNF) gene are strongly associated with obsessive-compulsive disorder. Am J Hum Genet 73:370–376, 2003

Halmi KA, Tozzi F, Thornton LM, et al: The relation among perfectionism, obsessive-compulsive personality disorder and obsessive-compulsive disorder in individuals with eating disorders. Int J Eat Disord 38:371–374, 2005

Hanna G, Veenstra-VanderWeele J, Cox N, et al: Genome-wide linkage analysis of families with obsessive-compulsive disorder ascertained through pediatric probands. Am J Med Genet B Neuropsychiatr Genet 114:541–552, 2002

Hanna G, Fingerlin TE, Himle JA, et al: Complex segregation analysis of obsessive-compulsive disorder in families with pediatric probands. Hum Hered 60:1–9, 2005a

Hanna G, Fischer DJ, Chadha KR, et al: Familial and sporadic subtypes of early onset obsessive-compulsive disorder. Biol Psychiatry 57:895–900, 2005b

Hanna G, Himle JA, Curtis GC, et al: A family study of obsessive-compulsive disorder with pediatric probands. Am J Med Genet B Neuropsychiatr Genet 134:13–19, 2005c

Hemmings SM, Kinnear CJ, Niehaus DJ, et al: Investigating the role of dopaminergic and serotonergic candidate genes in obsessive-compulsive disorder. Eur Neuropsychopharmacol 13:93–98, 2003

Hemmings SM, Kinnear CJ, Lochner C, et al: Early versus late-onset obsessive-compulsive disorder: investigating genetic and clinical correlates. Psychiatr Res 128:175–182, 2004

Hettema JM, Neale MC, Kendler KS: A review and meta-analysis of the genetic epidemiology of anxiety disorders. Am J Psychiatry 158:1568–1578, 2001

Hollander E, Kim S, Khanna S, et al: Obsessive-compulsive disorder and obsessive-compulsive spectrum disorders: diagnostic and dimensional issues. CNS Spectr 2(suppl):5–13, 2007

Hu XZ, Lipsky RH, Zhu G, et al: Serotonin transporter promoter gain-of-function genotypes are linked to obsessive-compulsive disorder. Am J Hum Genet 78:815–826, 2006

Hudziak JJ, Van Beijsterveldt CE, Althoff RR, et al: Genetic and environmental contributions to the Child Behavior Checklist Obsessive-Compulsive Scale: a cross-cultural twin study. Arch Gen Psychiatry 61:608–616, 2004

Joel D, Zohar O, Afek M, et al: Impaired procedural learning in obsessive-compulsive disorder and Parkinson's disease, but not in major depressive disorder. Behav Brain Res 157:253–263, 2005

Jonnal AH, Gardner CO, Prescott CA, et al: Obsessive and compulsive symptoms in a general population sample of female twins. Am J Med Genet 96:791–796, 2000

Karayiorgou M, Altemus M, Galke BL, et al: Genotype determining low catechol-O-methyltransferase activity as a risk factor for obsessive-compulsive disorder. Proc Natl Acad Sci 94:4572–4575, 1997

Karayiorgou M, Sobin C, Blundell ML, et al: Family based association studies support a sexually dimorphic effect of COMT and MAOA on genetic susceptibility to obsessive-compulsive disorder. Biol Psychiatry 45:1178–1189, 1999

Kuelz AK, Hohagen F, Voderholzer U: Neuropsychological performance in obsessive-compulsive disorder: a critical review. Biol Psychol 65:185–236, 2004

Leckman JF, Pauls DL, Zhang H, et al: Obsessive-compulsive symptom dimensions in affected sibling pairs diagnosed with Gilles de la Tourette syndrome. Am J Med Genet B Neuropsychiatr Genet 116:60–68, 2003

Levitan RD, Kaplan AS, Masellis M, et al: The serotonin-1Dbeta receptor gene and severity of obsessive-compulsive disorder in women with bulimia nervosa. Eur Neuropsychopharmacol 16:1–6, 2006

Lochner C, Hemmings SM, Kinnear CJ, et al: Gender in obsessive-compulsive disorder: clinical and genetic findings. Eur Neuropsychopharmacol 14:105–113, 2004

Lochner C, Kinnear CJ, Hemmings SM, et al: Hoarding in obsessive-compulsive disorder: clinical and genetic correlates. J Clin Psychiatry 66:1155–1160, 2005

Lougee L, Perlmutter SJ, Nicolson R, et al: Psychiatric disorders in first-degree relatives of children with pediatric autoimmune neuropsychiatric disorders associated with streptococcal infections (PANDAS). J Am Acad Child Adolesc Psychiatry 39:1120–1126, 2000

Mataix D, Pertusa A, Leckman JF: Issues for DSM-V: how should obsessive-compulsive and related disorders be classified? Am J Psychiatry 164:1313–1314, 2007

Mataix-Cols D, Wooderson S, Lawrence N, et al: Distinct neural correlates of washing, checking, and hoarding symptom dimensions in obsessive-compulsive disorder. Arch Gen Psychiatry 61:564–576, 2004

Meira-Lima I, Shavitt RG, Miguita K, et al: Association analysis of the catechol-O-methyl-transferase (COMT), serotonin transporter (5-HTT) and serotonin 2A receptor (5HT2A) gene polymorphisms with obsessive-compulsive disorder. Genes Brain Behav 3:75–79, 2004

Menzies L, Achard S, Chamberlain SR, et al: Neurocognitive endophenotypes of obsessive-compulsive disorder. Brain 130:3223–3236, 2007

Miguel EC, Leckman JF, Rauch S, et al: Obsessive-compulsive disorder phenotypes: implications for genetic studies. Mol Psychiatry 10:258–275, 2005

Millet B, Chabane N, Delorme R, et al: Association between the dopamine receptor D4 (DRD4) gene and obsessive-compulsive disorder. Am J Med Genet 116(suppl):55–59, 2003

Mossner R, Daniel S, Albert D, et al: Serotonin transporter function is modulated by brain-derived neurotrophic factor (BDNF) but not nerve growth factor (NGF). Neurochem Int 36:197–202, 2000

Mundo E, Richter MA, Sam F, et al: Is the 5-HT(1Dbeta) receptor gene implicated in the pathogenesis of obsessive-compulsive disorder? Am J Psychiatry 157:1160–1161, 2000

Mundo E, Richter MA, Zai G, et al: 5HT1dbeta receptor gene implicated in the pathogenesis of obsessive-compulsive disorder: further evidence from a family based association study. Mol Psychiatry 7:805–809, 2002

Nestadt G, Lan T, Samuels J, et al: Complex segregation analysis provides compelling evidence for a major gene underlying obsessive-compulsive disorder and for heterogeneity by sex. Am J Hum Genet 67:1611–1616, 2000a

Nestadt G, Samuels J, Riddle M, et al: A family study of obsessive-compulsive disorder. Arch Gen Psychiatry 57:358–363, 2000b

Nicolini H, Hanna G, Baxter L, et al: Segregation analysis of obsessive compulsive and associated disorders. Ursus Medicus Journal 1:25–28, 1991

Nicolini H, Cruz-Fuentes C, Camarena B, et al: DRD2, DRD3 and 5HT2A receptor genes polymorphisms in obsessive-compulsive disorder. Mol Psychiatry 1:461–465, 1996

Nicolini H, Cruz-Fuentes C, Camarena B, et al: Understanding the genetic basis of obsessive-compulsive disorder. CNS Spectr 4:32–48, 1999

Nicolini H, Urraca N, Camarena B, et al: Lack of association of apolipoprotein E polymorphism in obsessive-compulsive disorder. CNS Spectr 6:978–979, 992, 2001

Niehaus DJ, Kinnear CJ, Corfield VA, et al: Association between a catechol-O-methyltransferase polymorphism and obsessive-compulsive disorder in the Afrikaner population. J Affect Disord 65:61–65, 2001

Pauls DL: The genetics of obsessive compulsive disorder: a review of the evidence. Am J Med Genet 148:133–139, 2008

Pauls DL, Pakstis AJ, Kurlan R, et al: Segregation and linkage analyses of Tourette's syndrome and related disorders. J Am Acad Child Adolesc Psychiatry 29:195–203, 1990

Pauls DL, Alsobrook JP II, Goodman W, et al: A family study of obsessive-compulsive disorder. Am J Psychiatry 152:76–84, 1995

Pauls DL, Alsobrook JP II, Goodman W, et al: A family study of obsessive-compulsive disorder. Am J Psychiatry 152:76–84, 1999

Penades R, Catalan R, Andres S, et al: Executive function and nonverbal memory in obsessive-compulsive disorder. Psychiatr Res 133:81–90, 2005

Phillips KA, Menard W, Fay C, et al: Demographic characteristics, phenomenology, comorbidity, and family history in 200 individuals with body dysmorphic disorder. Psychosomatics 46:317–325, 2005

Pinto A, Greenberg BD, Grados MA, et al: Further development of YBOCS dimensions in the OCD Collaborative Genetics Study: symptoms vs. categories. Psychiatry Res 160:83–93, 2008

Poyurovsky M, Michaelovsky E, Frisch A, et al: COMT Val158Met polymorphism in schizophrenia with obsessive-compulsive disorder: a case-control study. Neurosci Lett 389:21–24, 2005

Rosario-Campos MC, Miguel EC, Quatrano S, et al: The Dimensional Yale–Brown Obsessive-compulsive Scale (DYBOCS): an instrument for assessing obsessive-compulsive symptom dimensions. Mol Psychiatry 11:495–504, 2006

Salema M, Sampaio A, Hounie A, et al: Prenatal, perinatal and postnatal risk factors for obsessive compulsive disorder. Biol Psychiatry 601:301–307, 2007

Samuels J, Nestadt G, Bienvenu OJ, et al: Personality disorders and normal personality dimensions in obsessive-compulsive disorder. Br J Psychiatry 177:457–462, 2000

Samuels J, Shugart YY, Grados MA, et al: Significant linkage to compulsive hoarding on chromosome 14 in families with obsessive-compulsive disorder: results from the OCD Collaborative Genetics Study. Am J Psychiatry 164:493–499, 2007

Santangelo SL, Pauls DL, Lavori PW, et al: Assessing risk for the Tourette spectrum of disorders among first-degree relatives of probands with Tourette syndrome. Am J Med Genet 67:107–116, 1996

Saxena S, Brody AL, Maidment KM, et al: Cerebral glucose metabolism in obsessive-compulsive hoarding. Am J Psychiatry 161:1038–1048, 2004

Shetti CN, Reddy YC, Kandavel T, et al: Clinical predictors of drug nonresponse in obsessive-compulsive disorder. J Clin Psychiatry 66:1517–1523, 2005

Shugart YY, Samuels J, Willour VL, et al: Genomewide linkage scan for obsessive-compulsive disorder: evidence for susceptibility loci on chromosomes 3q, 7p, 1q, 15q, and 6q. Mol Psychiatry 11:763–770, 2006

Stewart SE, Fagerness JA, Platko J, et al: Association of the SLC1A1 glutamate transporter gene and obsessive-compulsive disorder. Am J Med Genet B Neuropsychiatr Genet 144:1027–1033, 2007a

Stewart SE, Platko J, Fagerness J, et al: A genetic family based association study of OLIG2 in obsessive-compulsive disorder. Arch Gen Psychiatry 64:209–214, 2007b

Stewart SE, Rosario MC, Brown TA, et al: Principal components analysis of obsessive-compulsive disorder symptoms in children and adolescents. Biol Psychiatry 61:285–291, 2007c

Urraca N, Camarena B, Gomez-Caudillo L, et al: Mu opioid receptor gene as a candidate for the study of obsessive compulsive disorder with and without tics. Am J Med Genet 127B:94–96, 2004

Van Grootheest DS, Cath DC, Beekman AT, et al: Twin studies on obsessive-compulsive disorder: a review. Twin Res Hum Genet 8:450–458, 2005

Walitza S, Wewetzer C, Warnke A, et al: 5-HT2A promoter polymorphism-1438G/A in children and adolescents with obsessive-compulsive disorders. Mol Psychiatry 7:1054–1057, 2002

Walitza S, Wewetzer C, Gerlach M, et al: Transmission disequilibrium studies in children and adolescents with obsessive-compulsive disorders pertaining to polymorphisms of genes of the serotonergic pathway. J Neural Transm 111:817–825, 2004

Wang Y, Samuels JF, Chang YC, et al: Gender differences in genetic linkage and association on 11p15 in obsessive-compulsive disorder families. Am J Med Genet B Neuropsychiatr Genet 150B:30–40, 2009

Willour VL, Yao Shugart Y, Samuels J, et al: Replication study supports evidence for linkage to 9p24 in obsessive-compulsive disorder. Am J Hum Genet 75:508–513, 2004

Zai G, Bezchlibnyk YB, Richter MA, et al: Myelin oligodendrocyte glycoprotein (MOG) gene is associated with obsessive-compulsive disorder. Am J Med Genet B Neuropsychiatr Genet 129:64–68, 2004

Zai G, Arnold P, Burroughs E, et al: Evidence for the gamma-amino-butyric acid type B receptor 1 (GABBR1) gene as a susceptibility factor in obsessive-compulsive disorder. Am J Med Genet B Neuropsychiatr Genet 134:25–29, 2005a

Zai G, Arnold P, Strauss J, et al: No association between brain-derived neurotrophic factor gene and obsessive-compulsive disorder. Psychiatr Genet 15:235, 2005b

Zai G, Arnold PD, Burroughs E, et al: Tumor necrosis factor-alpha gene is not associated with obsessive-compulsive disorder. Psychiatr Genet 16:43–45, 2006

7

NEUROLOGICAL CONSIDERATIONS

Autism and Parkinson's Disease

Eric Hollander, M.D.
A. Ting Wang, Ph.D.
Ashley Braun, B.A.
Laura Marsh, M.D.

Neurological disorders are frequently complicated by behavioral disturbances that involve obsessive-compulsive and related phenomena. Two seemingly disparate disorders, autism and Parkinson's disease, provide insights into the nosology of obsessive-compulsive spectrum phenomena. Autism, a neurodevelopmental disorder with onset prior to 3 years of age, and Parkinson's disease, a neurodegenerative disorder that occurs with aging, both manifest a spectrum of behavioral symptoms including compulsive-impulsive disturbances. Other interesting parallels between core features of autism and Parkinson's, respectively, include impaired theory of mind (Saltzman et al. 2000) and parkinsonian gait disturbances (Vilensky et al. 1981), suggesting shared pathology in frontal systems and the basal ganglia. This review focuses on the commonalities between obsessive-compulsive-related phe-

---

This chapter was first published as "Neurological Considerations: Autism and Parkinson's Disease." *Psychiatry Research* 170:43–51, 2009. Copyright 2009. Used with permission.

nomena in autism and Parkinson's disease to the extent that they provide insight into the pathophysiology and treatment of obsessive-compulsive-related disorders.

Phenomenology

AUTISM

Autism spectrum disorders (ASD), including autism, Asperger's syndrome, and pervasive development disorder not otherwise specified (PDD-NOS), are characterized by significant impairments in social communication and the presence of repetitive behaviors and restricted interests (American Psychiatric Association 2000). The repetitive behavior domain comprises phenomena that overlap significantly with those observed in OCD and obsessive-compulsive spectrum disorders (OCSDs) and can be conceptualized as higher- and lower-order repetitive behaviors (Hollander et al. 1998). Disruption of higher-order behaviors often leads to anxiety, whereas lower-order behaviors are often thought to moderate arousal. Along these lines, converging evidence supports the existence of higher- and lower-order subtypes of repetitive behaviors across individual patients. For example, factor analyses of relevant items in the Autism Diagnostic Interview–Revised yield two dimensions, described as "insistence on sameness/resistance to change" and "repetitive sensory and motor behaviors" (Cuccaro et al. 2003; Shao et al. 2003; Szatmari et al. 2006), respectively. However, a recent factor analysis of responses on the Yale-Brown Obsessive Compulsive Scale checklist in autism revealed four subtypes of symptoms, including obsessions, higher-order repetitive behaviors, lower-order repetitive behaviors, and hoarding (Anagnostou et al. 2005). The higher-order repetitive factor included ordering, washing, repeating, checking, ritualistic eating behaviors, and rituals involving others, which are all similar to compulsive behaviors seen in OCD and OCSDs. These higher-order repetitive behaviors have been associated with higher cognitive abilities in autism (Militerni et al. 2002). Lower-order repetitive behaviors, such as self-injurious behaviors and the need to touch or rub, are not as common in OCD but in fact may not be specific to autism, because these behaviors are also seen in children with mental retardation (Bodfish et al. 2000) and individuals with frontal lobe degeneration (Ames et al. 1994).

In OCD, obsessions and compulsions related to hoarding may be associated with a distinct biological and genetic profile and resistance to treatment with serotonin reuptake inhibitors (Lochner et al. 2005). Likewise, in autism, hoarding behaviors also seem to fall along a separate dimension within the repetitive behaviors domain. Although there appears to be overlap between the repetitive behaviors observed in autism and OCD, obsessions and compulsions in patients with autism may not be ego-dystonic or recognized as excessive or senseless. In addition, assessment of these symptoms can be difficult in patients with autism given its frequent association with mental retardation (although estimates of association vary from 26% to 80% of individuals; Lord and Volkmar 2002) and the fact that even high-functioning individuals with ASD show impairments in recognizing and talking about their mental states (Baron-Cohen et al. 1999).

PARKINSON'S DISEASE

A fundamental motor feature of Parkinson's disease is the inability to perform voluntary motor acts automatically (bradykinesia and akinesia), suggesting that the underlying neuropathological processes of the disorder affect striatal circuits integral to the generation and execution of programmed motor acts or habits (Graybiel 2004; Ridley 1994). Cognitively, deficits in set-shifting in patients with Parkinson's disease are somewhat analogous to motor deficits, representing a form of perseveration or inflexibility of mental activity and suggesting the additional involvement of frontal systems (Ridley 1994). Whereas these cognitive and motor features involve reduced behavioral output, obsessive-compulsive spectrum behavioral disturbances in Parkinson's disease involve the pathological overproduction of repetitive behaviors, some of which appear related to the combined effects of dopaminergic medications in the context of the underlying Parkinson's disease neuropathological processes.

Punding

Phenomenological overlap between the repetitive behaviors of autism and Parkinson's is most evident with a phenomenon called *punding* that is reported to occur in 1.4%–14% of patient samples (Evans et al. 2004; Fernandez and Friedman 1999; Friedman 1994; Miyasaki et al. 2007). *Punding,* a term initially used to refer to stereotyped behaviors in amphetamine and cocaine addicts, is generally thought to be associated with an excess of dopaminergic therapy in Parkinson's disease. It is characterized by intense engagement in purposeless repetitive activities such as dismantling and reassembling equipment (flashlights, appliances), picking at oneself, or handling, sorting and arranging objects (buttons, paperwork, pocketbook items, books on shelves).

There are many similarities between punding and OCD, but there are also important differences. Most notable is that punding behaviors are also influenced by gender and personal history (Evans et al. 2004). For example, past work or hobbies shape the type of behavior, such as a retired carpenter who performs unneeded home repairs and a woman who moves items in and out of her purse (Evans et al. 2004; Miwa and Kondo 2005). As a consequence of the time spent punding, activities such as eating, sleeping, and social obligations may be neglected. Similar to OCD, punding behaviors may or may not be recognized as pointless and disruptive by the patient, and they are usually more upsetting to others. In addition, punding behavior is often calming, whereas stopping the behavior (by self or others) is associated with irritability and dysphoria. An important difference from OCD is that punding behaviors are generally not intrusive, ego-alien, or resisted. Another difference is that punding is not associated with obsessions or the goal of preventing unwanted events. Finally, the punding behaviors are not rule bound or done in a rigid manner (i.e., not compulsive).

Obsessive-Compulsive Symptoms and Obsessive-Compulsive Disorder

Although higher-order obsessive-compulsive symptoms are common in individuals with autism, only a few studies on Parkinson's disease have examined obsessive-compulsive symptoms and OCD, and prevalence rates are less clear. Encephalitis lethargica frequently involves parkinsonism and obsessive-compulsive symptoms (Cheyette and Cummings 1995), but there is no evidence for increased rates of classic OCD in Parkinson's relative to that in the general population, which is about 2% (Harbishettar et al. 2005; Maia et al. 2003; Muller et al. 1997). This is in contrast to other anxiety disturbances, such as panic disorder, that occur at higher rates in patients with PD (Marsh 2000a). There are some reports showing higher rates of obsessive-compulsive symptoms in patients with Parkinson's disease based on obsessive-compulsive rating scale scores relative to norms (Alegret et al. 2001; Tomer et al. 1993), although studies with direct comparisons to matched control samples have not found higher rates of obsessive-compulsive symptoms in patients with Parkinson's disease (Maia et al. 2003; Muller et al. 1997).

Impulse-Control Disorders

The occurrence of impulse-control disorders (ICDs) in patients with Parkinson's disease has been increasingly recognized over the past decade (Potenza et al. 2007). The core feature of an ICD is the inability to resist an impulse, drive, or temptation that is harmful to the individual or others. The behaviors typically involve pleasurable or hedonic behaviors such as gambling, sex, eating, or shopping and are performed repetitively, excessively, or compulsively to the point of causing emotional or functional impairments (Potenza et al. 2007). Although behaviors initially are reward driven, over time they can be regarded as addictive in nature, and it can be difficult to distinguish whether the behavior is reward driven versus a programmed motor act that is performed compulsively in certain contexts (Ridley 1994). Estimated prevalence is around 6%–7%, with pathological gambling and hypersexuality each occurring in 2%–4% of the patients with Parkinson's disease (Potenza et al. 2007). However, prevalence approaches 14% in patients taking dopamine agonist therapy (Pontone et al. 2006; Voon et al. 2006); other specific clinical features are also associated with ICDs, such as a younger age, earlier onset of Parkinson's, impulsive personality traits, and a family or personal history of alcoholism (Potenza et al. 2007). The pathophysiology of ICDs is not understood but may involve individual susceptibility factors, the neurodegenerative effects of Parkinson's disease on striatal dopaminergic systems and habit learning, antiparkinsonian treatments, and interactions between these factors (Voon et al. 2007a, 2007b).

Obsessive-Compulsive Spectrum Behaviors in Autism and Parkinson's Disease: Shared Phenomenology

Pathological repetition is a common feature of obsessive-compulsive spectrum behavioral disturbances in both autism and Parkinson's disease, although the types of behavior occur at many different levels of function, including rituals, preoccupations, or inflexible activity (Ridley 1994). Using the nomenclature from the autism literature, the higher-order and lower-order repetitive behaviors and punding are the most salient obsessive-compulsive spectrum behaviors shared by patients with autism and Parkinson's. Although punding behaviors in Parkinson's disease have not been subtyped as higher- or lower-order in character, these behaviors appear to be, in large part, calming and thus similar to the anxiolytic effect of the repetitive behaviors seen in autism. It has not been examined whether punding in Parkinson's involves lower-order behaviors that moderate arousal or if such behaviors develop with progression of the disease and further cognitive deterioration, but this is worthy of investigation to the extent that there may be shared phenomena and treatment approaches. The ICDs appear to fall into a different class of behaviors in that they are highly complex and reward driven and, in that regard, are dissimilar to the stereotyped repetitive behaviors of autism. However, over time, the ICD behaviors can become more habitual and stimulus related (Lawrence et al. 2003), taking on characteristics of a disorder in motor programming (Ridley 1994). By contrast, although obsessions and compulsions occur in both autism and Parkinson's disease, the occurrence of obsessive-compulsive symptoms or OCD in individuals with Parkinson's appears largely coincidental as opposed to their being a core and required feature of the presentation of ASD in DSM-IV-TR (American Psychiatric Association 2000).

Comorbid Psychopathology

AUTISM

Comparisons of rates of comorbid psychopathology with obsessive-compulsive spectrum behaviors in autism relative to Parkinson's disease are limited in that most studies on obsessive-compulsive symptoms and OCD in the Parkinson's literature have not ascertained formal psychiatric diagnoses. A subgroup of patients with ASD and prominent OCD symptomatology may also have comorbid motor/ vocal tics (Kerbeshian and Burd 1996) and attention-deficit/hyperactivity disorder (Goldstein and Schwebach 2004), as is also seen in pediatric OCD. These comorbid conditions are known to reflect underlying dopaminergic dysfunction. In general, the comorbid psychopathology associated with autism and Parkinson's disease is similar in that mood and anxiety disorders are relatively common in each condition.

Like OCD, autism is associated with comorbid anxiety (Kim et al. 2000), mood disorders (Green et al. 2000; Kim et al. 2000), obsessional disorders (Green et al. 2000; Kim et al. 2000), attention-deficit/hyperactivity disorder (Goldstein and Schwebach 2004), Tourette's syndrome (Kerbeshian and Burd 1996), schizophrenia (Clarke et al. 1989; Tantam 1988), and problems with eating (Rastam et al. 2003). There also appears to be a high rate of body dysmorphic disorder in individuals with Asperger's syndrome (E. Hollander, personal opinion).

PARKINSON'S DISEASE

Although depressive and anxiety disorders are also common in Parkinson's disease (Marsh 2000b), these conditions do not appear to occur at increased rates in patients with obsessive-compulsive spectrum behaviors. Rather, the psychiatric comorbidities associated with punding include complications of hyperdopaminergic states such as ICDs, psychosis, and excessive use of dopaminergic medications resembling an addiction as well as motoric side effects such as extreme on/off fluctuations and dyskinesias (Evans et al. 2004; Kurlan 2004; Potenza et al. 2007). Some case reports suggest that punding may not be related exclusively to medications; in some cases, it appears more related to an association with greater cognitive impairment, namely executive dysfunction or dementia (Kurlan 2004).

One study (Harbishettar et al. 2005) that examined rates of other psychiatric diagnoses along with OCD found no differences in rates of OCD, obsessive-compulsive symptoms, or other psychiatric conditions between patients with Parkinson's disease and age- and sex-matched medically ill control subjects.

Patients with ICDs not uncommonly experience more than one ICD (Potenza et al. 2007) as well as abuse or overuse of dopaminergic therapy (Lawrence et al. 2003). Although depressed mood, irritability, and appetite changes are greater in intensity than in non-ICD Parkinson's, mood and anxiety disorders are not found in higher rates than in non-ICD patients (Pontone et al. 2006). Psychosis may also be present, but the behaviors are generally unrelated to the behavioral disturbance (Potenza et al. 2007). Medication-induced hypomania has also been reported (Voon et al. 2006).

Course of Illness

AUTISM

The onset of autism occurs prior to the age of 3 years. Autism is thought to be present from birth, although a small minority of parents report near-normal development in their children prior to a loss of social and communicative skills between 15 and 24 months of age (Davidovitch et al. 2000; Goldberg et al. 2003). Autism affects more males than females at a ratio of approximately four to one (Fombonne 2005). Although parents report some symptom improvement in adolescence as compared to middle childhood (McGovern and Sigman 2005), the disorder is chronic and lifelong. Autism shares some similarities in course with early onset OCD, which has a more prolonged course, occurs more often in boys than girls, and is more often associated with tics than other OCSDs.

As far as the time course of repetitive thoughts and behaviors in autism, as well as other OCSDs, in patients with ASD there is a general progression from lower-order to higher-order behaviors over the course of development. For example, very young children tend to have self-stimulatory perseverative behaviors designed to regulate arousal, such as hand flapping, lining objects up, opening and closing doors, turning on and off light switches, and tantrums in response to changes in rigid routines. Comorbid OCSDs early on might include trichotillomania, or hair-pulling, designed to regulate arousal. As children age, there is an increase in the higher-order OCD-like behaviors designed to regulate anxiety, such as checking, washing, counting, and asking for reassurance. Comorbid OCSDs at this later age might include body dysmorphic disorder, with obsessional focus on body image, and rituals involving grooming and checking (E. Hollander, personal opinion).

PARKINSON'S DISEASE

Parkinson's disease typically begins in later life, with the average age of onset around age 60, although 5%–10% of patients may develop symptoms before age 40, defined as young-onset Parkinson's disease (Korell and Tanner 2005). The course of obsessive-compulsive spectrum behaviors in Parkinson's has not been examined comprehensively. For some disturbances, it appears that antiparkinsonian treatments can influence their course. A number of reports, including the original description of the disease by James Parkinson in 1817, describe the tendency for patients who develop Parkinson's disease to have premorbid personality traits of industriousness, punctuality, orderliness, inflexibility, cautiousness, and low novelty-seeking (Menza et al. 1990). Although the concept of a "Parkinsonian personality" remains controversial, and there is considerable variability in personality qualities among patients with the disorder, several studies, including a study of twins (Ward et al. 1984), provide general support for the presence of this personality profile both premorbidly and as persistent features after disease onset (Menza 2005). It is possible that such traits reduce the susceptibility to development of ICDs, given that impulsive personality traits are a reported risk factor for ICDs (Potenza et al. 2007).

In cases of punding, the course of disease in affected individuals has not been studied. It appears to be more common in patients taking higher dosages of dopaminergic medications (Evans et al. 2004). However, disparities in prevalence, lack of data on effective treatments, and the fact that the behavior is frequently unreported or unrecognized limit speculation on its overall course. However, personal observations suggest that punding behaviors tend to be chronic, with the intensity associated with circumstances and opportunity as well as the antiparkinsonian regimen. ICDs can develop into chronic conditions, although there is often improvement after adjusting the antiparkinsonian regimen (Mamikonyan et al. 2008).

Family History

AUTISM

Autism is one of the most heritable of all behavioral disorders. Twin studies show a concordance rate of 60%–90% in monozygotic twins, which drops to less than 5% for dizygotic twins (Bailey et al. 1995; Rutter et al. 1999). The risk of ASD in siblings of individuals with autism is estimated at 6% (Icasiano et al. 2004), whereas the risk for broader phenotype traits (including poor social language abilities, restricted interests/OCD type traits) in first-degree relatives is approximately 30% (Murphy et al. 2000; Pickles et al. 2000).

OCD has been noted to be significantly more common in relatives of autistic probands than in relatives of Down's syndrome probands (Bolton et al. 1998). With respect to repetitive behaviors in particular, one study found that parents of children with autism who scored high on the repetitive behavior domain were more likely to have obsessive-compulsive traits or OCD than parents of children who scored low on this domain (Hollander et al. 2003b). Similarly, Abramson et al. (2005) observed a positive correlation between obsessive-compulsive behaviors in parents and repetitive behaviors falling under an "insistence on sameness" factor based on the Autism Diagnostic Interview probands with autism. Finally, Silverman et al. (2000) found reduced variation within families for the severity of repetitive behaviors, particularly those associated with OCD (i.e., unusual preoccupations, verbal and nonverbal rituals and compulsions, circumscribed interests) as opposed to lower-level stereotypies.

PARKINSON'S DISEASE

The family history of psychiatric disturbances among patients with Parkinson's disease has not been extensively studied. A recent analysis suggests that depressive disorders and anxiety disorders may share familial susceptibility factors with Parkinson's (Arabia et al. 2007). A family history of alcoholism is associated with ICDs (Potenza et al. 2007), but there is no apparent increased rate of a family history of ICDs in Parkinson's patients.

Genetic Factors

AUTISM

In a subsample of individuals with more severe obsessive-compulsive behaviors, linkage analysis revealed evidence for an autism susceptibility gene on chromosomes 1, 6, and 19 (Buxbaum et al. 2004). As with OCD, there is some support for an association with the serotonin transporter gene *SLC6A/5-HTT.* Three recent genome scans have reported linkage evidence to 17q11–12, where *SLC6A* is located (Cantor et al. 2005; McCauley et al. 2004; Risch et al. 1999), but evidence for association with the *5-HTTLPR* polymorphism is mixed (Conroy et al. 2004; Devlin et al. 2005; Kim et al. 2002; Yirmiya et al. 2001) and negative (Maestrini et al. 1999; Ramoz et al. 2006; Wu et al. 2005; Zhong et al. 1999). Likewise, evidence for the involvement of GABA-A receptor subunit genes is inconsistent, with the most common positive findings within *GABRB3* (Buxbaum et al. 2002; McCauley et al. 2004). Overall, regions from chromosome 7q and 2q are the most frequently cited as having the strongest evidence for linkage across studies. Recently, Silverman et al. (2008) found that a mitochondrial aspartate/glutamate carrier polymorphism (chromosome 2) was associated with levels of routines and rituals in individuals with autism. With respect to chromosome 7, *NrCAM* is a candidate gene located on chromosome 7 with a specific haplotype that has been associated with substance abuse and is expressed in brain regions related to reward. Sakurai et al. (2006) observed a significant overtransmission of this haplotype in families with severe obsessive-compulsive behaviors.

PARKINSON'S DISEASE

Genetic factors associated with obsessive-compulsive spectrum disturbances in Parkinson's disease have not been studied. In patients with ICDs, genetic factors under consideration include functional polymorphisms of genes that regulate central dopaminergic transmission—for example, the catechol-O-methyltransferase gene (*COMT;* Foltynie et al. 2004)—and the role of genetic variation in the *DRD1* gene and interactions between genetic variants of dopamine receptor genes in addictive behaviors (Comings et al. 1997).

Brain Circuitry

The common occurrence of obsessive-compulsive spectrum behaviors in autism and Parkinson's disease as well as other neurological disorders involving the basal ganglia, such as Huntington's disease, provides support for the role of basal ganglia dysfunction in idiopathic OCD (Rauch et al. 1998) and suggests shared neural mechanisms, at least in part, across seemingly disparate conditions (Graybiel 2004). For example, both autism and Parkinson's disease involve multiple brain regions, and proposed models of dysfunctional neurocircuitry in both conditions implicate cortico-striatal-thalamic-cortical circuits, but how the various corticostriatal circuits mediate obsessive-compulsive spectrum behaviors in autism and Parkinson's disease is probably different (Graybiel 2004; Harbishettar et al. 2005).

The most obvious difference between autism and Parkinson's disease is the dynamic nature of the neuropathology of the latter, a neurodegenerative disorder in which there is a discrete and progressive deficit of dopamine production in the substantia nigra, leading to loss of striatal dopamine, and effective symptomatic treatment with exogenous dopamine. Conversely, autism occurs early in life, is nonprogressive, and lacks consistent evidence for microscopic pathological changes, discrete neurotransmitter deficits, or direct symptomatic treatments.

However, there is converging evidence that striatal dysfunction and hyperdopaminergic states play a role in certain repetitive behaviors seen in both disorders. Considerable evidence implicates the dorsal striatum and related interneurons in procedural learning and the establishment of behavioral routines (or habits) in mammals. That evidence supports hypotheses that functional deficits and abnormal activation of striatal circuits underlie behavioral disturbances along the obsessive-compulsive spectrum, ranging from stereotypies and rituals to addiction (Graybiel 2004; Ridley 1994).

AUTISM

Neuroimaging studies have shown abnormalities in many of the same areas in which differences have been described in OCD, including the basal ganglia, anterior cingulate, dorsolateral and orbitofrontal cortex, and thalamus. However, as with OCD, there is no single brain region identified as the primary structural or functional "lesion" site associated with autism. In a recent meta-analysis, Stanfield et al. (2008) found consistent evidence of increased size of the cerebral hemispheres, the cerebellum, and the caudate nucleus as well as an increase in total brain volume associated with autism. In contrast, the size of the corpus callosum was decreased in autism. Interestingly, repetitive behavior (but not social or communication dysfunction) appears to be correlated with caudate volume within individuals with autism (Hollander et al. 2005a; Sears et al. 1999). With respect to the anterior cingulate, both hypometabolism and reduced volume have been observed in this region in individuals with autism and Asperger's syndrome relative to healthy control subjects using positron emission tomography (PET), magnetic resonance imaging, and single-photon emission computed tomography (Haznedar et al. 1997, 2000; Ohnishi et al. 2000). Additionally, functional magnetic resonance imaging during a response inhibition task yielded reduced activity in the anterior cingulate in high-functioning individuals with autism compared with control subjects (Anagnostou et al. 2006). Moreover, using diffusion tensor imaging, disruption of white matter in the anterior cingulate has been observed (Barnea-Goraly et al. 2004), similar to that recently found in OCD (Szeszko et al. 2005). In prefrontal regions, activation differences have been detected in the orbitofrontal cortex during a theory of mind task (Baron-Cohen et al. 1999) as well as the dorsolateral prefrontal cortex during a spatial working memory task (Luna et al. 2002) and various executive functioning tasks (Schmitz et al. 2006). Chugani et al. (1997) found abnormalities in the frontal cortex, thalamus, and dentate nucleus in seven autistic boys relative to unaffected siblings using PET. Abnormality in thalamic activity compared with control subjects has also been observed during language and emotion processing tasks (Hall et al. 2003; Muller et al. 1999).

Taken together, the evidence discussed here is consistent with dysfunction of the cortico-striato-thalamic neural pathway underlying executive functioning and proposed to be aberrant in models of OCD. That abnormalities in these brain regions are associated with repetitive behaviors in autism and OCD (as well as Tourette's syndrome) further suggests that dysfunction in this circuitry may be important for the expression of repetitive behaviors across disorders. However, it should be noted that the direction of the abnormalities noted (i.e., increases or decreases in size and activation of the implicated brain regions) is inconsistent both within and across disorders. A complete model of the neuropathology underlying repetitive behaviors will need to be able to explain these differences.

PARKINSON'S DISEASE

Neuroimaging studies of idiopathic OCD have identified consistent metabolic abnormalities in the orbitofrontal cortex, anterior cingulate, caudal medial prefrontal cortex, and striatum (Rauch et al. 1998). Orbitofrontal dysfunction in OCD is supported by direct impairments on tasks that assess orbitofrontal functions. By contrast, evidence for striatal dysfunction in OCD is based on PET studies showing relative increases in hippocampal metabolism, rather than the striatum, during a procedural (implicit) learning task, suggesting recruitment of brain regions involved in explicit memory functions in order to complete the task (Graybiel and Rauch 2000). Patients with Parkinson's disease are also impaired on procedural learning tasks for which explicit processing probably impairs, rather than assists, acquisition (Joel et al. 2005) However, this deficit in Parkinson's disease most likely reflects a defective procedural learning mechanism resulting from degeneration of the nigrostriatal dopaminergic pathway. In addition, whereas increased indirect activation via the sensorimotor loop, with projections from sensorimotor cortex to the putamen, is thought to underlie Parkinsonian motor features in the setting of a dopamine deficit, the addition of dopaminergic medications in this setting influences the balance of direct (stimulatory) and indirect (inhibitory) stimulation to the thalamus (Rauch and Savage 1997). The emergence of problematic obsessive-compulsive spectrum behaviors in patients with Parkinson's may thus be associated with excess dopaminergic stimulation via the direct path, relative to the indirect pathway, within the limbic loop.

The neural circuitry underlying punding is thought to involve disordered motor programming in basal ganglia and the development of behavioral stereotypies related to interactions between ventral and dorsal striatal systems (Evans et al. 2004). A leading theory is that hyperdopaminergic stimulation in Parkinson's disease results in indiscriminate activation of the direct versus indirect pathway, which leads to these compulsive-like behaviors (Kurlan 2004). However, greater neurodegeneration in cases of punding is also suspected because behaviors frequently persist even after dopaminergic therapy is reduced. It is possible this observation involves hippocampal degeneration in patients with Parkinson's disease, in contrast to patients with idiopathic OCD, who show compensatory increases in hippocampal activity in the setting of normal performance on procedural learning tasks (Rauch and Savage 1997).

Although two reports describe associations between obsessive-compulsive symptoms and greater left-sided Parkinson's disease symptoms, implicating a role for right hemispheric dysfunction (Maia et al. 2003; Tomer et al. 1993), the lack of an increased occurrence of obsessive-compulsive symptoms or OCD in patients with Parkinson's disease suggests that different corticostriatal pathways are involved in the underlying pathology of Parkinson's relative to idiopathic OCD (Harbishettar et al. 2005). This is in contrast to autism, in which the more classic obsessive-compulsive phenomena appear to have greater similarities with OCD in terms of the relevant neural circuitry (Hollander et al. 2005a) and pharmacological response (Hollander et al. 2005b).

Dysfunction in different corticostriatal circuits for the OCD phenomena in PD versus punding and ICD behaviors in Parkinson's disease is further supported by two separate reports describing improvement of OCD after bilateral deep brain stimulation (Fontaine et al. 2004; Mallet et al. 2002). Mallet et al. (2002) described rapid resolution of compulsions and improvement in obsessions in two patients with Parkinson's disease and longstanding primary OCD who underwent bilateral deep brain stimulation with electrodes placed in the anteromedial subthalamic nucleus and zona incerta. Although dopaminergic medications were also reduced postoperatively, the authors suggested that the improvement of OCD symptoms was related to stimulatory effects that inhibited limbic striato-pallido-subthalamo-pallido-thalamo-cortical circuits. Specifically, the inhibitory effects on the medial limbic tip of the subthalamic nucleus (part of the indirect pathway within the corticostriatal-thalamic-cortical circuit) had a greater influence than stimulatory effects on serotonergic fibers to the frontal cortex from the zona incerta (Mallet et al. 2002). In these cases, thus, it appears that the locations of the surgical lesions, rather than primary Parkinson's disease–related pathology, are related to the development and improvement of OCD phenomena.

A number of corticostriatal systems and neurotransmitters are implicated in the development of ICDs (Sood et al. 2003). Particularly implicated is dysfunction of the mesolimbic dopaminergic system, which is associated with cognitive and reward-related processing, and its related limbic-corticostriatal-thalamic circuit, specifically orbitofrontal cortex in mood state. Serotonergic dysfunction is implicated because of its role in harm avoidance and impulsivity; the noradrenergic system has a role in arousal and novelty-seeking behaviors that may also be relevant to development or maintenance of ICDs.

Although reduced novelty-seeking and increased harm avoidance are more common among Parkinson's disease patients (Czernecki et al. 2002), treatment-induced stimulation of mesolimbic dopamine receptors appears to influence novelty- and reward-seeking behaviors, including impulsivity. In experimental studies, dopamine replacement therapy improves or impairs neuropsychological functioning, depending on the nature of the task and the basal level of dopamine function in corticostriatal circuitry (Cools et al. 2003), and may underlie fluctuating effects of dopaminergic medications on cognitive and behavioral functions. A PET study of patients with compulsive use of dopaminergic medications suggests sensitization to levodopa effects, because there was enhanced levodopa-induced ventral striatal dopamine release compared with levodopa-treated patients with Parkinson's disease not compulsively taking dopaminergic drugs (Evans et al. 2006). Other brain regions in the limbic corticostriatal–thalamic circuit that interact with the mesolimbic dopamine pathway are also involved in ICDs (Chau et al. 2004). For example, the orbitofrontal cortex is implicated in decision making and emotional-related learning and is involved in the representation of abstract rewards and punishments, such as winning and losing money.

Pharmacological Dissection

AUTISM

Some commonalities exist between OCD and autism in terms of neurotransmitter function and pharmacological response. Hollander et al. (2000) observed that the severity of repetitive behaviors in adults with autism or Asperger's syndrome was linked to serotonin function as measured by 5-HT_{1D} receptor sensitivity. In addition, PET revealed an increase in 5-HT_{2A} receptors in patients with autism relative to control subjects (E. Hollander and M. Laruelle, unpublished data). Clearly, dopaminergic dysfunction may also play a prominent role both in OCD (Hollander et al. 2003a) and autism (McCracken et al. 2002), because both conditions have a favorable response to atypical antipsychotic agents such as risperidone. Overall, selective serotonin reuptake inhibitors (SSRIs) appear to be effective in decreasing repetitive behaviors and anxiety and improving global functioning in autism spectrum disorders. Thus far, randomized, controlled clinical trials have observed an improvement in overall functioning as well as in symptoms in the repetitive behavior domain following treatment with fluoxetine (Buchsbaum et al. 2001; Hollander et al. 2005b) and fluvoxamine (McDougle et al. 1996). Side effects were generally mild, although increased agitation occurred in some patients. Also similar to what has been observed in OCD, clomipramine appears to be more effective than desipramine in reducing stereotyped and repetitive behaviors (Gordon et al. 1993). In addition, consistent with a role for hyperdopaminergic dysfunction, McCracken et al. (2002) found that children treated with risperidone were more likely than those in the placebo group to have reductions in aggressive symptoms, as well as stereotypy and hyperactivity, but not in symptoms of social withdrawal. Lastly, divalproex treatment has also been associated with significant improvement in repetitive behaviors in children with ASD (Hollander et al. 2006).

PARKINSON'S DISEASE

Although the pathognomic neurotransmitter deficit in Parkinson's disease involves dopamine, the disease also involves changes in serotonergic and noradrenergic neurotransmission (Jellinger 1999). The pharmacology of OCD and obsessive-compulsive symptoms in Parkinson's, however, has not been specifically studied. Although SSRIs can be used to treat obsessive-compulsive symptoms in Parkinson's disease, dopamine antagonists, used for idiopathic obsessive-compulsive symptoms, would not be tolerated in Parkinson's patients (Marsh 2000b). Given its appearance in amphetamine or cocaine abusers, punding appears most associated with excessive dopaminergic tone related to dopamine replacement therapy. Similarly, ICDs are associated with all antiparkinsonian treatments, particularly dopamine agonists, suggesting that a fundamental feature of both punding and ICDs in Parkinson's disease is hyperdopaminergic tone. In contrast to the stereotypies of autism, however, there is an apparent lack of response to SSRIs in patients with punding or ICDs (Evans et al. 2004; Potenza et al. 2007), suggesting a diminished pathophysiological role of serotonin when these repetitive behaviors occur in patients with Parkinson's disease.

Interventional Treatments
AUTISM

Vagus nerve stimulation, repetitive transcranial magnetic stimulation (rTMS), and deep brain stimulation have all been examined as treatment options for OCD. A couple of preliminary studies with small numbers of subjects suggest that participants with "autistic behaviors" may show behavioral improvements following vagus nerve stimulation (Park 2003), but the subjects in these studies were poorly characterized. With regard to rTMS, because of a couple of reports of the effectiveness of rTMS for treating catatonia combined with a link to serotonergic autoreceptor activity in the rat brain, it has been theorized that rTMS may be effective for autism (Tsai 2005), but there is no direct evidence yet to support this suggestion. Moreover, rTMS does not seem to be effective for treating OCD. Likewise, deep brain stimulation has not yet been examined as a treatment option for autism, although there are reports of success with this approach for treatment-resistant OCD. Mayberg et al. (2005) have successfully used deep brain stimulation for treatment-resistant depression, targeting the subgenual cingulate region (BA 25). Interestingly, hyperactivation of the subgenual cingulate relative to healthy control subjects has been noted during a response inhibition task (Anagnostou et al. 2006), which suggests that this region could potentially be a target for treatment-resistant autism.

PARKINSON'S DISEASE

Pharmacological and psychotherapeutic interventions for OCD in Parkinson's disease have not been studied explicitly. Treatment of obsessive-compulsive symptoms in Parkinson's disease is generally not indicated, unless the symptoms are clinically significant or there is a primary mood disorder, in which case the treatments would involve similar strategies as for idiopathic OCD or mood syndromes (Marsh 2000a and personal observation). Recommended treatments for punding include education about the role of high doses of dopaminergic medications, adjustments in the antiparkinsonian regiment, rationing of Parkinson's medications, and behavioral and pharmacological treatments aimed at improving associated insomnia (Evans et al. 2004). There is little empirical evidence on treatment of ICDs in Parkinson's disease (Potenza et al. 2007). Recommended strategies include adjustments in antiparkinsonian medications, with reductions in dopamine agonists if used; psychotherapeutic approaches; and various pharmacological treatments, including atypical antipsychotic agents, opioid antagonists, and SSRIs (Potenza et al. 2007). Reports on the effectiveness of SSRIs for repetitive behaviors in Parkinson's disease have not been favorable (Kurlan 2004).

Cross-National/Ethnic

AUTISM

Cross-cultural issues have not yet been well studied, but autism appears to occur across all ethnicities and nationalities. Although it has been theorized that autism is more prevalent among immigrant families (e.g., Gillberg et al. 1987), these reports have relied on a very small sample size. A large epidemiological survey in the United Kingdom found no differences for ethnicity in the prevalence of pervasive developmental disorders, including autism (Fombonne 2005).

PARKINSON'S DISEASE

Published reports from multiple nations indicate that all of the OCSDs (punding, obsessive-compulsive symptoms, OCD, and ICDs) are present cross-nationally with common features, including in Canada (Miyasaki et al. 2007; Voon et al. 2007a, 2007b), France (Mallet et al. 2002), Great Britain (Evans et al. 2004), Spain (Alegret et al. 2001), Brazil (Maia et al. 2003), Germany (Muller et al. 1997), and the United States (Pontone et al. 2006; Tomer et al. 1993).

Conclusion

Obsessive-compulsive spectrum behaviors occur in Parkinson's disease and in autism and the ASDs, including Asperger's syndrome and PDD-NOS. The phenomenological similarities in repetitive behaviors occurring across conditions, especially punding in Parkinson's disease and stereotypies in the autistic disorders, suggest shared pathology with idiopathic OCD and the obsessive-compulsive spectrum. For autism, other important similarities with OCD are seen in the areas of comorbidity, course of illness, family history, pathophysiology, and treatment response, suggesting a close relationship between these disorders, which include serotonergic dysfunction. In Parkinson's disease, however, the obsessive-compulsive spectrum disturbances that occur at an increased rate, namely punding and ICDs, are primarily related to hyperdopaminergic states and striatal dysfunction. Accordingly, shared neural mechanisms underlying these disturbances in Parkinson's disease, autism, and OCD are probably limited to dopaminergic dysfunction and discrete aspects of cortico-striatal-thalamic circuitry.

References

Abramson R, Ravan S, Wright H, et al: The relationship between restrictive and repetitive behaviors in individuals with autism and obsessive compulsive symptoms in parents. Child Psychiatry Hum Dev 36:155–165, 2005

Alegret M, Junqué C, Valldeoriola F, et al: Obsessive-compulsive symptoms in Parkinson's disease. J Neurol Neurosurg Psychiatry 70:394–396, 2001

American Psychiatric Association: Diagnostic and Statistical Manual of Mental Disorders, 4th Edition, Text Revision. Washington, DC, American Psychiatric Association, 2000

Ames D, Cummings JL, Wirshing WC, et al: Repetitive and compulsive behavior in frontal lobe degenerations. J Neuropsychiatry Clin Neurosci 6:100–113, 1994

Anagnostou E, ChaplinW, Watner D, et al: Factor analysis of repetitive behaviors as measured by the Y-BOCS in autism. Neuropsychopharmacology 30:S153, 2005

Anagnostou E, Fan J, Soorya LV, et al: fMRI of response inhibition in ASD. Paper presented at the International Meeting for Autism Research, Montreal, Canada, June 2006

Arabia G, Grossardt BR, Geda YE, et al: Increased risk of depressive and anxiety disorders in relatives of patients with Parkinson disease. Arch Gen Psychiatry 64:1385–1392, 2007

Bailey A, Le Couteur A, Gottesman I, et al: Autism as a strongly genetic disorder: evidence from a British twin study. Psychol Med 25:63–77, 1995

Barnea-Goraly N, Kwon H, Menon V, et al: White matter structure in autism: preliminary evidence from diffusion tensor imaging. Biol Psychiatry 55:323–326, 2004

Baron-Cohen S, Ring HA, Wheelwright S, et al: Social intelligence in the normal and autistic brain: an fMRI study. Eur J Neurosci 11:1891–1898, 1999

Bodfish JW, Symons FJ, Parker DE, et al: Varieties of repetitive behavior in autism: comparisons to mental retardation. J Autism Dev Disord 30:237–243, 2000

Bolton PF, Pickles A, Murphy M, et al: Autism, affective and other psychiatric disorders: patterns of familial aggregation. Psychol Med 28:385–395, 1998

Buchsbaum MS, Hollander E, Haznedar MM, et al: Effect of fluoxetine on regional cerebral metabolism in autistic spectrum disorders: a pilot study. Int J Neuropsychopharmacol 4:119–125, 2001

Buxbaum JD, Silverman JM, Smith CJ, et al: Association between a GABRB3 polymorphism and autism. Mol Psychiatry 7:311–316, 2002

Buxbaum JD, Silverman J, Keddache M, et al: Linkage analysis for autism in a subset families with obsessive-compulsive behaviors: evidence for an autism susceptibility gene on chromosome 1 and further support for susceptibility genes on chromosome 6 and 19. Mol Psychiatry 9:144–150, 2004

Cantor RM, Kono N, Duvall JA, et al: Replication of autism linkage: fine-mapping peak at 17q21. Am J Hum Genet 76:1050–1056, 2005

Chau DT, Roth RM, Green AI: The neural circuitry of reward and its relevance to psychiatric disorders. Curr Psychiatry Rep 6:391–399, 2004

Cheyette SR, Cummings JL: Encephalitis lethargica: lessons for contemporary neuropsychiatry. J Neuropsychiatry Clin Neurosci 7:125–134, 1995

Chugani DC, Muzik O, Rothermel R, et al: Altered serotonin synthesis in the dentatothalamocortical pathway in autistic boys. Ann Neurol 42:666–699, 1997

Clarke DJ, LittleJohns CS, Corbett JA, et al: Pervasive developmental disorders and psychoses in adult life. Br J Psychiatry 155:692–699, 1989

Comings DE, Gade R, Wu S, et al: Studies of the potential role of the dopamine D1 receptor gene in addictive behaviors. Mol Psychiatry 2:44–56, 1997

Conroy J, Meally E, Kearney G, et al: Serotonin transporter gene and autism: a haplotype analysis in an Irish autistic population. Mol Psychiatry 9:587–593, 2004

Cools R, Barker RA, Sahakian BJ, et al: L-Dopa medication remediates cognitive inflexibility, but increases impulsivity in patients with Parkinson's disease. Neuropsychologia 41:1431–1441, 2003

Cuccaro ML, Shao Y, Grubber J, et al: Factor analysis of restricted and repetitive behaviors in autism using the Autism Diagnostic Interview-R. Child Psychiatry Hum Dev 34:3–17, 2003

Czernecki V, Pillon B, Houeto JL, et al: Motivation, reward, and Parkinson's disease: influence of dopatherapy. Neuropsychologia 40:2257–2267, 2002

Davidovitch M, Glick L, Holtzman G, et al: Developmental regression in autism: maternal perception. J Autism Dev Disord 30:113–119, 2000

Devlin B, Cook EH Jr, Coon H, et al: Autism and the serotonin transporter: the long and short of it. Mol Psychiatry 10:1110–1116, 2005

Evans AH, Katzenshlager R, Paviour D, et al: Punding in Parkinson's disease: its relation to the dopamine dysregulation syndrome. Mov Disord 19:397–405, 2004

Evans AH, Pavese N, Lawrence AD, et al: Compulsive drug use linked to sensitized ventral striatal dopamine transmission. Ann Neurol 59:852–858, 2006

Fernandez HH, Friedman J: Punding on L-dopa. Mov Disord 14:836–838, 1999

Foltynie T, Goldberg TE, Lewis SG, et al: Planning ability in Parkinson's disease is influenced by the COMT val158met polymorphism. Mov Disord 19:885–891, 2004

Fombonne E: Epidemiology of autistic disorder and other pervasive developmental disorders. J Clin Psychiatry 66(suppl):3–8, 2005

Fontaine D, Mattei V, Borg M, et al: Effect of subthalamic nucleus stimulation on obsessive-compulsive disorder in a patient with Parkinson disease: case report. J Neurosurg 100:1084–1086, 2004

Friedman JH: Punding on levodopa. Biol Psychiatry 36:350–351, 1994

Gillberg C, Steffenburg S, Borjesson B, et al: Infantile autism in children of immigrant parents: a population-based study from Goteborg, Sweden. Br J Psychiatry 150:856–858, 1987

Goldberg WA, Osann K, Filipek PA, et al: Language and other regression: assessment and timing. J Autism Dev Disord 33:607–616, 2003

Goldstein S, Schwebach AJ: The comorbidity of pervasive developmental disorder and attention deficit hyperactivity disorder: results of a retrospective chart review. J Autism Dev Disord 34:329–339, 2004

Gordon CT, State RC, Nelson JE, et al: A double-blind comparison of clomipramine, desipramine, and placebo in the treatment of autistic disorder. Arch Gen Psychiatry 50:441–447, 1993

Graybiel AM: Network-level neuroplasticity in cortico-basal ganglia pathways. Parkinsonism Relat Disord 10:293–296, 2004

Graybiel AM, Rauch SL: Toward a neurobiology of obsessive-compulsive disorder. Neuron 28:343–347, 2000

Green J, Gilchrist A, Burton D, et al: Social and psychiatric functioning in adolescents with Asperger syndrome compared with conduct disorder. J Autism Dev Disord 30:279–293, 2000

Hall GB, Szechtman H, Nahmias C: Enhanced salience and emotion recognition in autism: a PET study. Am J Psychiatry 160:1439–1441, 2003

Harbishettar V, Pal PK, Janardhan Reddy YC, et al: Is there a relationship between Parkinson's disease and obsessive-compulsive disorder? Parkinsonism Relat Disord 11:85–88, 2005

Haznedar MM, Buchsbaum MS, Metzger M, et al: Anterior cingulate gyrus volume and glucose metabolism in autistic disorder. Am J Psychiatry 154:1047–1050, 1997

Haznedar MM, Buchsbaum MS, Wei TC, et al: Limbic circuitry in patients with autism spectrum disorders studied with positron emission tomography and magnetic resonance imaging. Am J Psychiatry 157:1994–2001, 2000

Hollander E, Cartwright C, Wong C, et al: A dimensional approach to the autism spectrum. CNS Spectr 3:22–39, 1998

Hollander E, Novotny S, Allen A, et al: The relationship between repetitive behaviors and growth hormone response to sumatriptan challenge in adult autistic disorder. Neuropsychopharmacology 22:163–167, 2000

Hollander E, Baldini Rossi N, Sood E, et al: Risperidone augmentation in treatment-resistant obsessive compulsive disorder: a double-blind, placebo controlled trial. Int J Neuropsychopharmacol 6:397–400, 2003a

Hollander E, King A, Delaney K, et al: Obsessive-compulsive behaviors in parents of multiplex autism families. Psychiatry Res 117:11–16, 2003b

Hollander E, Anagnostou E, Chaplin W, et al: Striatal volume on magnetic resonance imaging and repetitive behaviors in autism. Biol Psychiatry 58:226–232, 2005a

Hollander E, Phillips A, Chaplin W, et al: A placebo controlled crossover trial of liquid fluoxetine on repetitive behaviors in childhood and adolescent autism. Neuropsychopharmacology 30:582–589, 2005b

Hollander E, Soorya L, Wasserman S, et al: Divalproex sodium vs. placebo in the treatment of repetitive behaviours in autism spectrum disorder. Int J Neuropsychopharmacol 9:209–213, 2006

Icasiano F, Hewson P, Machet P, et al: Childhood autism spectrum disorder in the Barwon region: a community based study. J Paediatr Child Health 40:696–701, 2004

Jellinger KA: Neuropathological correlates of mental dysfunction in Parkinson's disease: an update, in Mental Dysfunction in Parkinson's Disease. Edited by Wolters EC, Scheltens PH, Berendse HW. Utrecht, The Netherlands, Academic Pharmaceutical Productions BV, 1999, pp 82–105

Joel D, Zohar O, Afek M, et al: Impaired procedural learning in obsessive-compulsive disorder and Parkinson's disease, but not in major depressive disorder. Behav Brain Res 157:253–263, 2005

Kerbeshian J, Burd L: Case study: comorbidity among Tourette's syndrome, autistic disorder, and bipolar disorder. J Am Acad Child Adolesc Psychiatry 35:681–685, 1996

Kim J-A, Szatmari P, Bryson S-E, et al: The prevalence of anxiety and mood problems among children with autism and Asperger syndrome. Autism 4:117–132, 2000

Kim SJ, Cox N, Courchesne R, et al: Transmission disequilibrium mapping at the serotonin transporter gene (slc6a4) region in autistic disorder. Mol Psychiatry 7:278–288, 2002

Korell M, Tanner CM: Epidemiology of Parkinson's disease: an overview, in Parkinson's Disease. Edited by Ebadi MPR. Boca Raton, FL, CRC Press, 2005, pp 39–50

Kurlan R: Disabling repetitive behaviors in Parkinson's disease. Mov Disord 19:433–469, 2004

Lawrence AD, Evans AH, Lees AJ: Compulsive use of dopamine replacement therapy in Parkinson's disease: reward systems gone awry? Lancet Neurol 2:595–604, 2003

Lochner C, Kinnear CJ, Hemmings SM, et al: Hoarding in obsessive-compulsive disorder: clinical and genetic correlates. J Clin Psychiatry 66:1155–1160, 2005

Lord C, Volkmar F: Genetics of childhood disorders, XLII. Autism, part 1: diagnosis and assessment in autistic spectrum disorders. J Am Acad Child Adolesc Psychiatry 41:1134–1136, 2002

Luna B, Minshew NJ, Garver KE, et al: Neocortical system abnormalities in autism: an fMRI study of spatial working memory. Neurology 59:834–840, 2002

Maestrini E, Lai C, Marlow A, et al: Serotonin transporter (5-HTT) and gamma-aminobutyric acid receptor subunit beta3 (gabrb3) gene polymorphisms are not associated with autism in the IMGSA families. The International Molecular Genetic Study of Autism Consortium. Am J Med Genet 88:492–496, 1999

Maia AF, Pinto AS, Barbosa ER, et al: Obsessive-compulsive symptoms, obsessive-compulsive disorder related disorders in Parkinson's disease. J Neuropsychiatry Clin Neurosci 15:371–374, 2003

Mallet L, Mesnage V, Houeto JL, et al: Compulsions, Parkinson's disease, and stimulation. Lancet 360:1302–1304, 2002

Mamikonyan E, Siderowf AD, Dusa JE, et al: Long-term follow-up of impulse control disorders in Parkinson's disease. Mov Disord 23:75–80, 2008

Marsh L: Anxiety disorders in Parkinson's disease. Int Rev Psychiatry 12:307–318, 2000a

Marsh L: Neuropsychiatric aspects of Parkinson's disease. Psychosomatics 41:15–23, 2000b

Mayberg HS, Lozano AM, Voon V, et al: Deep brain stimulation for treatment-resistant depression. Neuron 45:651–660, 2005

McCauley JL, Olson LM, Dowd M, et al: Linkage and association analysis at the serotonin transporter (slc6a4) locus in a rigid-compulsive subset of autism. Am J Med Genet B Neuropsychiatr Genet 127:104–112, 2004

McCracken JT, McGough J, Shah B, et al: Risperidone in children with autism and serious behavioral problems. N Engl J Med 347:314–321, 2002

McDougle CJ, Naylor ST, Cohen DJ, et al: A double-blind, placebo-controlled study of fluvoxamine in adults with autistic disorder. Arch Gen Psychiatry 53:1001–1008, 1996

McGovern CW, Sigman M: Continuity and change from early childhood to adolescence in autism. J Child Psychol Psychiatry 46:401–408, 2005

Menza M: Personality issues, in Psychiatric Issues in Parkinson's Disease: A Practical Guide. Edited by Menza M, Marsh L. London, England, Taylor and Francis, 2005, pp 249–256

Menza M, Forman NE, Goldstein HS, et al: Parkinson's disease, personality, and dopamine. J Neuropsychiatry Clin Neurosci 2:282–287, 1990

Militerni R, Bravaccio C, Falco C, et al: Repetitive behaviors in autistic disorder. Eur Child Adolesc Psychiatry 11:210–218, 2002

Miwa H, Kondo T: Increased writing activity in Parkinson's disease: a punding-like behavior? Parkinsonism Relat Disord 11:323–325, 2005

Miyasaki JM, Al Hassan K, Lang AE, et al: Punding prevalence in Parkinson's disease. Mov Disord 22:1179–1181, 2007

Muller N, Putz A, Kathmann N, et al: Characteristics of obsessive–compulsive symptoms in Tourette's syndrome, obsessive-compulsive disorder, and Parkinson's disease. Psychiatry Res 70:105–114, 1997

Muller RA, Behen ME, Rothermel RD, et al: Brain mapping of language and auditory perception in high-functioning autistic adults: a PET study. J Autism Dev Disord 29:19–31, 1999

Murphy M, Bolton PF, Pickles A, et al: Personality traits of the relatives of autistic probands. Psychol Med 30:1411–1424, 2000

Ohnishi T, Matsuda H, Hashimoto T, et al: Abnormal regional cerebral blood flow in childhood autism. Brain 123:1838–1844, 2000

Park YD: The effects of vagus nerve stimulation therapy on patients with intractable seizures and either Landau-Kleffner syndrome or autism. Epilepsy Behav 4:286–290, 2003

Pickles A, Starr E, Kazak S, et al: Variable expression of the autism broader phenotype: findings from extended pedigrees. J Child Psychol Psychiatry 41:491–502, 2000

Potenza MN, Voon V, Weintraub D: Drug insight: impulse control disorders and dopamine therapies in Parkinson's disease. National Clinical Practice Neurology 3:664–672, 2007

Pontone G, Williams JR, Bassett SS, et al: Clinical features associated with impulse control disorders in Parkinson disease. Neurology 67:1258–1261, 2006

Ramoz N, Reichert JG, Corwin TE, et al: Lack of evidence for association of the serotonin transporter gene slc6a4 with autism. Biol Psychiatry 60:189–191, 2006

Rastam M, Gillberg C, Wentz E: Outcome of teenage-onset anorexia nervosa in a Swedish community-based sample. Eur Child Adolesc Psychiatry 12(suppl):I78–I90, 2003

Rauch SL, Savage CR: Neuroimaging and neuropsychology of the striatum: bridging basic science and clinical practice. Psychiatr Clin North Am 20:741–768, 1997

Rauch SL, Whalen PJ, Dougherty D, et al: Neurobiologic models of obsessive-compulsive disorder, in Obsessive Compulsive Disorders: Practical Management. Edited by Jenike MA, Baer L, Minishiello WE. St. Louis, MO, Mosby, 1998, pp 222–253

Ridley RM: The psychology of perserverative and stereotyped behaviour. Prog Neurobiol 44:221–231, 1994

Risch N, Spiker D, Lotspeich L, et al: A genomic screen of autism: evidence for a multilocus etiology. Am J Hum Genet 65:493–507, 1999

Rutter M, Silberg J, O'Connor T, et al: Genetics and child psychiatry, II: empirical research findings. J Child Psychol Psychiatry 40:19–55, 1999

Sakurai T, Ramoz N, Reichert JG, et al: Association analysis of the NrCAM gene in autism and in subsets of families with severe obsessive-compulsive or self-stimulatory behaviors. Psychiatr Genet 16:251–257, 2006

Saltzman J, Strauss E, Hunter M, et al: Theory of mind and executive functions in normal human aging and Parkinson's disease. J Int Neuropsychol 6:781–788, 2000

Schmitz N, Rubia K, Daly E, et al: Neural correlates of executive function in autistic spectrum disorders. Biol Psychiatry 59:7–16, 2006

Sears LL, Vest C, Mohamed S, et al: An MRI study of the basal ganglia in autism. Prog Neuropsychopharmacol Biol Psychiatry 23:613–624, 1999

Shao Y, Cuccaro ML, Hauser ER, et al: Fine mapping of autistic disorder to chromosome 15q11-q13 by use of phenotypic subtypes. Am J Hum Genet 72:539–548, 2003

Silverman JM, Smith CJ, Schmeidler J, et al: Symptom domains in autism and related conditions: evidence for familiality. Am J Med Genet 114:64–73, 2000

Silverman JM, Buxbaum JD, Ramoz N, et al: Autism-related routines and rituals associated with a mitochondrial aspartate/glutamate carrier SLC25A12 polymorphism. Am J Med Genet B Neuropsychiatr Genet 147:408–410, 2008

Sood ED, Pallanti S, Hollander E: Diagnosis and treatment of pathologic gambling. Curr Psychiatry Rep 5:9–15, 2003

Stanfield AC, McIntosh AM, Spencer MD, et al: Towards a neuroanatomy of autism: a systematic review and meta-analysis of structural magnetic resonance imaging studies. Eur Psychiatry 23:289–299, 2008

Szatmari P, Georgiades S, Bryson S, et al: Investigating the structure of the restricted, repetitive behaviours and interests domain of autism. J Child Psychol Psychiatry 47:582–590, 2006

Szeszko PR, Ardekani BA, Ashtari M, et al: White matter abnormalities in obsessive-compulsive disorder: a diffusion tensor imaging study. Arch Gen Psychiatry 62:782–790, 2005

Tantam D: Asperger's syndrome. J Child Psychol Psychiatry 29:245–255, 1988

Tomer R, Levin BE, Weiner WJ: Obsessive-compulsive symptoms and motor asymmetries in Parkinson's disease. Neuropsychiatry Neuropsychol Behav Neurol 6:26–30, 1993

Tsai SJ: Could repetitive transcranial magnetic stimulation be effective in autism? Med Hypotheses 64:1070–1071, 2005

Vilensky JA, Damasio AR, Maurer RG: Gait disturbances in patients with autistic behavior: a preliminary study. Arch Neurol 10:646–649, 1981

Voon V, Hassan K, Zurowski M, et al: Prevalence of repetitive and reward-seeking behaviors in Parkinson disease. Neurology 67:1254–1257, 2006

Voon V, Potenza MN, Thomsen T: Medication-related impulse control and repetitive behaviors in Parkinson's disease. Curr Opin Neurol 20:484–492, 2007a

Voon V, Thomsen T, Miyasaki JM, et al: Factors associated with dopaminergic drug-related pathological gambling in Parkinson disease. Arch Neurol 64:212–216, 2007b

Ward CD, Duvoisin RC, Ince SE, et al: Parkinson's disease in twins. Adv Neurol 40:341–344, 1984

Wu S, Guo Y, Jia M, et al: Lack of evidence for association between the serotonin transporter gene (slc6a4) polymorphisms and autism in the Chinese trios. Neurosci Lett 381:1–5, 2005

Yirmiya N, Pilowsky T, Nemanov L, et al: Evidence for an association with the serotonin transporter promoter region polymorphism and autism. Am J Med Genet 105:381–386, 2001

Zhong N, Ye L, Ju W, et al: 5-HTTLPR variants not associated with autistic spectrum disorders. Neurogenetics 2:129–131, 1999

8

CROSS-SPECIES MODELS OF OBSESSIVE-COMPULSIVE SPECTRUM DISORDERS

Vasileios Boulougouris, B.Sc., M.Phil., Ph.D.
Samuel R. Chamberlain, M.D., Ph.D.
Trevor W. Robbins, Ph.D., FRS, FMedSci

Advances in our understanding of the genetic and neural substrates of obsessive-compulsive disorder (OCD) and related spectrum disorders such as trichotillomania, as well as their characteristic behavioral and cognitive symptoms, render the search and evaluation of appropriate animal models especially timely. Such modeling in neurology and neuropsychiatry generally occurs on at least two levels: the etiological, in terms of genetics and molecular pathology, and the symptomatic, in terms of identifying suitable neurocognitive endophenotypes that encompass the range of behavioral and psychiatric manifestations of particular disorders in the

This chapter was first published as "Cross-Species Models of OCD Spectrum Disorders." *Psychiatry Research* 170:15–21 2009. Copyright 2009. Used with permission.

This work was supported by a Programme Grant from the Wellcome Trust to TWR. The Behavioural and Clinical Neuroscience Institute (BCNI) is funded by a joint award from the Medical Research Council (MRC) and the Wellcome Trust. Dr. Boulougouris is supported by the Domestic Research Studentship, the Cambridge European Trusts and the Bakalas Foundation Scholarship. Dr. Chamberlain is supported by a priority research studentship from the MRC and by the School of Clinical Medicine, University of Cambridge.

context of altered brain circuitry. The former is generally difficult in psychiatry as distinct from neurogenetic disorders such as Huntington's disease or where the molecular pathology is well defined, as in the case of Alzheimer's disease. Although there are a number of candidate genes for obsessive-compulsive spectrum disorders (OCSDs), it is probable that multiple genes confer vulnerability, each with small effect, thus making it especially difficult to model disease in a suitable transgenic preparation. Even if such a preparation was feasible, there would be questions about the extent to which its behavioral phenotype in the mouse could simulate all of the subtleties of the clinical syndrome. Several studies have provided important information regarding the neural and neurochemical substrates of OCD, and the availability of somewhat effective pharmacological treatments (e.g., selective serotonin reuptake inhibitors [SSRIs], see Fineberg and Gale 2005) provides essential information that in combination with other evidence contributes to criteria to be set for model validation (discussed later).

This review focuses on animal models of OCD based on criteria for model evaluation. Hence, before reviewing these models, it is important to discuss the criteria by which the validity of an animal model might be assessed.

Assessing Animal Models

Validation criteria are general standards that are relevant to the evaluation of any model. Although there have been several attempts to discuss criteria for the evaluation of animal models (Geyer and Markou 1995; Matthysse 1986; McKinney and Bunney 1969; Segal and Geyer 1985), most of these discussions are based on the assumption that it is not always made explicit. Probably the most widespread classification system is the one proposed by Willner (1984). Willner grouped the different criteria for assessing animal models into criteria used to establish face, predictive, and construct validity. *Face validity* concerns the phenomenological similarity between the animal model and the disorder it models. The model should resemble the human phenomenon in terms of its etiology, symptomatology, treatment, and physiological basis. *Predictive validity* generally means that performance in the experimental test predicts performance in the modeled human phenomenon. Although predictive validity in principle can rely on etiological factors, physiological mechanism, and pharmacological isomorphism, Willner (1991) added that in practice predictive validity usually relies on the latter. *Construct validity* means that the model should be logical in itself and is based 1) on the degree of functional homology between the modeled behavior and the behavior in the model that depends on the two behaviors sharing a similar physiological basis, and 2) on the significance of the modeled behavior in the clinical setting.

Unfortunately, this validation system is very rigid in its definitions and is highly subjective. An additional attempt to describe and classify the criteria for evaluating the validity of animal models has been made by Geyer and Markou (1995, 2002). Working from Willner's definitions, Geyer and Markou restricted face validity to the phenomenological similarity between inducing conditions and specific symptoms of the human phenomenon, while defining predictive validity as the extent to which an animal model allows accurate predictions about the human phenomenon based on the performance of the model. Moreover, *reliability* means that the behavioral outputs of the model are robust and reliable between laboratories. Based on these definitions, Geyer and Markou (1995, 2002) concluded that the evaluation of experimental models in neurobiological research should rely solely on reliability and predictive validity, face similarity being considered a subjective, and therefore secondary, criterion. In other words, every proposed model has to offer a specific, measurable behavior that is pharmacologically analogous with the clinical disorder under study, in order to predict the response of the disorder to new pharmacological treatments.

Although there is a longstanding debate over terminology and classification, it is widely recognized that no one animal model can account for the psychiatric syndrome it mimics in its entirety and that the validation criteria that each model has to fulfill to demonstrate its validity are determined by the defined purpose of the model (Geyer and Markou 1995; Matthysse 1986; Willner 1991).

Clinical Profile and Neurobiological Substrate of Obsessive-Compulsive Disorder

OCD is characterized by intrusive and unwanted ideas, thoughts, urges, and images known as *obsessions,* together with repetitive ritualistic cognitive and physical activities comprising *compulsions.* OCD is heterogeneous in terms of its symptomatology, which appears to reflect different pathophysiological mechanisms. Based on specific analytic methods, OCD symptoms have been split into four categories (Cavallini et al. 2002; Leckman et al. 1997; Summerfeldt et al. 1999): 1) aggressive sexual and religious obsessions with checking compulsions; 2) symmetry obsessions with compulsions of classification, sorting, and repetitiveness; 3) obsessions of contamination with cleaning compulsions; and 4) hoarding. There is some evidence that these symptom clusters differ in terms of treatment response (Black et al. 1998; Mataix-Cols et al. 1999, 2002; Winsberg et al. 1999), comorbidity with other psychiatric disorders (Samuels et al. 2002), and genetic predisposition (Leckman et al. 2003).

The essential features of OCD and related spectrum disorders capable of being captured by animal models are the maladaptive and perseverative behavioral or cognitive output, mediated by dysfunctional nodes within the frontostriatal circuitry, probably modulated by altered dopaminergic or serotoninergic influences, for example, the repetitive rituals in OCD, or hair-pulling in trichotillomania. Human neuroimaging studies have implicated in particular the orbitofrontal cortex and the caudate nucleus in OCD, and cingulotomy has had a limited therapeutic success (see Baxter 1999). However, there may be grounds for considering OCSDs as reflecting impaired functioning of several distinct frontostriatal "loops" (Chamberlain et al. 2005, 2007a; Choi et al. 2007; Graybiel and Rauch 2000; Menzies et al. 2008; Nakao et al. 2005; Whiteside et al. 2006). Animal models of OCSDs have generally fulfilled the criteria of face validity but have sometimes been based on psychological theorizing about the nature of OCD, thus attempting the deeper level of modeling, construct validity. Predictive validity can therefore be employed to a limited extent in OCD, given the known but largely unexplained efficacy of the SSRIs (beginning with fluoxetine) and other less widely evaluated candidate treatments such as dopamine D_1 receptor antagonists and specific serotonin receptor agents.

Current Ethological and Laboratory Animal Models of Obsessive-Compulsive Disorder

ETHOLOGICAL ANIMAL MODELS

The animal literature has approached OCD from two angles, namely, ethological models and laboratory models (genetic, pharmacological, and behavioral). Ethological models (see Table 8–1) focus on spontaneous persistent behaviors with genetic components reminiscent of OCD, offering good face similarity and predictive validity but low practicality. Such behaviors include tail-chasing (Brown et al. 1987) and fur-chewing, acral lick dermatitis (paw licking) in dogs (Rapoport et al. 1992), psychogenic alopecia (hair-pulling) in cats (Swanepoel et al. 1998), feather picking in birds (Grindlinger and Ramsay 1991), cribbing in horses (Luescher et al. 1998), schedule-induced polydipsia (which can be considered as a form of displacement behavior in the face of the thwarting of goal-directed behavior, e.g., Robbins and Koob 1980; Woods et al. 1993) and food-restriction-induced hyperactivity (Altemus et al. 1996). Other responses in animals that have been likened to OCD-like behavior include wheel-running, allogrooming (or "barbering," cf. trichotillomania) in mice (Garner et al. 2004), and marble-burying (the use of bedding material to bury noxious/harmless objects, behavior that may be induced by basic fear avoidance mechanisms; Ichimaru et al. 1995). Some of these models have tested the effects of SSRIs and also compared them with the effects of drugs ineffective in OCD (Altemus et al. 1996; Nurnberg et al. 1997; Rapoport et al. 1992; Winslow and Insel 1991; Woods et al. 1993). It is worth noting that the reported efficacy of clomipramine in OCD and trichotillomania was predicated by observations of its remediating effects on canine lick dermatitis (Rapoport et al. 1992; Swedo et al. 1989) and similar abnormal behavior elicited in veterinary contexts. For example, psychogenic alopecia in cats (Swanepoel et al. 1998), cribbing in horses (Luescher et al. 1998), and repetitive pacing in several species, often elicited by stressful environments, continue to be a valid source of naturalistic stereotypies that may be informative about OCSDs (Stein et al. 1994). Both stereotypies and schedule-induced polydipsia have been considered as "coping responses" that hypothetically reduce stress. This hypothesis, however, has proved difficult to test experimentally and may well not apply to all forms of stereotypy.

GENETIC AND PHARMACOLOGICAL MODELS

In terms of genetic models (see Table 8–1), these have largely been based on face validity and include the *hoxb8* mutant (Greer and Cappechi 2002) as well as genetic manipulations of both dopamine and serotonin functioning leading to similar behavior. Greer and Cappechi (2002) reported that mice with mutations of the *hoxb8* gene (expressed in the orbital cortex, the striatum and the limbic system, all of which are implicated in OCD pathophysiology) groomed excessively to the point of hair removal and skin lesions compared with their control counterparts. In terms of genetic manipulations of dopamine and serotonin, boosting D_1 receptor function by a neuropotentiating cholera toxin expressed in the pyriform cortex and amygdala produces perseveration and repetitive jumping behavior in mice, named D1CT-7 mice, probably mediated ultimately via striatal mechanisms (Campbell et al. 1999a, 1999b, 1999c). It should also be noted that this repetitive jumping behavior was exacerbated by the administration of yohimbine, an anxiogenic drug (McGrath et al. 1999). Knockdown of the dopamine transporter (DAT) produces "sequential super-stereotypy" in mice, named "DAT KD" mice, with the perseverative performance of quite complex chains of grooming behavior (Berridge et al. 2005). A knockdown of the 5-HT_{2C} receptor similarly leads to perseverative "head-dipping" or the excessively orderly chewing of screen material (Chou-Green et al. 2003), a compulsive behavior (accompanied by other like responses such as stereotypic locomotion and excessive self-aggressive grooming) that has also been shown in rats following chronic lesions of median raphe nucleus (Hoshino et al. 2004). Some of these responses obviously have clear superficial parallels to some of the elaborative rituals in OCD, possibly related to hygiene and checking. However, it is of course essentially impossible to know in fact how closely related they are. It seems likely that these examples of stereotyped behavior are mediated by striatal structures, given the known role of the caudate–putamen in stereotyped behavior produced by psychomotor stimulant drugs (Creese and Iversen 1975) and in normal grooming sequences (Aldridge and Berridge 1998).

It is tempting to utilize pharmacological models based on the stereotypy produced by stimulants such as amphetamine at high dosages (Lyon and Robbins 1975). Although stereotypies in rodents typically consist of gnawing and licking with repetitive sideways movements of the head that may represent vestiges of orienting

TABLE 8–1. Animal models of obsessive-compulsive disorder (OCD)

Model		Modeled behavior (face validity)	Neuroanatomical/ neurochemical substrate (construct validity)	Predictive validity
Ethological models	Tail-chasing (Brown et al. 1987), acral lick dermatitis (paw licking) in dogs (Rapoport et al. 1992), psychogenic alopecia (hair pulling) in cats (Swanepoel et al. 1998), feather picking in birds (Grindlinger and Ramsay 1991), cribbing in horses (Luescher et al. 1998), schedule induced polydipsia (Woods et al. 1993), food-restriction-induced hyperactivity (Altemus et al. 1996)	Spontaneous persistent behaviors with genetic components reminiscent of OCD	Although these models offer good face similarity and predictive validity, construct validity is difficult to be tested mainly due to the fact that they focus on spontaneous persistent behaviors	The effects of SSRIs have been tested and compared with the effects of drugs ineffective in OCD, e.g., remediating effects of clomipramine on canine lick dermatitis
Genetic models	*hoxb8* mutant mice (Greer and Cappechi 2002)	Excessive grooming similar to that seen in trichotillomania and OCD	*hoxb8* gene is expressed in orbitofrontal cortex, the anterior cingulate, and the limbic system, all of which are implicated in OCD	There are no reports on the isomorphic response of these models with clinical compulsive behavior

TABLE 8–1. Animal models of obsessive-compulsive disorder (OCD) *(continued)*

Model	Modeled behavior (face validity)	Neuroanatomical/ neurochemical substrate (construct validity)	Predictive validity
Genetic models *(continued)*			
D1CT-7 mice (Campbell et al. 1999b, 1999c; McGrath et al. 1999)	Perseveration and repetitive leaping Tourette's syndrome-like behaviors	Transgene expression in neural systems hyperactive in human OCD, e.g., amygdala, somatosensory/ insular and orbitofrontal cortical regions	
DAT KD mice (Berridge et al. 2005)	Sequential super-stereotypy apparent in OCD/ Tourette's syndrome patients in the form of rigid patterns of actions, language, or thought	Dopaminergic involvement in OCD. Basal ganglia are implicated in grooming and OCD	
5-HT$_{2c}$ KO mice (Chou-Green et al. 2003)	Perseverative "head dipping" and excessively orderly chewing of screen material similar to human obsessive-compulsive symptoms such as ordering, washing, etc.	5-HT$_{2C}$ receptors involvement in OCD pathophysiology	

TABLE 8–1. Animal models of obsessive-compulsive disorder (OCD) *(continued)*

Model	Modeled behavior (face validity)	Neuroanatomical/ neurochemical substrate (construct validity)	Predictive validity
Pharmacological models Quinpirole-induced compulsive checking (Szechtman et al. 1998)	Compulsive checking in OCD patients (e.g., ritual-like motor activities)	Dopaminergic involvement in OCD pathophysiology	Quinpirole-induced compulsive checking is reduced following treatment with clomipramine
8-OHDPAT-induced spontaneous alternation (Yadin et al. 1992)		5-HT_{1A} receptors involvement in OCD pathophysiology	Administration of fluoxetine (chronic) and clomipra-mine (subacute), but not desipramine, offers protection from the 8-OHDPAT-induced decrease in spontaneous alternation
m-CPP-induced directional persistence in reinforced spatial alternation (Tsaltas et al. 2005)		5-HT_{2C} receptor involvement in OCD pathophysiology	Chronic treatment with fluoxetine, but not with diazepam or desipramine, blocks the mCPP-induced directional persistence

TABLE 8–1. Animal models of obsessive-compulsive disorder (OCD) *(continued)*

	Model	Modeled behavior (face validity)	Neuroanatomical/ neurochemical substrate (construct validity)	Predictive validity
Behavioral models	Barbering (Garner et al. 2004)	Compulsive hair plucking in humans (trichotillomania)	Spontaneous development	No reports
	Marble burying (Ichimaru et al. 1995)	Inability to achieve a sense of task completion	No reports	Marble burying is sensitive to SSRIs and diazepam. However, the effects of diazepam disappear following repeated administration, which is not the case with SSRIs, e.g., fluvoxamine. No response to desipramine
	Signal attenuation (Joel and Avisar 2001; Joel et al. 2004)	Compulsive lever-pressing is both excessive and unreasonable, as are compulsions in OCD patients	1. Similarities in the compulsivity-inducing mechanism (i.e., attenuation of an external feedback and a deficient response feedback mechanism, respectively) 2. Orbital, but not medial prefrontal or amygdala, lesions induce compulsive lever-pressing	Acute administration of fluoxetine, but not diazepam, desipramine or haloperidol, reduces compulsive lever pressing

TABLE 8–1.   Animal models of obsessive-compulsive disorder (OCD) *(continued)*

Model	Modeled behavior (face validity)	Neuroanatomical/ neurochemical substrate (construct validity)	Predictive validity
Other possible behavioral models			
Reversal learning (Boulougouris et al. 2007; Chudasama and Robbins 2003; Clarke et al. 2004)	Inability to withhold, modify, or sustain adaptive behavior in response to changing situational demands	Lesions to the orbitofrontal cortex as well as serotonin depletion in this brain region heavily implicated in OCD disrupt reversal learning, manifested as increased perseverative responding to the prepotent stimulus	The isomorphic response of these models with clinical compulsive behavior needs to be tested
Attentional set-shifting (Extradimensional shift) (Birrell and Brown 2000; Clarke et al. 2007)		Sensitive to lateral frontal lesions and catecholamine but not serotonin depletion in monkeys and medial prefrontal cortical lesions in rats	
Extinction		No reports but see signal attenuation model	

TABLE 8–1. Animal models of obsessive-compulsive disorder (OCD) *(continued)*

Model		Modeled behavior (face validity)	Neuroanatomical/ neurochemical substrate (construct validity)	Predictive validity
Other possible behavioral models *(continued)*	Habit-learning (Killcross and Coutureau 2003; Yin and Knowlton 2006)	This behavior is controlled by stimulus–response links with a generally weakened influence of the ultimate goal	Habit learning is mediated by specific sectors of the striatum and can be influenced by prefrontal cortical mechanisms	
	SSRT (Aron et al 2003a, 2003b, 2003c; Eagle and Robbins 2003; Eagle et al. 2008)	"Impulsive" responding particularly as it is impaired in ADHD	Studies in human patients with frontal lobe damage have localized the critical zone for SSRT to the right inferior gyrus whereas others have localized it to the striatum	SSRT is insensitive to serotoninergic manipulations both in rats and humans

Note. 8-OHDPAT = 8-hydroxy-2-(di-ni-popylamino)-tetralin hydrobromide; ADHD = Attention-deficit/hyperactivity disorder; D1CT mice: transgenic mice expressing a neuropotentiating protein (cholera toxin A1 subunit) within a cortical-limbic subset of dopamine D_1-receptor expressing (D_{1+}) neurons; DAT KD mice: dopamine transporter *(DAT)* knockdown (KD) mice, expressing 10% of wild-type *DAT* levels and exhibiting elevated extracellular dopamine concentration; KO = knockout; m-CPP = meta-chlorophenylpiperazine; SSRI = selective serotonin reuptake inhibitor; SSRT = stop-signal reaction time task.

behavior, they can be elaborated in many ways, for example, to include grooming (including allogrooming, Sahakian and Robbins 1975) and perseverative operant behavior in which rats may continue to work for food they do not eat (Robbins and Sahakian 1983). These responses are dopamine mediated, but it may be a mistake to consider them as being directly related to OCSD because, for example, treatment of mice receiving the D_1 receptor potentiation treatment actually exhibit reduced stereotypy after treatment with cocaine, showing that drug-induced stereotypy and the behavior produced by enhanced D_1 receptor overexpression do not necessarily lie on the same continuum (Campbell et al. 1999b). This may also be reflected in clinical experience. For example, D-amphetamine has actually been shown to ameliorate OCD symptoms in certain circumstances (Insel et al. 1983). Nevertheless, Szechtman et al. (1998) have shown that the D_2/D_3 agonist quinpirole leads to behavior that can be analyzed as a form of repetitive "checking" behavior in rats. Specifically, after drug administration (0.5 mg/kg twice weekly for 5 weeks), rats were placed individually into an open field with four objects at fixed locations, and their activity was recorded for 55 minutes. Analysis of quinpirole- and saline-treated rats revealed that quinpirole-treated rats stopped at two locales more frequently than control rats and exhibited a "ritual-like" set of motor activities at these places (Szechtman et al. 1998). This behavior is reduced by treatment with clomipramine.

As mentioned earlier, *perseveration* is a term that can be applied to a variety of behavioral outputs ranging from relatively simple to complex. The "complex" category is where it is not a motor output that is performed repetitively but an approach to a particular goal or the persistence in complex sequences of behavior. We also include in the "complex" category trained operant behavior (in which rats keep on working for food they do not eat) and also both spontaneous (Yadin et al. 1992) and reinforced delayed alternation behavior (Tsaltas et al. 2005), which can become perseverative if the animal continues to make the previous choice following treatment, for example, with dopaminergic or serotoninergic agents. At yet higher levels of organization, we can consider impairments of object reversal behavior to reflect a "higher order" form of perseveration because the animal may perseverate in responding to a formerly reinforced stimulus, even though its spatial position is shifted across trials. Such behavior occurs when serotonin depletion is effected in the orbitofrontal cortex (Clarke et al. 2004, 2005, 2007) in marmoset monkeys. Moreover, this behavior is truly perseverative in the sense that reversal learning is normal if the previously rewarded stimulus is substituted by a novel one (Clarke et al. 2007). However, this form of perseverative responding is probably not the same as that produced by perseveration of a learned rule in the Wisconsin Card Sort Test, following, for example, frontal lobe damage (or OCD), which involves a so-called "extra-dimensional shift." This form of attentional shifting is impaired by lateral frontal lesions in the marmoset and by catecholamine, but not serotonin, depletion (Clarke et al. 2005, 2007; for a review, see also Robbins 2005).

SIGNAL ATTENUATION AND EXTINCTION: BEHAVIORAL MODELS

Another sophisticated model is that of "signal attenuation" (see Table 8–1) in which it is postulated that OCD results when behavior receives weakened response feedback (whether kinaesthetic in nature or in terms of conditioned reinforcers, analogous to sub-goals) that signal when the required contingency has been completed. Joel et al. (2004) developed this model perhaps more fully than any other extant model of OCD. Rats are trained to respond for food that they retrieve at a food magazine, accompanied by a conditioned stimulus functioning as a conditioned reinforcer. The magazine response is then separately extinguished (i.e., undergoes signal attenuation) before the animal is allowed again to respond on the lever, but during extinction. The critical consequence of the signal attenuation procedure is that the rat may continue to respond on the lever but fail to complete the sequence by moving on to the food magazine. The instrumental lever-pressing thus has a perseverative quality that is sensitive to reductions produced by virtually all of the drugs used therapeutically in OCD, but not to those that are less effective, such as diazepam or desipramine. This behavior is also enhanced by lesions of the rat orbitofrontal cortex and sensitive to manipulations of the medial striatum, to which the orbitofrontal cortex projects. Joel and colleagues have thus established many of the validating criteria for a successful model of OCD, although the exact theoretical explanation in terms of signal attenuation may perhaps be queried.

Signal attenuation appears to resemble a special form of extinction in which pavlovian associations of a conditioned stimulus are extinguished differentially with respect to instrumental responding. The perseveration in instrumental behavior arises because the terminal links in the response chain leading to food are extinguished. Extinction itself also depends on an inhibitory process that suppresses associations, which in fact remain intact (Rescorla 2001). Another example of this form of perseveration has been reported in the performance of an attentional task for rats that requires the animals to visit the food magazine after a nose-poke response to detect a target visual stimulus. Perseverative nose-poking, possibly caused by a failure to detect response feedback cues, can arise from lesions to the orbitofrontal cortex in rats (Chudasama et al. 2003).

PUTATIVE BEHAVIORAL ANIMAL MODELS

It would be parsimonious to describe all of these examples of perseverative responding from the level of single response elements to complicated sequences of behavior, to a perseverative attentional focus, as resulting from failures of "behavioral inhibition." However, the fact that they are mediated by both striatal and different prefrontal cortical sectors suggests that these are not the same forms of inhibition and that a generic explanation in terms of behavioral inhibition may lack explanatory power. However, it is possible that particular forms of behavioral inhibition are impaired in OCSDs. There are several other theoretical positions that may be especially useful in explaining certain forms of OCD while capturing some of the clinical observations of patients exhibiting these disorders (see Table 8–1). Thus, one set of theoretical constructs suggests that anxiety (e.g., Mowrer 1960) is the prime trigger of OCD, as posited, for example, by Rachman and Hodgson (1980). Active avoidance behavior in animals is well known to be very persistent because it so rarely has the opportunity for extinction, and drugs such as D-amphetamine exacerbate this perseverative tendency. Thus behavior that initially has some adaptive value, for example, in avoiding shocks, apparently loses its rationale after thousands of trials in which shock is never presented. We have previously alluded to the possibility that stereotyped behavior acts as a coping response to reduce stress, and this is essentially the same contingency. A more recent formulation is that by Szechtman and Woody (2004) that OCD-like behavior arises as an aberrant excess of behavior motivated by the need for security. These theories are of obvious clinical interest and will ultimately depend on their validation by the importance assigned to anxiety in producing the persistent symptoms of OCD. A related concept is that of exaggerated habit learning, in which behavior is controlled by stimulus–response links with a generally weakened influence of the ultimate goal. Recent evidence (e.g., Yin and Knowlton 2006) strongly supports the hypothesis that habit learning in the rat is mediated by specific sectors of the rat striatum (those probably homologous to the putamen). However, we have to consider what types of mechanism are brought into play to turn habits into compulsions (for a discussion of compulsive drug taking, which may be governed by similar mechanisms, see Everitt and Robbins 2005). Evidence also indicates that habit learning in the striatum can be influenced by prefrontal cortical mechanisms (see, e.g., Killcross and Coutureau 2003).

The clinical concept of a continuum of impulsive and compulsive behavior is highly relevant to OCSD, where different aspects of behavior can perhaps be thought of as having impulsive or compulsive features (Hollander and Rosen 2000; Stein and Hollander 1995), or even that impulsive behavior is converted into compulsive responding as a function of its repetition (see Everitt and Robbins 2005). This counterbalancing of impulsive and compulsive responding brings us back to sophisticated notions of behavioral inhibition, which might become disrupted in both cases, possibly while engaging different neural circuitry. These notions have been recruited previously by Gray (2000) in his extensive theory based on behavioral inhibition, in which OCD symptoms are accredited to an overactive "checking" mechanism that compares intended actions with their outcomes: if the hypothetical comparator is constantly detecting mismatches, the "checking" mechanism will be continuously engaged, possibly dependent on anterior cingulate influences.

The Stop-Signal Reaction Time Task

Another way of explaining this form of perseveration is to suggest that in OCD or related forms there is a failure of "stop-signal inhibition"—an inability to stop an already-initiated response. This notion is compatible with the proposed lateral orbitofrontal cortex dysfunction in OCD, and OCD patients do show decreased behavioral and cognitive inhibition in a variety of tasks (Bannon et al. 2002; Enright and Beech 1993; Rosenberg et al. 1997; Tien et al. 1992; for review, see Chamberlain et al. 2005) in addition to the increased errors they show on the alternation learning task (Abbruzzese et al. 1995; Cavedini et al. 1998). Moreover, Logan and Cowan (1984) have devised a way of measuring the stop-signal reaction time in humans by measuring the response latency required to successfully cancel a response in a choice-reaction time procedure. This can also be conceived as measuring "impulsive" responding, particularly as it is impaired in attention-deficit/hyperactivity disorder (ADHD) and it has been shown for example that methylphenidate normalizes stop-signal reaction time in adult ADHD patients (Aron et al. 2003b). A recent comparative study of OCD and trichotillomania (Chamberlain et al. 2006a) shows an interesting dissociation in which trichotillomania patients had greatly lengthened stop-signal reaction times and that OCD patients were also significantly slowed on this measure, as compared with age- and IQ-matched control subjects. By contrast OCD patients were significantly impaired on the extra-dimensional shift test, whereas trichotillomania patients were not. These data suggest that whereas OCD is accompanied by a general problem in cognitive flexibility, trichotillomania is associated more specifically with a failure to stop motor output. Moreover, recent studies of first-degree relatives of OCD patients (Chamberlain et al. 2007a; Menzies et al. 2008) identified behavioral deficits on these tasks in "at risk" relatives of patients linked with structural abnormalities of frontostriatal circuitry.

In terms of neural substrates, studies of human patients with frontal lobe damage have localized the critical zone for stop-signal reaction time to the right inferior frontal gyrus (Aron et al. 2003a), and other data implicate the striatum in this inhibitory process (Aron et al. 2003c). It is intriguing that precisely the same structure is implicated in the extra-dimensional shift test, according to a recent functional magnetic resonance imaging study (Hampshire and Owen 2006). A method of measuring stop-signal reaction time in rats has been developed that is dependent on possibly homologous structures in the lateral orbitofrontal cortex and medial striatum (Eagle and Robbins 2003; Eagle et al. 2008). Intriguingly, however, the stop-signal reaction time is insensitive to serotoninergic manipulations in both rats (Eagle et al. 2009) and humans (Chamberlain et al. 2006b, 2007b; Clark et al. 2005).

Conclusion

We are thus intriguingly close to providing useful theoretically motivated models of OCSDs, particularly with regard to repetitive motoric habits and inhibitory failures. Nonetheless, significant puzzles still remain (Table 8–1). For example, two of the most sensitive of the human tests used to highlight deficits in OCD (the stop-signal and extradimensional shift tests) appear to be more dependent on the integrity of the inferior frontal cortex rather than the orbitofrontal cortex. Moreover, OCD patients are not markedly impaired on simple reversal learning, which has been associated in animal studies with damage to the orbitofrontal cortex (Boulougouris et al. 2007) and which is sensitive to serotonin manipulations (Boulougouris et al. 2008). Neuroimaging versions of these tasks may yet identify subtle brain dysfunction in patients and unaffected relatives at risk of OCSDs, in the absence of overt behavioral deficits. OCD has received the most research attention to date; it would be of considerable interest to determine whether the more obvious motor manifestations of other conditions such as trichotillomania are associated with structural and/or functional impairments of similar corticostriatal loops, possibly more at striatal than cortical nodes, or whether, as seems likely, these are associated with impairments in other frontostriatal pathways, for example, related to the putamen and its role in the control of motor output.

References

Abbruzzese M, Bellodi L, Ferri S, et al: Frontal lobe dysfunction in schizophrenia and obsessive-compulsive disorder: a neuropsychological study. Brain Cogn 27:202–212, 1995

Aldridge JW, Berridge KC: Coding of serial order by neostriatal neurons: a "natural action" approach to movement sequence. J Neurosci 18:2777–2787, 1998

Altemus M, Glowa JR, Galliven E, et al: Effects of serotonergic agents on food-restriction-induced hyperactivity. Pharmacol Biochem Behav 53:123–131, 1996

Aron AR, Dowson JH, Sahakian BJ, et al: Methylphenidate improves response inhibition in adults with attention-deficit/hyperactivity disorder. Biol Psychiatry 54:1465–1468, 2003a

Aron AR, Fletcher PC, Bullmore ET, et al: Stop-signal inhibition disrupted by damage to right inferior frontal gyrus in humans. Nat Neurosci 6:115–116, 2003b

Aron AR, Watkins L, Sahakian BJ, et al: Task set switching deficits in early stage Huntington's disease: implications for basal ganglia function. J Cogn Neurosci 15:629–642, 2003c

Bannon S, Gonsalvez CJ, Croft RJ, et al: Response inhibition deficits in obsessive-compulsive disorder. Psychiatry Res 110:165–174, 2002

Baxter L: Functional imaging of brain systems mediating obsessive-compulsive disorder, in Neurobiology of Mental Illness. Edited by Charney DS, Nestler EJ, Bunney BS. New York, Oxford University Press, 1999, pp 534–547

Berridge KC, Aldridge JW, Houchard KR, et al: Sequential superstereotypy of an instinctive fixed action pattern in hyper-dopaminergic mutant mice: a model of obsessive compulsive disorder and Tourette's. BMC Biology 3:4, 2005

Birrell JM, Brown VJ: Medial frontal cortex mediates perceptual attentional set shifting in the rat. J Neurosci 20:4320–4324, 2000

Black DW, Monahan P, Gable J, et al: Hoarding and treatment response in 38 non-depressed subjects with obsessive-compulsive disorder. J Clin Psychiatry 59:420–425, 1998

Boulougouris V, Dalley JW, Robbins TW: Effects of orbitofrontal, infralimbic and prelimbic cortical lesions on serial spatial reversal learning in the rat. Behav Brain Res 179:219–228, 2007

Boulougouris V, Glennon JC, Robbins TW: Dissociable effects of selective 5-HT (2A) and 5-HT(2C) receptor antagonists on serial spatial reversal learning in rats. Neuropsychopharmacology 33:2007–2019, 2008

Brown SA, Crowell-Davis S, Malcolm T, et al: Naloxone-responsive compulsive tail chasing in a dog. J Am Vet Med Assoc 190:884–886, 1987

Campbell KM, de Lecea L, Severynse DM, et al: OCD-Like behaviors caused by a neuropotentiating transgene targeted to cortical and limbic D1+ neurons. J Neurosci 19:5044–5053, 1999a

Campbell KM, McGrath MJ, Burton FH: Behavioral effects of cocaine on a transgenic mouse model of cortical-limbic compulsion. Brain Res 833:216–224, 1999b

Campbell KM, McGrath MJ, Burton FH: Differential response of cortical-limbic neuro-potentiated compulsive mice to dopamine D1 and D2 receptor antagonists. Eur J Pharmacol 371:103–111, 1999c

Cavallini MC, Di Bella D, Siliprandi F, et al: Exploratory factor analysis of obsessive-compulsive patients and association with 5-HTTLPR polymorphism. Am J Med Genet 114:347–355, 2002

Cavedini P, Ferri S, Scarone S, et al: Frontal lobe dysfunction in obsessive-compulsive disorder and major depression: a clinical-neuropsychological study. Psychiatry Res 78:21–28, 1998

Chamberlain SR, Blackwell AD, Fineberg NA, et al: The neuropsychology of obsessive compulsive disorder: the importance of failures in cognitive and behavioural inhibition as candidate endophenotypic markers. Neurosci Biobehav Rev 29:399–419, 2005

Chamberlain SR, Fineberg NA, Blackwell AD, et al: Motor inhibition and cognitive flexibility in obsessive-compulsive disorder and trichotillomania. Am J Psychiatry 163:1282–1284, 2006a

Chamberlain SR, Muller U, Blackwell AD, et al: Neurochemical modulation of response inhibition and probabilistic learning in humans. Science 311:861–863, 2006b

Chamberlain SR, Fineberg NA, Menzies LA, et al: Impaired cognitive flexibility and motor inhibition in unaffected first-degree relatives of patients with obsessive-compulsive disorder. Am J Psychiatry 164:335–338, 2007a

Chamberlain SR, Müller U, Deakin JB, et al: Lack of deleterious effects of buspirone on cognition in healthy male volunteers. J Psychopharmacol 21:210–215, 2007b

Choi JS, Kim SH, Yoo SY, et al: Shape deformity of the corpus striatum in obsessive-compulsive disorder. Psychiatry Res 155:257–264, 2007

Chou-Green JM, Holscher TD, Dallman MF, et al: Compulsive behavior in the 5-HT2C receptor knockout mouse. Physiol Behav 785:641–649, 2003

Chudasama Y, Robbins TW: Dissociable contribution of the orbitofrontal and infralimbic cortex to pavlovian autoshaping and discrimination reversal learning: further evidence for the functional heterogeneity of the rodent frontal cortex. J Neurosci 23:8771–8780, 2003

Chudasama Y, Passetti F, Rhodes SE, et al: Dissociable aspects of performance on the 5-choice serial reaction time task following lesions of the dorsal anterior cingulate, infralimbic and orbitofrontal cortex in the rat: differential effects on selectivity, impulsivity and compulsivity. Behav Brain Res 146:105–119, 2003

Clark L, Roiser JP, Cools R, et al: Stop signal response inhibition is not modulated by tryptophan depletion or the serotonin transporter polymorphism in healthy volunteers: implications for the 5-HT theory of impulsivity. Psychopharmacology 182:570–578, 2005

Clarke HF, Dalley JW, Crofts HS, et al: Cognitive inflexibility after prefrontal serotonin depletion. Science 304:878–880, 2004

Clarke HF, Walker SC, Crofts HS, et al: Prefrontal serotonin depletion affects reversal learning but not attentional set shifting. J Neurosci 25:532–538, 2005

Clarke HF, Walker SC, Dalley JW, et al: Cognitive inflexibility after prefrontal serotonin depletion is behaviorally and neurochemically specific. Cereb Cortex 17:18–27, 2007

Creese I, Iversen SD: The pharmacological and anatomical substrates of the amphetamine response in the rat. Brain Res 83:419–436, 1975

Eagle DM, Robbins TW: Inhibitory control in rats performing a stop-signal reaction-time task: effects of lesions of the medial striatum and D-amphetamine. Behav Neurosci 117:1302–1317, 2003

Eagle DM, Baunez C, Hutcheson DM, et al: Stop-signal reaction time task performance: role of prefrontal cortex and subthalamic nucleus. Cereb Cortex 18:178–188, 2008

Eagle DM, Lehmann O, Theobald DEH, et al: Serotonin depletion impairs waiting but not stop-signal reaction time in rats: implications for theories of the role of 5-HT in behavioral inhibition. Neuropsychopharmacology 34:1311–1321, 2009

Enright SJ, Beech AR: Reduced cognitive inhibition in obsessive-compulsive disorder. Br J Clin Psychol 32:67–74, 1993

Everitt BJ, Robbins TW: Neural systems of reinforcement for drug addiction: from actions to habits to compulsion. Nat Neurosci 8:1481–1489, 2005

Fineberg NA, Gale TM: Evidence-based pharmacotherapy of obsessive-compulsive disorder. Int J Neuropsychopharmacol 8:107–129, 2005

Garner JP, Dufour B, Gregg LE, et al: Social and husbandry factors affecting the prevalence and severity of barbering ("whisker trimming") by laboratory mice. Appl Anim Behav Sci 89:263–282, 2004

Geyer MA, Markou A: Animal models of psychiatric disorders, in Psychopharmacology: The Fourth Generation of Progress. Edited by Bloom FE, Kupfer DJ. New York, Raven Press, 1995, pp 787–798

Geyer MA, Markou A: Role of preclinical models in the development of psychotropic drugs, in Psychopharmacology: The Fifth Generation of Progress. Edited by Davis KL, Coyle JT, Nemeroff C. Philadelphia, PA, Lippincott, Williams & Wilkins, 2002, pp 445–455

Gray JA: The Neuropsychology of Anxiety. New York, Oxford University Press, 2000

Graybiel AM, Rauch SL: Toward a neurobiology of obsessive-compulsive disorder. Neuron 28:343–347, 2000

Greer JM, Cappechi MR: Hoxb8 is required for normal grooming behaviour in mice. Neuron 33:23–34, 2002

Grindlinger HM, Ramsay E: Compulsive feather picking in birds. Arch Gen Psychiatry 48:857, 1991

Hampshire A, Owen AM: Fractionating attentional control using event-related fMRI. Cereb Cortex 16:1679–1689, 2006

Hollander E, Rosen J: Impulsivity. J Psychopharmacol 14:S39–S44, 2000

Hoshino K, Uga DA, de Paula HM: The compulsive-like aspect of the head dipping emission in rats with chronic electrolytic lesion in the area of the medial raphé nucleus. Braz J Med Biol Res 37:245–250, 2004

Ichimaru Y, Egawa T, Sawa A: 5-HT1A-receptor subtype mediates the effect of fluvoxamine, a selective serotonin reuptake inhibitor, on marble-burying behavior in mice. J Pharmacol 68:65–70, 1995

Insel TR, Hamilton JA, Guttmacher LB, et al: D-amphetamine in obsessive-compulsive disorder. Psychopharmacology 80:231–235, 1983

Joel D, Avisar A: Excessive lever pressing following post-training signal attenuation in rats: a possible animal model of obsessive compulsive disorder? Behav Brain Res 123:77–87, 2001

Joel D, Ben-Amir E, Doljansky J, et al: "Compulsive" lever-pressing in rats is attenuated by the serotonin re-uptake inhibitors paroxetine and fluvoxamine but not by the tricyclic antidepressant desipramine or the anxiolytic diazepam. Behav Pharmacol 15:241–252, 2004

Killcross S, Coutureau E: Coordination of actions and habits in the medial prefrontal cortex of rats. Cereb Cortex 13:400–408, 2003

Leckman JF, Grice DE, Boardman J, et al: Symptoms of obsessive-compulsive disorder. Am J Psychiatry 154:911–917, 1997

Leckman JF, Pauls DL, Zhang H, et al: Obsessive-compulsive symptom dimensions in affected sibling pairs diagnosed with Gilles de la Tourette syndrome. Am J Med Genet 116B:60–68, 2003

Logan G, Cowan W: On the ability to inhibit thought, and action: a theory of an act of control. Psychol Rev 91:295–327, 1984

Luescher UA, McKeown DB, Dean H: A cross-sectional study on compulsive behaviour (stable vices) in horses. Equine Vet J Suppl 27:14–18, 1998

Lyon M, Robbins TW: The action of central nervous system stimulant drugs: a general theory concerning amphetamine effects, in Current Developments in Psychopharmacology, Vol 4. Edited by Essman W, Valzelli L. New York, Spectrum, 1975, pp 79–163

Mataix-Cols D, Rauch SL, Manzo PA, et al: Use of factor analyzed symptom dimensions to predict outcome with serotonin reuptake inhibitors and placebo in the treatment of obsessive-compulsive disorder. Am J Psychiatry 156:1409–1416, 1999

Mataix-Cols D, Marks IM, Greist JH, et al: Obsessive-compulsive symptom dimensions as predictors of compliance with and response to behaviour therapy: results from a controlled trial. Psychother Psychosom 71:255–262, 2002

Matthysse S: Animal models in psychiatric research. Prog Brain Res 65:259–270, 1986

McGrath MJ, Campbell KM, Veldman MB, et al: Anxiety in transgenic mouse model of corti-cal-limbic neuro-potentiated compulsive behaviour. Behav Pharmacol 10:435–443, 1999

McKinney WT, Bunney WE: Animal model of depression: a review of evidence: implications for research. Arch Gen Psychiatry 21:240–248, 1969

Menzies L, Chamberlain SR, Laird AR, et al: Integrating evidence from neuroimaging and neuropsychological studies of obsessive-compulsive disorder: the orbitofronto-striatal model revisited. Neurosci Biobehav Rev 32:525–549, 2008

Mowrer OH: Learning Theory and Behavior. New York, Wiley, 1960

Nakao T, Nakagawa A, Yoshiura T, et al: A functional MRI comparison of patients with obsessive-compulsive disorder and normal controls during a Chinese character Stroop task. Psychiatry Res 139:101–114, 2005

Nurnberg HG, Keith SJ, Paxton DM: Consideration of the relevance of ethological animal models for human repetitive behavioral spectrum disorders. Biol Psychiatry 411:226–229, 1997

Rachman SJ, Hodgson RJ: Obsessions and Compulsions. Englewood Cliffs, NJ, Prentice-Hall, 1980

Rapoport JL, Ryland DH, Kriete M: Drug treatment of canine acral lick: an animal model of obsessive-compulsive disorder. Arch Gen Psychiatry 49:517–521, 1992

Rescorla RA: Experimental extinction, in Handbook of Contemporary Learning Theories. Edited by Mowrer RR, Klein S. Hillsdale, NJ, Erlbaum, 2001, pp 119–154

Robbins TW: Chemistry of the mind: neurochemical modulation of prefrontal cortical function. J Comp Neurol 493:140–146, 2005

Robbins TW, Koob GF: Selective disruption of displacement behaviour by lesions of the mesolimbic dopamine system. Nature 285:409–412, 1980

Robbins TW, Sahakian BJ: Behavioural effects of psychomotor stimulant drugs: clinical and neuropsychological implications, in Stimulants, Neurochemical, Behavioral and Clinical Perspectives. Edited by Creese I. New York, Raven Press, 1983, pp 301–338

Rosenberg DR, Dick EL, O'Hearn KM, et al: Response-inhibition deficits in obsessive-compulsive disorder: an indicator of dysfunction in frontostriatal circuits. J Psychiatry Neurosci 22:29–38, 1997

Sahakian BJ, Robbins TW: The effects of test environment and rearing condition on amphetamine-induced stereotypy in the guinea-pig. Psychopharmacologia 45:S115–S117, 1975

Samuels J, Bienvenu OJ, Riddle MA, et al: Hoarding in obsessive-compulsive disorder: results from a case-control study. Behav Res Ther 40:517–528, 2002

Segal DS, Geyer MA: Animal models of psychopathology, in Psychobiological Foundations of Clinical Psychiatry. Edited by Judd LL, Groves PM. Philadelphia, PA, JB Lippincott, 1985, pp 1–14

Stein DJ, Hollander E: Obsessive-compulsive spectrum disorders. J Clin Psychiatry 56:265–266, 1995

Stein DJ, Dodman NH, Borchelt P, et al: Behavioral disorders in veterinary practice: relevance to psychiatry. Compr Psychiatry 35:275–285, 1994

Summerfeldt LJ, Richter MA, Antony MM, et al: Symptom structure in obsessive-compulsive disorder: a confirmatory factor-analytic study. Behav Res Ther 37:297–311, 1999

Swanepoel N, Lee E, Stein DJ: Psychogenic alopecia in a cat: response to clomipramine. J S Afr Vet Assoc 69:22, 1998

Swedo SE, Leonard HL, Rapoport JL, et al: A double-blind comparison of clomipramine and desipramine in the treatment of trichotillomania (hair pulling). N Engl J Med 321:497–501, 1989

Szechtman H, Woody E: Obsessive-compulsive disorder as a disturbance of security motivation. Psychol Rev 111:111–127, 2004

Szechtman H, Sulis W, Eilam D: Quinpirole induces compulsive checking behavior in rats: a potential animal model of obsessive-compulsive disorder (OCD). Behav Neurosci 112:1475–1485, 1998

Tien AY, Pearlson GD, Machlin SR, et al: Oculomotor performance in obsessive-compulsive disorder. Am J Psychiatry 149:641–646, 1992

Tsaltas E, Kontis D, Chrysikakou S, et al: Reinforced spatial alternation as an animal model of obsessive-compulsive disorder (OCD): investigation of 5-HT2C and 5-HT1D receptor involvement in OCD pathophysiology. Biol Psychiatry 57:1176–1185, 2005

Whiteside SP, Port JD, Deacon BJ, et al: A magnetic resonance spectroscopy investigation of obsessive-compulsive disorder and anxiety. Psychiatry Res 146:137–147, 2006

Willner P: The validity of animal models of depression. Psychopharmacology (Berl) 83:1–16, 1984

Willner P: Behavioural models in psychopharmacology, in Behavioural Models in Psychopharmacology: Theoretical, Industrial and Clinical Perspectives. Edited by Willner P. Cambridge, United Kingdom, Cambridge University Press, 1991, pp 3–18

Winsberg ME, Cassic KS, Koran LM: Hoarding in obsessive-compulsive disorder: a report of 20 cases. J Clin Psychiatry 60:591–597, 1999

Winslow JT, Insel TR: Neuroethological models of obsessive-compulsive disorder, in The Psychobiology of Obsessive-Compulsive Disorder. Edited by Zohar J, Insel T, Rasmussen S. New York, Springer, 1991, pp 208–226

Woods A, Smith C, Szewczak M, et al: Selective serotonin re-uptake inhibitors decrease schedule-induced polydipsia in rats: a potential model for obsessive compulsive disorder. Psychopharmacology 112:195–198, 1993

Yadin E, Friedman E, Bridger WH: Spontaneous alternation behavior: an animal model for obsessive-compulsive disorder? Pharmacol Biochem Behav 40:311–315, 1992

Yin HH, Knowlton BJ: The role of the basal ganglia in habit formation. Nat Rev Neurosci 7:464–476, 2006

9

OBSESSIVE-COMPULSIVE SPECTRUM DISORDERS

Cross-National and Ethnic Issues

Hisato Matsunaga, M.D., Ph.D.
Soraya Seedat, Ph.D., MBChB, FCPsych

Culture traditionally refers to the sum total of learned behaviors of a group that are generally considered to be a tradition of that people and are transmitted from generation to generation. Culturally prescribed ritual behaviors are not of themselves indicative of obsessive-compulsive disorder (OCD) unless they exceed cultural norms and occur at times and in places judged inappropriate by others who belong to the same group (American Psychiatric Association 2000). It has been well demonstrated that obsessive and compulsive symptoms are not limited to one specific culture but are universal phenomena that extend beyond cultural and ethnic boundaries (de Silva 2006; Eisen and Rasmussen 2002; Sasson et al. 1997). Indeed, clinical descriptions of OCD are available in the literature not only from Western countries but from many other parts of the world, such as Nepal, India, Egypt, Saudi Arabia, Turkey, Brazil, and Japan (Fontenelle et al. 2004; Honjo et al. 1989; Khanna and Channabasavanna 1988; Mahgoub and Abdel-Hafeiz 1991; Okasha

This chapter was first published as "Obsessive-Compulsive Spectrum Disorders: Cross-National and Ethnic Issues." *CNS Spectrums* 12:392–387, 2007. Copyright 2009. Used with permission.

205

et al. 1994; Shama 1968; Tukel et al. 2002). The international acceptance of DSM-IV-TR (American Psychiatric Association 2000), along with the development of standardized and reliable instruments for the assessment of diagnosis and symptom status provide further support for the clinical and epidemiological studies that have been conducted cross-culturally.

In general, studies to date suggest that OCD and some of the obsessive-compulsive spectrum disorders (OCSDs; Hollander and Wong 1995) exhibit a certain degree of transcultural homogeneity, with sociodemographic features and core symptoms largely independent of cultural, ethnic, religious, and geographical differences (Sasson et al. 1997). In general, the most common obsessions and compulsions, respectively, are fears of contamination followed by pathological doubt and washing and checking compulsions (Eisen and Rasmussen 2002; Sasson et al. 1997). Where standard instruments are used, similar symptoms of OCD have been documented in the United States, Canada, Puerto Rico, Germany, Taiwan, Korea, and New Zealand (Weissman et al. 1994). Although cultural factors are unlikely to lead to OCD and OCSDs, per se, the symptoms, themes, and course of these disorders may be influenced by culture, ethnicity, and religion. People within a particular culture or living in a particular era may share concerns, and these concerns are reflected in the obsessions and compulsions that manifest (de Silva 2006). For instance, obsessional themes of HIV/AIDS usually associated with contamination fears and washing compulsions have recently been described in OCD patients in Western countries as well as in Japan (de Silva 2006; Matsunaga et al. 2002a). Moreover, cultural differences observed cross-nationally have mostly been related to the religious shaping of contamination concerns and scrupulosity (de Silva 2006; Eisen and Rasmussen 2002; Sasson et al. 1997). Specific environmental contexts and settings, such as high levels of inner-city violence, may also exert certain influences on the expression of OCD symptoms (Fontenelle et al. 2004).

On the other hand, there is a growing recognition that OCD is a heterogeneous disorder with clinical subtypes characterized by differing neurobiological mechanisms and treatment outcomes (Hollander and Wong 2000; Pigott et al. 1994). One robust approach for subtyping OCD is to consider comorbidity. Indeed, the presence of a specific comorbid condition, such as chronic tic disorder or schizotypal personality disorder, may be important in determining treatment strategies and also in predicting outcome (Baer et al. 1992; McDougle et al. 1993). Even though in OCD patients, comorbid depression or anxiety disorders are considered consistently common beyond cultural confounds (Eisen and Rasmussen 2002; Okasha et al. 1994; Pigott et al. 1994; Sasson et al. 1997; Tukel et al. 2002), few systematic investigations regarding cross-cultural aspects of comorbidity have been performed. In particular, it should be noted that both psychosocial and cultural contexts and conditions during childhood might have a crucial role in the pathogenesis of personality disorders, together with the contribution of constitutional disposition (Derkesen 1995). Thus, little is known about the extent and mechanisms through which culture, ethnicity, and religion may affect the nuclear phenotype of OCD or OCSDs. In this review, we seek to examine the epidemiological, phenomenological, psychopathological (comorbidity), and treatment aspects of OCD and OCSDs from a cross-cultural perspective.

Epidemiology

The frequency with which the diagnosis of OCD was made increased markedly during the 1980s. This might be related to the growth of information and evidence of OCD and the availability of effective treatments, such as drug and behavioral therapies (Stoll et al. 1992), along with the development of both objective criteria and more comprehensive and reliable structured interview methods (Eisen and Rasmussen 2002; Fontenelle et al. 2006). Since the early 1980s, accordingly, there has been a growing interest in the descriptive epidemiology of OCD in the general population. The results of a first large, psychiatric epidemiological study, the National Epidemiological Catchment Area Survey, conducted using the Diagnostic Interview Schedule (Robins et al. 1985) in 1984, revealed that OCD was the fourth most common psychiatric disorder after phobias, substance use disorders, and major depression, with a 6-month point prevalence of 1.6%, and a lifetime prevalence of 2.5% (Myers et al. 1984; Robins et al. 1984). Weissman et al. (1994), using the Diagnostic Interview Schedule, found that prevalence rates of OCD in seven international communities, including Puerto Rico, Canada, Germany, Taiwan, New Zealand, and Korea ranged from 1.9% to 2.5% for lifetime prevalence and from 1.1% to 1.8% for annual prevalence. There was remarkable consistency across sites, with the exception of Taiwan, where much lower lifetime and annual prevalence rates were documented (0.7% and 0.4%, respectively). In other studies using the Diagnostic Interview Schedule, the reported lifetime prevalence rates of OCD were as follows: 2.0% in Iceland (Stefansson et al. 1991), 1.1% in Hong Kong (Chen et al. 1993), and 2.7% in Hungary (Nemeth et al. 1997). On the other hand, epidemiological studies using the Composite International Diagnostic Instrument (Robins et al. 1988) to investigate DSM-IV-TR or ICD-10 (World Health Organization 1992) OCD conducted in Canada (Stein et al. 1997), The Netherlands (Bijl et al. 1998), Germany (Grabe et al. 2000), Australia (Henderson et al. 2000), Brazil (Andrade et al. 2002), and Turkey (Cillicilli et al. 2004) revealed 1-month prevalence ranging from 0.3% to 3.1% and lifetime prevalence rates ranging from 0.5% to 2.0%. Similarly, across studies using the Composite International Diagnostic Instrument (Andrade et al. 2002; Bijl et al. 1998; Cillicilli et al. 2004; Grabe et al. 2000; Henderson et al. 2000; Stein et al. 1997), no remarkable cross-country differences were observed. Data from prevalence studies employing other instruments, such as the Schedule for Affective Disorders and Schizophrenia (Endicott and Spitzer 1978), have been somewhat limited and preclude transcultural comparisons. In a study conducted using the Schedule for Affective Disorders and Schizophrenia in Iran (Mohammadi et al. 2004), the lifetime prevalence rate for OCD was 1.8%.

In general, cross-national epidemiological data on OCD have been consistent, irrespective of the diagnostic instruments used. Arguably, there may be little cultural or economic influence on OCD prevalence in developed and developing countries (Sasson et al. 1997). However, this is still tentative because there are few epidemiological data available from regions such as Central Asia, Eastern Europe, and sub-Saharan Africa. Additionally, it should be cautioned that prevalence rates in epidemiological studies vary not only according to the timeframe of measurement (1-month, 12-month, or lifetime) and diagnostic instruments used but are also influenced by factors such as interviewers (mental health professionals vs lay personnel), the setting of the evaluation (face to face vs by telephone), and the diagnostic criteria employed (e.g., DSM-IV-TR or ICD-10) (Fontenelle et al. 2006). In order to improve reliability and cross-cultural validity, it is necessary to establish a global consensus practice for the assessment of OCD that includes the standardization of instruments and interview techniques.

Regarding other epidemiological features of OCD, women typically seem to develop OCD slightly more frequently than men, even though juvenile onset of OCD is common in males (Eisen and Rasmussen 2002). Age at onset in OCD has a bimodal distribution; in some patients, OCD starts at puberty or earlier, whereas others have a later onset, such as after pregnancy, miscarriage, or at parturition (Eisen and Rasmussen 2002). In adult-onset OCD, incident cases have been shown to occur in men after 30 years of age, whereas incident cases among women are more frequent at a younger age (Nestadt et al. 1998). Thus, in general, men have earlier age of OCD onset, whereas women with OCD are more likely to be married and to have children. Men are more likely to present with sexual and symmetry obsessions, checking, and ordering and arranging compulsions, whereas women are more likely to have obsessions of contamination and dirt and washing compulsions (Karadag et al. 2006; Mataix-Cols et al. 1999; Matsunaga et al. 2000; Shooka et al. 1998). These trends seem to be similar across cultures, including Taiwan (Juang and Liu 2001), Japan (Matsunaga et al. 2000), and Turkey (Tukel et al. 2002). In the Cross National Collaborative Study (Weissman et al. 1994), for instance, the age at onset along with the female-to-male ratio of OCD were consistent across countries. However, in an Egyptian study (Okasha et al. 1994), males seemed to outnumber females (69% vs. 31%, respectively), which did not reflect the rate of comorbidity in the population but rather sociocultural variables related to the pattern of referrals to the psychiatric clinic. Possible bias associated with sociocultural background, therefore, needs to taken into account when assessing epidemiological and clinical aspects of OCD transculturally.

Phenomenology

The core symptoms of OCD seem to be relatively independent of cultural influence, with studies in the West and in the East indicating that dirt and contamination obsessions (cleaning compulsions) and aggressive or harm obsessions (checking compulsions) are the most frequently occurring themes (Fontenelle et al. 2004). The heterogeneity in clinical symptoms, the changing symptoms over time within the same individual, and the waxing and waning course of illness occur with remarkable consistency across cultures. In clinical samples the presence of mixed obsessions and compulsions predominates, whereas in epidemiological samples the obsessive subtype has been more frequently documented (Horwath and Weissman 2000). A four- or five-factor model of symptoms also seems to hold true across countries (Denys et al. 2004a; Lochner et al. 2005a) providing support for distinct clinical phenotypes (subtypes) in OCD (e.g., contamination/cleaning, somatic obsessions/checking, symmetry/arranging compulsions, and pure aggressive/sexual/religious obsessions).

Cultural factors may be important in shaping the content of obsessions and compulsions, and people afflicted with OCD often adopt cultural themes (e.g., HIV/AIDS and kosher rules). However, concerns about these themes and responses to them in people with OCD are inconsistent with cultural norms and, as such, considered culturally inappropriate (Fiske and Haslam 1997). For example, religious themes often prevail in countries where religion has an important role in society (e.g., Middle Eastern, Muslim, and Jewish cultures) (Ghassemzadeh et al. 2002; Shooka et al. 1998), such that the content of obsessions and compulsions (e.g., washing and cleanliness rituals) may be consonant with specific religious beliefs and practices. Okasha et al. (1996) proposed that religious and contamination concerns and repeating compulsions may be more common in Muslims than Christians due the emphasis on religious cleansing rituals and the practices of repeating religious phrases (to ward off sin and blasphemous thought) that forms an integral component of Islamic religion and culture. It has also been found that patients with religious obsessions may have more severe OCD, may remain underdiagnosed, and may delay seeking professional help (Karadag et al. 2006; Okasha et al. 1996). Karadag et al. (2006) suggested that this may be attributable, in part, to culturally sanctioned practice in which doubts about the completion of religious rituals may be viewed in a positive light (i.e., seen as reflecting faithfulness, due diligence, and orderliness).

Another example of this is body dysmorphic disorder (BDD). Like OCD, BDD has been reported in North America, the United Kingdom, Europe, Africa, Australia, the Middle and Far East, China, Japan, and South America. Although no significant transcultural variations in the sociodemographic aspects of BDD have been noted, there are notable differences in the concept of physical attractiveness and on the importance placed on it. Americans, for example, rely more on appearance and attractiveness in their perception of human differences than do their Japanese and Chinese counterparts. It is also likely that there are cultural differences in the concern and emphasis placed on different body parts (Cansever et al. 2003). In one cross-cultural study (Bohne et al. 2002), the prevalence of symptoms of BDD was compared in nonclinical student samples in America and Germany. Body image concerns and resulting preoccupation with body image occurred more frequently in American than German students. These differences, however, remained on a subclinical level, and the prevalence of probable BDD was not higher in American (4%) than German (5.3%) students. The authors attributed the subclinical findings to differences in the value placed on appearance and the resulting sociocultural pressures.

Comorbidity

Recently, a number of studies using structured clinical interviews, such as the Structured Clinical Interview for DSM (Gibbon et al. 1996), have investigated comorbidity of other psychiatric disorders in patients with OCD (Eisen and Rasmussen 2002; Pigott et al. 1994). Across studies conducted in Western countries, major depressive disorder (MDD) was the most common coexisting disorder, with prevalence rates ranging from 20% to 31% and from 54% to 67% for current and lifetime comorbidity, respectively (Brown et al. 2001; Denys et al. 2004b; Eisen and Rasmussen 2002; Fireman et al. 2001; LaSalle et al. 2004; Nestadt et al. 2001). It has been noted that OCD more often precedes rather than follows MDD, suggesting that MDD is likely to be secondary, with a minority of subjects presenting with a concurrent onset of OCD symptoms with their depressive episode (Denys et al. 2004b; Eisen and Rasmussen 2002). There is also significant overlap with other anxiety disorders, including panic disorder with or without agoraphobia, social phobia, and generalized anxiety disorder (Eisen and Rasmussen 2002; Pigott et al. 1994). Among comorbid anxiety disorders, social phobia was most commonly diagnosed, with prevalence rates ranging from 3.6% to 26% for current diagnosis and from 18% to 36% for lifetime diagnosis. The prevalence rates for the other anxiety disorders reported ranged from 0% to 12% for current diagnosis and from 1% to 23% for lifetime diagnosis (see Brown et al. 2001; Denys et al. 2004b; Eisen and Rasmussen 2002; Fireman et al. 2001; LaSalle et al. 2004; Nestadt et al. 2001).

In addition, among patients with primary diagnosis of OCD, OCSDs such as hypochondriasis (lifetime prevalence: 8.2% to 13%), BDD (6.3% to 12.9%), eating disorders (4.7% to 9.6%), trichotillomania (9.6% to 12.9%), and Tourette's syndrome (2.4% to 3.9%) have also frequently been diagnosed (Denys et al. 2004b; du Toit et al. 2001; LaSalle et al. 2004). As for prevalence rates of comorbid Tourette's syndrome or tic disorder, studies of adults with OCD, which have included both child- and adult-onset cases, have generally found lower rates of tic disorders than in children with OCD; the comorbidity of tic disorders in children or in childhood-onset OCD varies across studies from 20% to 59% (Eichstedt and Arnold 2001). A study investigating the relation between OCD and OCSDs (Denys et al. 2004b) found that about 58% of OCD patients currently met criteria for at least one OCSD and about 67% had a lifetime history of at least one comorbid OCSD. In the aforementioned study (du Toit et al. 2001), the OCSDs with the highest prevalence rates were compulsive self-injury (22.4%), compulsive buying (10.6%), and intermittent explosive disorder (10.6%). Similarly, in a study that examined comorbid impulse-control disorders among OCD patients (Grant et al. 2006), 16.4% of patients had a lifetime impulse-control disorder, and current impulse-control disorders were found in 11.6% of patients. Skin-picking was the most common lifetime (10.4%) and current (7.8%) impulse-control disorder, followed by nail-biting (4.8% and 2.4%, respectively). OCD subjects with current impulse-control disorders showed significantly worse OCD symptoms and poorer functioning and quality of life.

Such a relatively higher prevalence of OCSDs in OCD seems to be differential phenomenon compared with other anxiety disorders and may be representative of an essential linkage of OCD with OCSDs (Bartz and Hollander 2006; Richter et al. 2003). Some studies of OCSDs in OCD suggest that these might be distinct entities, whereas others suggest that they might lie on a number of different dimensions (Hasler et al. 2005; Lochner et al. 2005b; Nestadt et al. 2003). These views are supported by studies that have found higher prevalence rates of OCD in patients with primary OCSDs. For instance, patients with Tourette's syndrome have a high rate of comorbid OCD, with 30%–40% reporting obsessive-compulsive symptoms (Leckman et al. 1993). About one third of eating disorder subjects met current or lifetime diagnostic criteria for OCD on the basis of symptoms not related to dieting and body image (Thiel et al. 1995). In addition, eating disorder patients with comorbid OCD have often been characterized by both elevated frequencies of symptoms related to "symmetry and ordering" and an obsessional personality, including obsessive-compulsive personality disorder (OCPD), which may be related to an underlying biological diathesis that places them at risk for developing eating disorders (Kaye 1997). Indeed, family studies of eating disorders have found a common vulnerability for developing these disorders, OCSDs, and obsessional personality traits (Lilenfeld et al. 1998).

On the other hand, there have been relatively few studies on OCD comorbidity reported from non-Western countries. However, similar to Western countries, MDD and anxiety disorders are most commonly diagnosed. In one Egyptian study (Okasha et al. 1994), for example, MDD was most frequently assigned as a comorbid diagnosis (at the prevalence rate of 35.6%) followed by phobic disorder (6.7%), panic disorder (6.7%), impulse-control disorder (6.7%), and eating disorder (3.3%). In Turkey, comorbid disorders comprised depressive and anxiety disorders to a great extent; the disorder occurring at the highest frequency was MDD (39.5%), followed by dysthymia (20.4%), simple phobia (17.7%), generalized anxiety disorder (12.2%), and panic disorder (9.5%) (Tukel et al. 2002). In this study, about 4% of participants were diagnosed as having comorbid hypochondriasis. In Japanese patients with OCD, MDD is also the most prevalent Axis I disorder; more than one-third of subjects demonstrate current comorbidity of MDD, and the majority (>70%) develop MDD after the onset of OCD (Matsui et al. 2001).

As for the relationship between OCD and OCSDs, results from an Indian study in OCD patients suggested that tic-related disorders were most commonly comorbid (16%), followed by hypochondriasis (13%), BDD (3%), trichotillomania (3%), Tourette's syndrome (3%), and any eating disorder (0.4%) (Jaisoorya et al. 2003). In a Japanese study of 153 OCD subjects (Matsunaga et al. 2005), 45 (29%) were assessed to have any impulse-control disorder, impulsive personality disorder, or impulse-control symptoms. Among the impulse-control disorders, intermittent explosive disorder was most frequent (7%), followed by kleptomania (6%) and trichotillomania (5%). Fourteen subjects (9%) met DSM-IV-TR criteria for borderline personality disorder, and five subjects (3%) met criteria for antisocial personality disorder. Of 19 subjects with either of these comorbid personality disorders, 15 (79%) additionally met criteria for one or other impulse-control disorder. Self-injurious behaviors were the most prevalent impulse-control problem. Impulsive patients were differentiated from other patients with OCD on a range of demographic features (e.g., younger age at onset, lower level of functioning, more pervasive and severe psychopathology, and poorer treatment outcomes). These findings are consistent with those from the Western world, including North American and South American patients (Fontenelle et al. 2005; Grant et al. 2006). The findings seem to support the notion that OCD patients with highly impulsive features constitute a certain subtype, which is consistent with other studies (Grant et al. 2006; Lochner and Stein 2006). In another Japanese study on eating disorders (Matsunaga et al. 1999a), on the other hand, ~40% of restricting anorexia nervosa subjects met criteria for current OCD, even after excluding the core obsessional symptoms typical of anorexia nervosa. OCPD as well as more obsessive concerns with symmetry/exactness and ordering/arranging compulsions were more common in anorexia nervosa patients with OCD compared with age- and gender-matched patients with OCD alone. Similar trends were also found in Japanese subjects with bulimia and OCD (Matsunaga et al. 1999b). Genetic or familial vulnerability factors may underlie the association of OCD or OCPD with eating disorders in Japanese patients rather than culturally specific factors, per se, but this is deserving of further investigation.

In Western countries, comorbidity of Axis II disorders (personality disorders) in OCD have also been well investigated using structured interview methods (Baer et al. 1992; Black and Noyes 1997; Denys et al. 2004b; Eisen and Rasmussen 2002; Pigott et al. 1994). Across studies, Cluster C personality disorders, such as dependent, avoidant, and OCPD, were most commonly diagnosed, followed by Cluster A and Cluster B personality disorders, although it is controversial whether comorbid personality disorders, especially Cluster C personality disorders, are responsive to treatments for OCD (Ricciardi et al. 1992). Cluster A personality disorders (e.g., schizotypal personality disorder, paranoid personality, and borderline personality disorder) are found less commonly in OCD but seem to be associated with poorer outcome (Baer et al. 1992). In most studies (Black and Noyes 1997; Eisen and Rasmussen 2002; Pigott et al. 1994), a specific relationship between OCD and OCPD, as expected from psychodynamically driven theories of OCD, has not be found.

A smaller number of studies investigating personality disorder comorbidity in OCD patients have been conducted in non-Western countries. Comorbid personality disorders in patients with OCD seem to occur at similar rates cross-culturally; personality disorders in the Cluster C category (avoidant, dependent, OCPD) are more common than Cluster A or Cluster B (Black and Noyes 1997). As suggested in the Western literature (Matsunaga et al. 1998, 2002b), some types of comorbid personality disorder, such as schizotypal personality disorder, may impact on the clinical manifestation or course of OCD, such as more severe social maladaptation, poorer insight, or poorer treatment outcome. The frequency of comorbidity with OCPD is also relatively low in patients with OCD in the non-Western world (Matsunaga et al. 1998; Okasha et al. 1994), even though in an Egyptian study (Okasha et al. 1996), a relatively higher prevalence of OCPD was observed in OCD patients compared with other anxiety disorder groups. Consistently, prevalence of OCPD was the same as that reported in the Western world. That said, compulsiveness associated with perfectionism has traditionally been described as a common characteristic in Japanese samples (Matsunaga et al. 1998). However, it should be noted that the prevalence of personality disorders in developing countries may be significantly lower than those in developed countries, and this difference may be due to cultural tolerance for certain personality traits (Okasha et al. 1996).

Taken together, even though there are still limited data on comorbidity with Axis I disorders (Richter et al. 2003) in OCD, especially in non-Western countries, a certain transcultural consistency in prevalence and content is observed when standardized diagnostic assessments such as the Structured Clinical Interview for DSM are used. For instance, the discontinuity of OCD and OCPD rather consistently suggested in the Western world has been further supported from a cross-cultural perspective (Denys et al. 2004b; du Toit et al. 2001; Matsunaga et al. 1998). Such a possible universal consistency in respect of comorbidity provides an argument for further validating the extent of overlap of the OCSDs in contributing to the heterogeneity of OCD. It also lends support to the hypothesis that there may be specific vulnerabilities, including a genetic one, that lead to a clustering of specific phenomena, regardless of the influence of cultural, ethnic, or environmental factors (Richter et al. 2003). This is an area in which work is needed, particularly in regions such as Central Asia, Eastern Europe, and sub-Saharan Africa, where few systematic studies have been conducted.

Neurobiology: Brain Circuitry and Family and Genetic Factors

Neurobiological theories of OCD implicate specific frontal-subcortical circuits in the symptoms and cognitive deficits associated with the disorder (Mataix-Cols and van den Heuvel 2006). After improvement of OCD with either selective serotonin reuptake inhibitors (SSRIs) or behavioral therapy, the finding of decreased metabolism in frontostriatal circuits has also been consistent across studies conducted in different countries (Ho Pian et al. 2005; Nakao et al. 2005). In respect of familial and genetic factors, although a positive family history of OCD and impulse-control disorders has been widely reported in first-degree relatives of probands with OCD and impulse-control disorders, to our knowledge no systematic family studies have been conducted cross-nationally. In several different populations (namely, Italians, Korean, Swiss, Afrikaner), an association has been found with functional polymorphisms in monoaminergic genes, for example, with the serotonin transporter gene (Cavallini et al. 2000; Hasler et al. 2006; Kim et al. 2005) and the catechol-O-methyl transferase gene (Cavallini et al. 2000; Karayiorgou et al. 1999; Kinnear et al. 2001). However, one study in South African Afrikaners (Lochner et al. 2005a) found a lack of association with several monoaminergic genotypes in patients with OCD and comorbid OCSD, using cluster analysis. Furthermore, in Afrikaner patients with OCD with hoarding, the L/L genotype of the catechol-O-methyl transferase Val158Met polymorphism was found to occur more frequently compared with non-hoarding patients and healthy control subjects (Lochner et al. 2005a).

Treatment Issues

As has been noted, in non-Western cultures nonmedical belief systems may influence help-seeking for OCD. For example, among Egyptian and Turkish patients with severe OCD (especially those with religious and sexual obsessions), treatment was considerably delayed, arguably on account of the shame, guilt, and cultural taboo associated with these symptoms (Karadag et al. 2006; Okasha et al. 1994).

Across countries, exposure and response prevention is arguably the most effective psychological treatment for OCD currently available (50%–60%), but no systematic cross-cultural comparative studies exist. Exposure and response prevention is effective in reducing OCD symptoms and producing durability of gains following treatment discontinuation (Braga et al. 2005; Fisher and Wells 2005). When "asymptomatic" is used as the index of outcome, exposure and response prevention and cognitive therapy have been found to have low but equivalent recovery rates, in the order of 25% (Huppert and Franklin 2005). Other types of cognitive-behavioral therapy involving pacing, prompting, modeling, and shaping may be preferable for OCD patients with primary obsessional slowness. Long-term (5 years) outcome does not seem to differ between exposure and response prevention, cognitive therapy alone, and cognitive-behavioral therapy combined with an SSRI (van Oppen et al. 2005).

There are no published cross-cultural comparative studies of drug response in OCD. SSRIs and clomipramine, with potent serotonin reuptake blocking activity, constitute the first-line pharmacotherapy for OCD internationally. Exposure and response prevention combined with an SSRI may be additive and useful in clinical practice in patients who have not responded to an SSRI alone (Kampman et al. 2002). Neuroleptic augmentation (i.e., with atypical antipsychotics) represents one of the most promising strategies for patients with SSRI-resistant OCD (Bloch et al. 2006; Fineberg et al. 2005; Marazziti et al. 2005; Schruers et al. 2005). Several studies (Billett et al. 1997; Di Bella et al. 2002) have found no association between allele/genotype distribution of the serotonin transporter gene and SSRI response, although there have been no studies to date exploring ethnogenetic differences in response.

Conclusion

To ensure the diagnostic reliability and validity of OCD and the OCSDs, further studies are needed that use internationally reliable instruments aimed specifically at comparing transcultural aspects (sociodemographic, clinical, and prognostic features) of OCD and the OCSDs and cross-cultural treatment designs that allow for ethno-specific analyses (e.g., pharmacogenetics). Little is known about the mechanisms through which culture and ethnicity shape the content and expression of OCD symptoms, and this is also an area in which more work is needed. Future neurobiological and genetic approaches to studying OCSDs should incorporate assessment of the interactions between culture and biology to allow for a better understanding of their impact on the development and maintenance of these disorders.

References

American Psychiatric Association: Diagnostic and Statistical Manual of Mental Disorders, 4th Edition, Text Revision. Washington, DC, American Psychiatric Association, 2000

Andrade L, Walters EE, Gentil V, et al: Prevalence of ICD-10 mental disorders in a catchment area in the city of Sao Paulo, Brazil. Soc Psychiatry Psychiatr Epidemiol 37:316–325, 2002

Baer L, Jenike MA, Black DW, et al: Effect of Axis II disorders on treatment outcome with clomipramine in 55 patients with obsessive-compulsive disorder. Arch Gen Psychiatry 49:862–866, 1992

Bartz JA, Hollander E: Is obsessive-compulsive disorder an anxiety disorder? Prog Neuropsychopharmacol Biol Psychiatry 30:338–352, 2006

Bijl RV, Ravelli A, van Zessen G: Prevalence of psychiatric disorder in the general population: results of The Netherlands Mental Health Survey and Incidence Study (NEMESIS). Soc Psychiatry Psychiatr Epidemiol 33:587–595, 1998

Billett EA, Richter MA, King N, et al: Obsessive compulsive disorder, response to serotonin reuptake inhibitors and the serotonin transporter gene. Mol Psychiatry 2:403–406, 1997

Black DW, Noyes R: Obsessive-compulsive disorder and Axis II. Int Rev Psychiatry 9:111–118, 1997

Bloch MH, Landeros-Weisenberger A, Kelmendi B, et al: A systematic review: antipsychotic augmentation with treatment refractory obsessive-compulsive disorder. Mol Psychiatry 11:622–632, 2006

Bohne A, Keuthen NJ, Wilhelm S, et al: Prevalence of symptoms of body dysmorphic disorder and its correlates: a cross-cultural comparison. Psychosomatics 43:486–490, 2002

Braga DT, Cordioli AV, Niederauer K, et al: Cognitive-behavioral group therapy for obsessive-compulsive disorder: a 1-year follow-up. Acta Psychiatr Scand 112:180–186, 2005

Brown TA, Campbell LA, Lehman CL, et al: Current and lifetime comorbidity of the DSM-IV anxiety and mood disorders in a large clinical sample. J Abnorm Psychol 110:585–599, 2001

Cansever A, Uzun O, Donmez E, et al: The prevalence and clinical features of body dysmorphic disorder in college students: a study in a Turkish sample. Compr Psychiatry 44:60–64, 2003

Cavallini MC, Di Bella D, Catalano M, et al: An association between 5-HTTLPR polymorphism, COMT polymorphism, and Tourette's syndrome. Psychiatry Res 97:93–100, 2000

Chen CN, Wong J, Lee N, et al: The Shatin community mental health survey in Hong Kong II major findings. Arch Gen Psychiatry 50:125–133, 1993

Cillicilli AS, Telcioglu M, Askin R, et al: Twelve-month prevalence of obsessive-compulsive disorder in Konya, Turkey. Compr Psychiatry 45:367–374, 2004

de Silva P: Culture and obsessive-compulsive disorder. Psychiatry 5:402–404, 2006

Denys D, de Geus F, van Megen HJ, et al: Use of factor analysis to detect potential phenotypes in obsessive-compulsive disorder. Psychiatry Res 128:273–280, 2004a

Denys D, Tenney N, van Megen HJ, et al: Axis I and II comorbidity in a large sample of patients with obsessive-compulsive disorder. J Affect Disord 80:155–162, 2004b

Derkesen J: Sociocultural and economic backgrounds of personality disorders, in Personality Disorders: Clinical and Social Perspectives. Edited by Derkesen J. Chichester, United Kingdom, John Wiley and Sons, 1995, pp 279–305

Di Bella D, Cavallini MC, Bellodi L: No association between obsessive-compulsive disorder and the 5-HT(1Dbeta) receptor gene. Am J Psychiatry 159:1783–1785, 2002 du Toit PL, van Kradenburg J, Niehaus D, et al: Comparison of obsessive-compulsive disorder patients with and without comorbid putative obsessive-compulsive spectrum disorders using a structured clinical interview. Compr Psychiatry 42:291–300, 2001

Eichstedt JA, Arnold SL: Childhood-onset obsessive-compulsive disorder: a tic-related subtype of OCD? Clin Psychol Rev 21:137–157, 2001

Eisen JL, Rasmussen SA: Phenomenology of obsessive-compulsive disorder, in The American Psychiatric Publishing Textbook of Anxiety Disorders. Edited by Stein DJ, Hollander E. Washington, DC, American Psychiatric Publishing, 2002, pp 173–189

Endicott J, Spitzer RL: A diagnostic interview: the schedule for affective disorders and schizophrenia. Arch Gen Psychiatry 35:837–844, 1978

Fineberg NA, Sivakumaran T, Roberts A, et al: Adding quetiapine to SRI in treatment-resistant obsessive-compulsive disorder: a randomized controlled treatment study. Int Clin Psychopharmacol 20:223–226, 2005

Fireman B, Koran LM, Leventhal JL, et al: The prevalence of clinically recognized obsessive-compulsive disorder in a large health maintenance organization. Am J Psychiatry 158:1904–1910, 2001

Fisher PL, Wells A: How effective are cognitive and behavioral treatments for obsessive-compulsive disorder? A clinical significance analysis. Behav Res Ther 43:1543–1558, 2005

Fiske AP, Haslam N: Is obsessive-compulsive disorder a pathology of the human disposition to perform socially meaningful rituals? Evidence of similar content. J Nerv Ment Dis 185:211–222, 1997

Fontenelle LF, Mendlowicz MV, Marques C, et al: Transcultural aspects of obsessive-compulsive disorder: a description of a Brazilian sample and a systematic review of international clinical studies. J Psychiatr Res 38:403–411, 2004

Fontenelle LF, Mendlowicz MV, Versiani M: Impulse control disorders in patients with obsessive-compulsive disorder. Psychiatry Clin Neurosci 59:30–37, 2005

Fontenelle LF, Mendlowicz MV, Versiani M: The descriptive epidemiology of obsessive-compulsive disorder. Prog Neuropsychopharmacol Biol Psychiatry 30:327–337, 2006

Ghassemzadeh H, Mojtabai R, Khamseh A, et al: Symptoms of obsessive-compulsive disorder in a sample of Iranian patients. Int J Soc Psychiatry 48:20–28, 2002

Gibbon M, Spitzer RL, Williams J, et al (eds): Structured Clinical Interview for DSM-IV Axis I Disorders. Clinician Version. Washington, DC, American Psychiatric Press, 1996

Grabe HJ, Meyer C, Hapke U, et al: Prevalence, quality of life and psychosocial function in obsessive-compulsive disorder and subclinical obsessive-compulsive disorder in northern Germany. Eur Arch Psychiatry Clin Neurosci 250:262–268, 2000

Grant JE, Mancebo MC, Pinto A, et al: Impulse control disorders in adult with obsessive-compulsive disorder. J Psychiatr Res 40:494–501, 2006

Hasler G, LaSalle-Ricci VH, Ronquillo JG, et al: Obsessive-compulsive disorder symptom dimensions show specific relationships to psychiatric comorbidity. Psychiatr Res 135:121–132, 2005

Hasler G, Kazuba D, Murphy DL: Factor analysis of obsessive-compulsive disorder Y-BOCS-SC symptoms and association with 5-HTTLPR SERT polymorphism. Am J Med Genet B Neuropsychiatr Genet 141:403–408, 2006

Henderson S, Andrews G, Hall W: Australia's mental health: an overview of the general population survey. Aust N Z J Psychiatry 34:197–205, 2000

Ho Pian KL, van Megen HJ, Ramsey NF, et al: Decreased thalamic blood flow in obsessive-compulsive disorder patients responding to fluvoxamine. Psychiatry Res 138:89–97, 2005

Hollander E, Wong CM: Obsessive-compulsive spectrum disorders. J Clin Psychiatry 56(suppl):3–6, 1995

Hollander E, Wong CM: Spectrum, boundary, and subtyping issues: implications for treatment refractory obsessive-compulsive disorder, in Obsessive-Compulsive Disorder: Contemporary Issues in Treatment. Edited by Goodman WK, Rudorfer MV, Maser JD. Mahwah, NJ, Lawrence Erlbaum, 2000, pp 3–22

Honjo S, Hirano C, Murase S, et al: Obsessive-compulsive symptoms in childhood and adolescence. Acta Psychiatr Scand 80:83–91, 1989

Horwath E, Weissman MM: The epidemiology and cross-national presentation of obsessive-compulsive disorder. Psychiatr Clin North Am 23:493–507, 2000

Huppert JD, Franklin ME: Cognitive behavioral therapy for obsessive-compulsive disorder: an update. Curr Psychiatry Rep 7:268–273, 2005

Jaisoorya TS, Reddy YC, Srinath S: The relationship of obsessive-compulsive disorder to putative spectrum disorders: results from an Indian study. Compr Psychiatry 44:317–323, 2003

Juang YY, Liu CY: Phenomenology of obsessive-compulsive disorder in Taiwan. Psychiatry Clin Neurosci 55:623–627, 2001

Kampman M, Keijsers GP, Hoogduin CA, et al: Addition of cognitive-behaviour therapy for obsessive-compulsive disorder patients non-responding to fluoxetine. Acta Psychiatr Scand 106:314–319, 2002

Karadag F, Oguzhanoglu NK, Ozdel O, et al: OCD symptoms in a sample of Turkish patients: a phenomenological picture. Depress Anxiety 23:145–152, 2006

Karayiorgou M, Sobin C, Blundell ML, et al: Family based association studies support a sexually dimorphic effect of COMT and MAOA on genetic susceptibility to obsessive-compulsive disorder. Biol Psychiatry 45:1178–1189, 1999

Kaye WH: Neurobiology and genetics-anorexia nervosa, obsessional behavior, and serotonin. Psychopharmacol Bull 33:335–344, 1997

Khanna S, Channabasavanna SM: Phenomenology of obsessions in obsessive-compulsive neurosis. Psychopathology 21:12–18, 1988

Kim SJ, Lee HS, Kim CH: Obsessive-compulsive disorder, factor-analyzed symptom dimensions and serotonin transporter polymorphism. Neuropsychobiology 52:176–182, 2005

Kinnear C, Niehaus DJ, Seedat S, et al: Obsessive-compulsive disorder and a novel polymorphism adjacent to the oestrogen response element (ERE 6) upstream to the COMT gene. Psychiatr Genet 11:85–87, 2001

LaSalle VH, Cromer KR, Nelson KN, et al: Diagnostic interview assessed neuropsychiatric disorder comorbidity in 334 individuals with obsessive-compulsive disorder. Depress Anxiety 19:163–173, 2004

Leckman JF, Walker DE, Cohen DJ: Premonitory urges in Tourette's syndrome. Am J Psychiatry 150:98–102, 1993

Lilenfeld LR, Kaye WH, Greeno CG, et al: A controlled family study of anorexia nervosa and bulimia nervosa: psychiatric disorders in first-degree relatives and effects of proband comorbidity. Arch Gen Psychiatry 55:603–610, 1998

Lochner C, Stein DJ: Does work on obsessive-compulsive spectrum disorders contribute to understanding the heterogeneity of obsessive-compulsive disorder? Prog Neuropsychopharmacol Biol Psychiatry 30:353–361, 2006

Lochner C, Hemmings SMJ, Kinnear CJ, et al: Cluster analysis of obsessive-compulsive spectrum disorders in patients with obsessive-compulsive disorder; clinical and genetic correlates. Compr Psychiatry 46:14–19, 2005a

Lochner C, Kinnear CJ, Hemmings SM, et al: Hoarding in obsessive-compulsive disorder: clinical and genetic correlates. J Clin Psychiatry 66:1155–1160, 2005b

Mahgoub OM, Abdel-Hafeiz HB: Pattern of obsessive-compulsive disorder in Eastern Saudi Arabia. Br J Psychiatry 158:840–842, 1991

Marazziti D, Pfanner C, Del'Osso B, et al: Augmentation strategy with olanzapine in resistant obsessive compulsive disorder: an Italian long-term open-label study. J Psychopharmacol 19:392–394, 2005

Mataix-Cols D, van den Heuvel OA: Common and distinct neural correlates of obsessive-compulsive and related disorders. Psychiatr Clin North Am 29:391–410, 2006

Mataix-Cols D, Rauch SL, Manzo PA, et al: Use of factor-analyzed symptom dimensions to predict outcome with serotonin reuptake inhibitors and placebo in the treatment of obsessive-compulsive disorder. Am J Psychiatry 156:1409–1416, 1999

Matsui T, Matsunaga H, Iwasaki Y, et al: Comorbid major depression in Japanese patients with obsessive-compulsive disorder. Seishin Igaku (Clin Psychiatry) 43:957–962, 2001

Matsunaga H, Kiriike N, Miyata A, et al: Personality disorders in patients with obsessive compulsive disorder in Japan. Acta Psychiatr Scand 98:128–134, 1998

Matsunaga H, Kiriike N, Iwasaki Y, et al: Clinical characteristics in patients with anorexia nervosa and obsessive-compulsive disorder. Psychol Med 29:407–414, 1999a

Matsunaga H, Kiriike N, Miyata A, et al: Prevalence and symptomatology of comorbid obsessive-compulsive disorder among bulimic patients. Psychiatr Clin Neurosci 53:661–666, 1999b

Matsunaga H, Kirrike N, Matsui T, et al: Gender difference in social and interpersonal features and personality disorders among Japanese patients with obsessive-compulsive disorder. Compr Psychiatry 41:266–272, 2000

Matsunaga H, Kiriike N, Matsui T, et al: Obsessive-compulsive disorder patients with poor insight. Compr Psychiatry 43:150–157, 2002a

Matsunaga H, Matsui T, Ohya K, et al: An examination of homogeneity in patients with contamination obsessions and washing compulsions using a manifest symptom-based typology [Japanese]. Seishin Igaku (Clin Psychiatry) 44:885–892, 2002b

Matsunaga H, Kiriike N, Matsui T, et al: Impulsive-control disorders in Japanese adult patients with obsessive-compulsive disorder. Compr Psychiatry 46:43–49, 2005

McDougle CJ, Goodman WK, Leckman JF, et al: The efficacy of fluvoxamine in obsessive compulsive disorder; effects of comorbid chronic tic disorder. J Clin Psychopharmacol 13:354–358, 1993

Mohammadi MR, Ghanizadeh A, Rahgozar M, et al: Prevalence of obsessive-compulsive disorder in Iran. BMC Psychiatry 4:2, 2004

Myers JK, Weissman MM, Tischler GL, et al: Six-month prevalence of psychiatric disorders in three communities 1980 to 1982. Arch Gen Psychiatry 41:959–967, 1984

Nakao T, Nakagawa A, Yoshiura T, et al: Brain activation of patients with obsessive-compulsive disorder during neuropsychological and symptom provocation tasks before and after symptom improvement: a functional magnetic resonance imaging study. Biol Psychiatry 57:901–910, 2005

Nemeth A, Szadoczky E, Teuer T, et al: Epidemiology of OCD in Hungary. Eur Neuropsychopharmacol 7(suppl):S234, 1997

Nestadt G, Bienvenu OJ, Cai G, et al: Incidence of obsessive-compulsive disorder in adults. J Nerv Ment Dis 186:401–406, 1998

Nestadt G, Samuels J, Riddle MA, et al: The relationship between obsessive-compulsive disorder and anxiety and affective disorders; results from the Johns Hopkins OCD family study. Psychol Med 31:481–487, 2001

Nestadt G, Addington A, Samuels J, et al: The identification of OCD-related sub-groups based on comorbidity. Biol Psychiatry 53:914–920, 2003

Okasha A, Saad A, Khalil AH, et al: Phenomenology of obsessive compulsive disorder: a transcultural study. Compr Psychiatry 35:191–197, 1994

Okasha A, Omar AM, Lotaief F, et al: Comorbidity of axis I and axis II diagnoses in a sample of Egyptian patients with neurotic disorders. Compr Psychiatry 37:95–101, 1996

Pigott TA, L'Heureux F, Dubbert B, et al: Obsessive compulsive disorder: comorbid conditions. J Clin Psychiatry 55(suppl):15–27, 1994

Ricciardi JN, Baer L, Jenike MA, et al: Changes in DSM-III-R Axis II diagnoses following treatment of obsessive-compulsive disorder. Am J Psychiatry 149:829–831, 1992

Richter MA, Summerfeldt LJ, Antony MM, et al: Obsessive-compulsive spectrum conditions in obsessive-compulsive disorder and other anxiety disorders. Depress Anxiety 18:118–127, 2003

Robins LN, Helzer JE, Weissman MM, et al: Lifetime prevalence of specific psychiatric disorders in three sites. Arch Gen Psychiatry 41:949–958, 1984

Robins LN, Helzer JE, Orvaschel H, et al: The Diagnostic Interview Schedule, in Epidemiologic Field Methods in Psychiatry: The NIMH Epidemiologic Catchment Area Program. Edited by Eaton WW, Kessler LG. Orlando, FL, Academic Press, 1985, pp 143–168

Robins LN, Wing J, Wittchen HU, et al: The Composite International Diagnostic Interview: an epidemiologic instrument suitable for use in conjunction with different diagnostic systems and in different cultures. Arch Gen Psychiatry 45:1069–1077, 1988

Sasson Y, Zohar J, Chopra M, et al: Epidemiology of obsessive-compulsive disorder: a world view. J Clin Psychiatry 58(suppl):7–10, 1997

Schruers K, Koning K, Luermans J, et al: Obsessive-compulsive disorder: a critical review of therapeutic perspectives. Acta Psychiatr Scand 111:261–271, 2005

Shama BP: Obsessive-compulsive neurosis in Nepal. Transcult Psychiatr Res Rev 5:38–41, 1968

Shooka A, Al-haddad MK, Raees A: OCD in Bahrain: a phenomenological profile. Int J Soc Psychiatry 44:147–154, 1998

Stefansson JG, Lindal E, Bjornsson JK, et al: Lifetime prevalence of specific mental disorders among people born in Island in 1931. Acta Psychiatr Scand 84:142–149, 1991

Stein MB, Forde DR, Anderson G, et al: Obsessive-compulsive disorder in the community: an epidemiologic survey with clinical reappraisal. Am J Psychiatry 154:1120–1126, 1997

Stoll AL, Tohen M, Baldessarini RJ: Increasing frequency of the diagnosis of obsessive-compulsive disorder. Am J Psychiatry 149:638–640, 1992

Thiel A, Broocks A, Ohlmeier M, et al: Obsessive-compulsive disorder among patients with anorexia nervosa and bulimia nervosa. Am J Psychiatry 152:72–75, 1995

Tukel R, Polat A, Ozdemir O, et al: Comorbid conditions in obsessive-compulsive disorder. Compr Psychiatry 43:204–209, 2002

van Oppen P, van Balkom AJ, de Haan E, et al: Cognitive therapy and expo-sure in vivo alone and in combination with fluvoxamine in obsessive-compulsive disorder: a 5-year follow-up. J Clin Psychiatry 66:1415–1422, 2005

Weissman MM, Bland RC, Canino GJ, et al: The cross national epidemiology of obsessive-compulsive disorder. The Cross National Collaborative Group. J Clin Psychiatry 55(suppl):5–10, 1994

World Health Organization: International Statistical Classification of Diseases and Related Health Problems, 10th Revision. Geneva, Switzerland, World Health Organization, 1992

INDEX

*Page numbers printed in **boldface** type refer to tables or figures.*

223